Handbook of Muscle Regeneration and Homeostasis

Handbook of Muscle Regeneration and Homeostasis

Editor: Keith Seibert

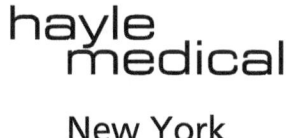

New York

Hayle Medical,
750 Third Avenue, 9th Floor,
New York, NY 10017, USA

Visit us on the World Wide Web at:
www.haylemedical.com

ISBN 978-1-64647-591-9 (Hardback)

Cataloging-in-Publication Data

Handbook of muscle regeneration and homeostasis / edited by Keith Seibert.
    p. cm.
Includes bibliographical references and index.
ISBN 978-1-64647-591-9
1. Muscles--Regeneration. 2. Homeostasis. 3. Regeneration (Biology). 4. Muscles.
5. Physiology. 6. Rheumatology. I. Seibert, Keith.
QP321 .H36 2023
612.74--dc23

Contents

Preface

Over the recent decade, advancements and applications have progressed exponentially. This has led to the increased interest in this field and projects are being conducted to enhance knowledge. The main objective of this book is to present some of the critical challenges and provide insights into possible solutions. This book will answer the varied questions that arise in the field and also provide an increased scope for furthering studies.

Homeostasis refers to the ability of an organism to keep the body's internal environment within bounds that enable the organism to survive. Chemical regulation, thermoregulation and osmoregulation are the primary types of homeostatic regulations that occur in the body. Muscle regeneration is the ability of an adult muscle to regenerate damaged fibers and it represents an essential homeostatic function. It is an extremely coordinated program, which partly mimics the embryonic developmental program. It also includes the activation of the muscle compartment of stem cells, specifically satellite cells as well as other precursor cells. The activities of these cells are dependent on environmental signals. Muscle regeneration can be hampered by a number of pathological conditions either because of the increasing loss of stem cell populations or due to the absence of signals that prevent damaged tissues from effectively activating a regenerative program. Thus, it is possible that losing control over these cells will result in pathological cell differentiation. The topics included herein on muscle regeneration and homeostasis is of utmost significance and bound to provide incredible insights to readers. Those in search of information to further their knowledge will be greatly assisted by this book.

I hope that this book, with its visionary approach, will be a valuable addition and will promote interest among readers. Each of the authors has provided their extraordinary competence in their specific fields by providing different perspectives as they come from diverse nations and regions. I thank them for their contributions.

Editor

Expression and Functional Analyses of Dlk1 in Muscle Stem Cells and Mesenchymal Progenitors during Muscle Regeneration

Lidan Zhang [1,2]**, Akiyoshi Uezumi** [3]**, Takayuki Kaji** [1]**, Kazutake Tsujikawa** [2]**,
Ditte Caroline Andersen** [4,5]**, Charlotte Harken Jensen** [4]⑩ **and So-ichiro Fukada** [1,*]⑩

[1] Project for Muscle Stem Cell Biology, Graduate School of Pharmaceutical Sciences, Osaka University, 1–6 Yamadaoka, Suita, Osaka 565–0871, Japan
[2] Laboratory of Molecular and Cellular Physiology, Graduate School of Pharmaceutical Sciences, Osaka University, 1–6 Yamadaoka, Suita, Osaka 565–0871, Japan
[3] Muscle Aging and Regenerative Medicine, Tokyo Metropolitan Institute of Gerontology, Itabashi-ku, Tokyo 173–0015, Japan
[4] Laboratory of Molecular and Cellular Cardiology, Department of Clinical Biochemistry and Pharmacology, Odense University Hospital, Winsloewparken 21 3rd, 5000 Odense C, Denmark
[5] Clinical Institute, University of Southern Denmark, Winsloewparken 21 3rd, 5000 Odense C, Denmark
* Correspondence: fukada@phs.osaka-u.ac.jp;

Abstract: Delta like non-canonical Notch ligand 1 (*Dlk1*) is a paternally expressed gene which is also known as preadipocyte factor 1 (*Pref–1*). The accumulation of adipocytes and expression of Dlk1 in regenerating muscle suggests a correlation between fat accumulation and Dlk1 expression in the muscle. Additionally, mice overexpressing Dlk1 show increased muscle weight, while Dlk1-null mice exhibit decreased body weight and muscle mass, indicating that Dlk1 is a critical factor in regulating skeletal muscle mass during development. The muscle regeneration process shares some features with muscle development. However, the role of Dlk1 in regeneration processes remains controversial. Here, we show that mesenchymal progenitors also known as adipocyte progenitors exclusively express Dlk1 during muscle regeneration. Eliminating developmental effects, we used conditional depletion models to examine the specific roles of Dlk1 in muscle stem cells or mesenchymal progenitors. Unexpectedly, deletion of Dlk1 in neither the muscle stem cells nor the mesenchymal progenitors affected the regenerative ability of skeletal muscle. In addition, fat accumulation was not increased by the loss of Dlk1. Collectively, Dlk1 plays essential roles in muscle development, but does not greatly impact regeneration processes and adipogenic differentiation in adult skeletal muscle regeneration.

Keywords: Dlk1; muscle regeneration; muscle stem cells; mesenchymal progenitors

1. Introduction

The delta like non-canonical Notch ligand 1 (*Dlk1*)-iodothyronine deiodinase 3 (*Dio3*) gene cluster is paternally expressed and involved in metabolism switching, stem cell maintenance, and cell differentiation [1,2]. The best known phenotype of the accelerated expression of the *Dlk1-Dio3* gene cluster is skeletal muscle hypertrophy in sheep, known as *callipyge* sheep [3]. Additionally, mice overexpressing Dlk1 show increased muscle weight [4], while Dlk1-null mice exhibit growth retardation including decreased body weight and skeletal muscle mass [5–7], indicating that Dlk1 plays critical roles in skeletal muscle biology. In adult skeletal muscle, including in myofibers, Dlk1 expression is rarely detected [8]. However, the reappearance of Dlk1 expression is observed in Becker and Duchenne muscular dystrophies (DMD), in which the muscle regeneration and degeneration cycles are repeated [8]. Dlk1 expression is also detected in adult murine regenerating muscle, suggesting that Dlk1 is an important factor for muscle regeneration or degeneration.

Muscle regeneration ability depends on muscle stem cells marked with Pax7 [9], known as muscle satellite cells (MuSCs) [10–13]. A group of skeletal muscle-specific basic helix-loop-helix transcription factors including MyoD, Myf5, myogenin, and Mrf4 (also known as Myf6) are critical for MuSC activation, proliferation, and differentiation as well as skeletal muscle development [14,15]. Using conditional *Dlk1*-null mice inactivated by *Myf5*-Cre (*Myf5-Dlk1* cKO), Waddell et al. showed that Dlk1 is necessary for proper skeletal muscle development and regeneration [5]. *Myf5-Dlk1* cKO mice showed a reduced body weight and muscle mass because of their decreased myofiber numbers. Using cardiotoxin-injury model, muscle regeneration experiments revealed impaired regeneration processes in *Myf5-Dlk1* cKO mice, suggesting that muscle regeneration is limited due to the loss of Dlk1 in Myf5-positive myogenic-lineage cells. However, since the recombination activity of *Myf5*-Cre driver mice is active at an early embryonic stage (around E9.0), developmental defects may secondarily affect the regenerative process in the adult skeletal muscle of *Myf5-Dlk1* cKO mice. Andersen et al. also reported a development defect of skeletal muscle in *Dlk1*-null mice [7] but in contrast to *Myf5-Dlk1* cKO mice, they observed accelerated muscle regeneration in *Dlk1*-null mice in knife-cut lesion model, when myogenic program genes were induced. Thus, the role of Dlk1 in the muscle regenerative process remains controversial, and studies eliminating the effect of developmental Dlk1-defects are required.

Dlk1, which is also known as preadipocyte factor 1, has been reported to negatively regulate adipogenesis [16]. Importantly, accompanying the progression of the disease, the accumulation of adipocytes is increased in DMD patients [8], and Dlk1 is re-expressed in skeletal muscle of DMD and other muscular dystrophy patients, suggesting that Dlk1 expression level might be correlated with fat accumulation. Mesenchymal progenitors, also known as fibro/adipogenic progenitors, exhibit adipogenic differentiation ability in both humans and mice [17–19]. Although the cells expressing Dlk1 have not been fully characterized, perivascular and interstitial Dlk1-expressing cells were detected in regenerating muscle [8]. Because fat accumulation decreases skeletal muscle integrity, force, and function, numerous studies have been conducted to evaluate the molecular mechanism underlying the adipogenic differentiation of mesenchymal progenitors.

To investigate the requirement for Dlk1 in adult skeletal muscle regeneration, we identified Dlk1-expressing cells during muscle regeneration and depleted *Dlk1* in specific populations using $Pax7^{CreERT2/+}$ (for MuSCs) or $Pdgfra^{CreERT2/+}$ (for mesenchymal progenitors) in mice. These mice were used to analyze the roles of Dlk1 only in adult muscle regeneration processes because Cre activity can be controlled by injection of tamoxifen. Interestingly, Dlk1 expression was extremely specific to mesenchymal progenitors in the middle stage of the regeneration processes. However, unexpectedly, neither MuSC-specific conditional *Dlk1*-depletion mice nor mesenchymal progenitor-specific conditional mice showed abnormalities. Increased fat accumulation was not observed in mesenchymal progenitor-specific conditional knockout mice. These results indicate that mesenchymal progenitors exclusively express Dlk1 during muscle regeneration, but that Dlk1 is dispensable for skeletal muscle regeneration, suggesting that the requirement for Dlk1 in skeletal muscle biology is limited to developmental processes.

2. Results

2.1. Role of Dlk1 in Myogenic Cells during Regeneration

MuSCs are indispensable for muscle regeneration and are marked by the expression of Pax7 [9]. Dlk1 is also expressed in MuSCs during development and remodeling and therefore, to determine the roles of MuSC-Dlk1 in adult skeletal muscle regeneration, we generated $Pax7^{CreERT2/+}::Dlk1^{flox/flox}$ mice (P7-cKO) and compared them to control mice (P7-control: $Pax7^{+/+}::Dlk1^{flox/flox}$). This system allowed us to examine the role of Dlk1 in adult skeletal muscle regeneration because *Dlk1* depletion is controlled by the timing of tamoxifen (Tm) injection.

Two weeks after Tm injection, muscle regeneration was induced by cardiotoxin (CTX) treatment; the muscles were sampled at 4 or 14 days after CTX injection for the analyses of myotube formation or regenerated myofiber, respectively (Figure 1A). Since the Dlk1 expression is not detected in MuSCs, it is difficult to observe the depletion of *Dlk1* in MuSCs. However, efficient recombination by *Pax7^CreERT2/+* with Tm was confirmed using Rosa-YFP reporter mice [20]. As shown in Figure 1B, the area of new regenerating myotubes marked by embryonic myosin heavy chain (eMyHC) expression in P7-cKO was comparable to that in P7-control mice. The size of regenerated myofibers observed at 14 days after CTX injection was also similar between P7-cKO and control mice (Figure 1C,D). Thus, in contrast to the results using *Myf5*-Cre mice, specific-depletion of *Dlk1* in adult muscle stem cells showed no apparent phenotypes in myotube formation and myofiber generation.

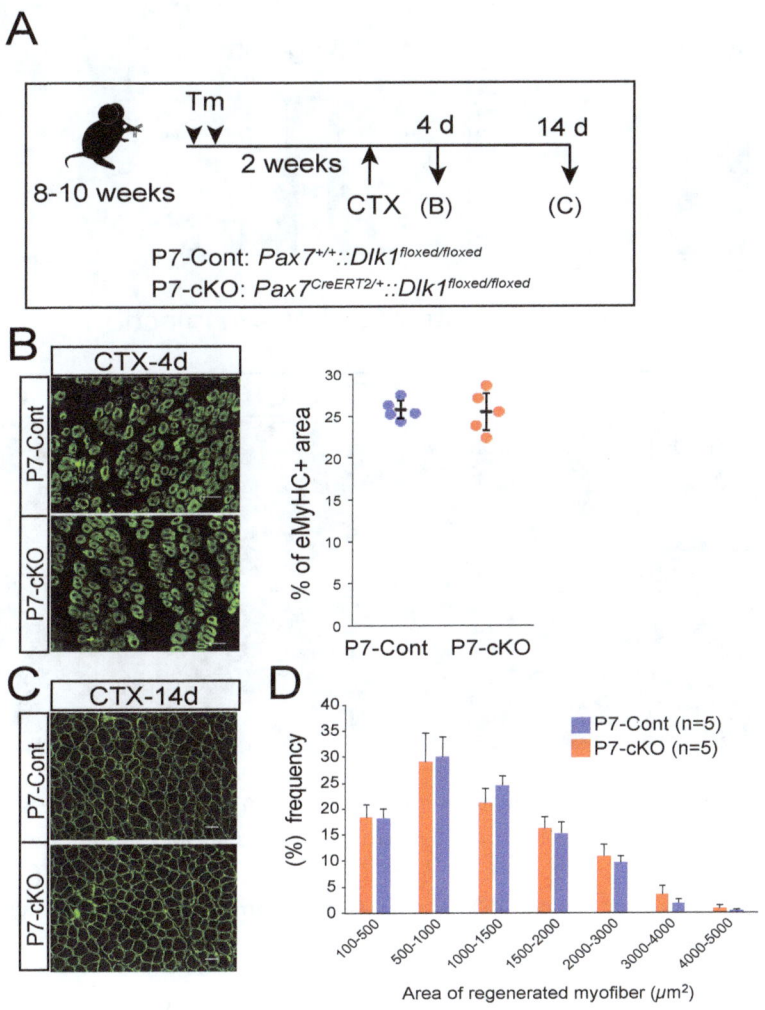

Figure 1. Role of Dlk1 in myogenic lineage cells. (**A**) Cardiotoxin (CTX) and tamoxifen (Tm) time scheme for analysis of the regenerative potential of P7-control and P7-cKO mice. (**B**) Immunostaining of embryonic myosin heavy chain (eMyHC, green) in injured TA muscle 4 days after CTX injection. The y-axis shows the eMyHC$^+$ area (percentage) in P7-control (blue circle, $n = 5$) and P7-cKO (red circle, $n = 5$) mice. Error bars indicate the mean with SD. Scale bar: 50 μm. (**C**) Immunostaining of laminin α2 (green) in P7-control and P7-cKO regenerated TA muscle 14 days after CTX injection. Scale bar: 50 μm. (**D**) Graphs indicate the quantitative analyses of the myofiber areas in P7-control (blue bar) and P7-cKO (red bar) mice. The y-axis represents the percentage of each myofiber size range. The x-axis indicates the size of the myofibers. Data show the average of five mice per group from two independent experiments with SD.

2.2. High Expression of Dlk1 in Mesenchymal Progenitors in the Middle Stage of Regeneration

Next, we characterized *Dlk1* expression during muscle regeneration. Compared to the expression pattern of *MyoD* and *myogenin* in regenerating muscle, *Dlk1* was expressed at a relatively late stage during muscle regeneration (Figure 2A). This result is consistent with those of Andersen et al. [7] who studied regeneration in a knife-cut lesion. We also examined Dlk1 protein expression in tissue sections. Using *Pax7::Rosa-YFP* mice, myogenic-lineage cells were labeled with yellow fluorescent protein (YFP). As observed by reverse transcription polymerase chain reaction (RT-PCR), a large number of Dlk1-expressing cells were detected in regenerating muscle five or seven days after CTX injection, while few cells were positive for Dlk1 at three days after injection (Figure 2B). Additionally, very low levels of Dlk1 staining were detected in myogenic cells (YFP$^+$ cells), indicating that the vast majority of Dlk1 expression originates from non-myogenic cells.

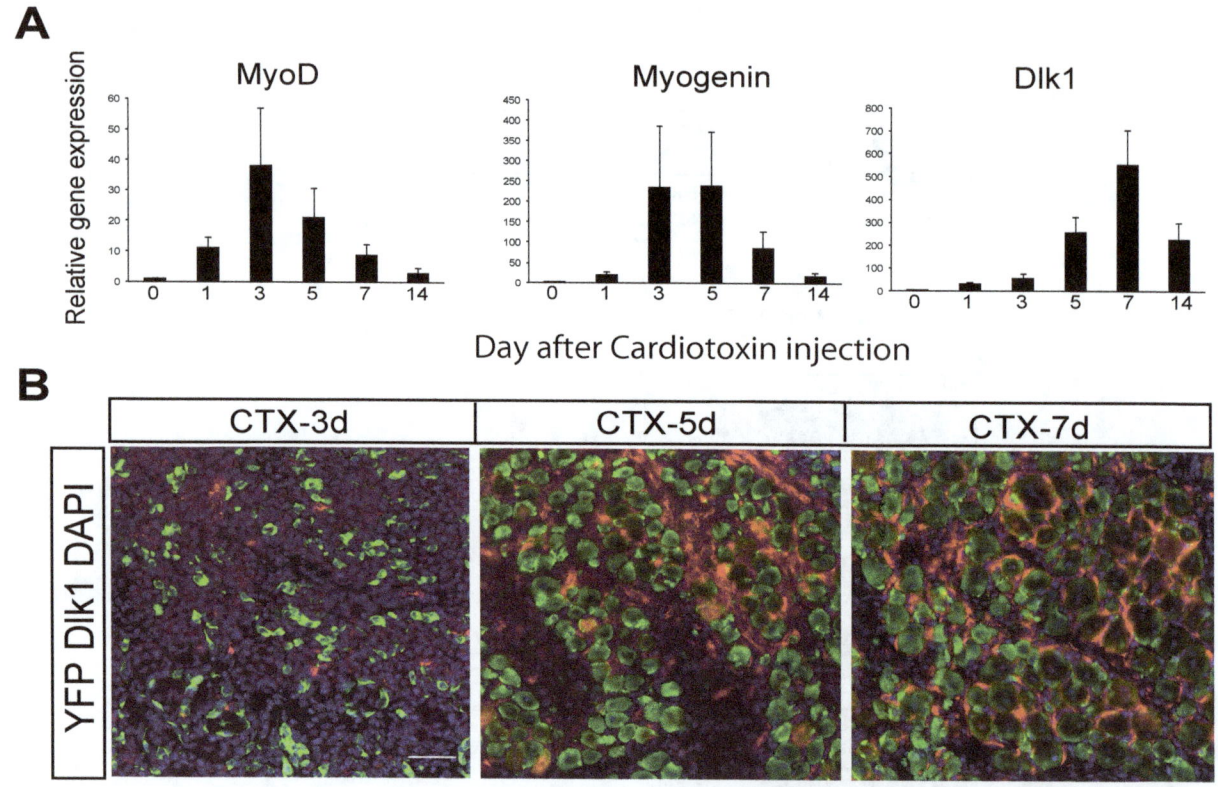

Figure 2. Dlk1 expression during muscle regeneration. (**A**) Relative expression level of MyoD, myogenin, or Dlk1 in intact and regenerating TA muscles. Data show the average of five independent experiments with the SD. (**B**) Immunostaining of Dlk1 (red), myogenic cells (green), and DAPI in regenerating muscle of *Pax7$^{CreERT2/+}$::Rosa-YFP* mice treated tamoxifen on the indicated days after CTX injection. Scale bar: 50 μm.

Although the characteristics of Dlk1$^+$ cells have not been fully identified, similarly to in a previous study [7], Dlk1$^+$ cells were found to reside in the interstitium of regenerating muscle (Figure 2B). To determine the type of cell expressing Dlk1, we isolated CD31/45, myogenic, and mesenchymal progenitor (Sca−1$^+$CD31$^-$CD45$^-$) fractions from regenerating muscle five days after CTX injection (Figure 3A) and evaluated the expression of *Dlk1* compared to in positive controls. Each positive control (*F4/80*; for macrophages, *Pax7*; for myogenic cells, and *Pdgfrα*; for mesenchymal progenitors) was specifically expressed in each fraction. Using these samples, we found that the *Dlk1* expression was highly enriched in mesenchymal progenitors (Figure 3B). We obtained similar results for samples isolated from regenerating muscle at seven days after CTX injection.

Next, we examined the protein expression of Dlk1 in regenerating muscles using tissues sections. Consistent with the results of mRNA expression, Dlk1 staining overlapped with Pdgfrα-staining

(Figure 3C). Collectively, these data indicate that mesenchymal progenitors almost exclusively express Dlk1 in the middle stage of adult skeletal muscle regeneration.

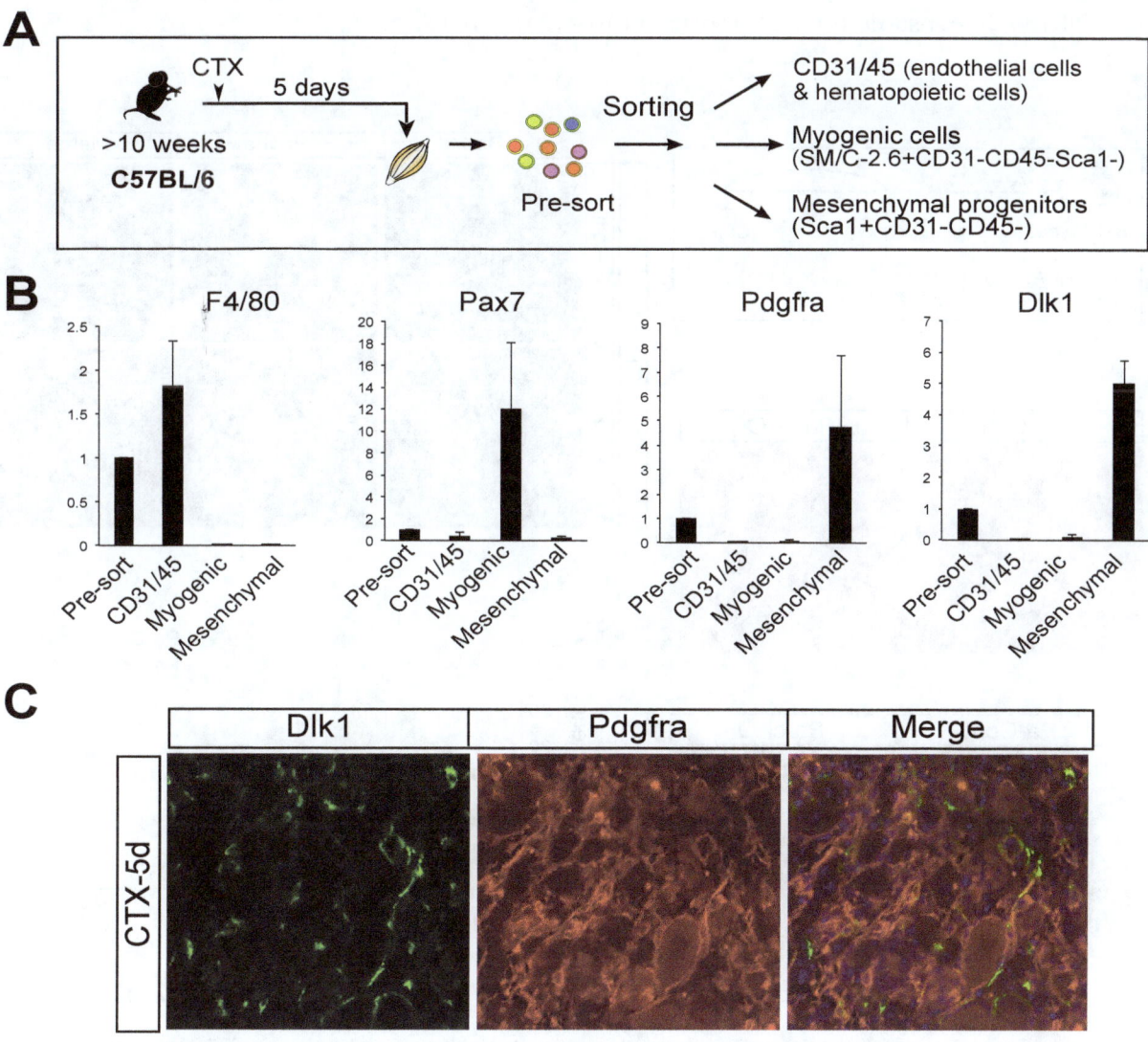

Figure 3. Specific expression of Dlk1 in mesenchymal progenitors. (**A**) Experimental scheme for analyses of Dlk1 in mononuclear cells from regenerating hindlimb muscle. (**B**) Relative mRNA expression levels of Dlk1, macrophage (F4/80), myogenic cells (Pax7), and mesenchymal progenitor marker (Pdgfra) in each cell fraction. Data show the average of three independent sorting experiment with SD. Three mice were used in this study. (**C**) Immunostaining of Dlk1 (green), Pdgfrα (red), and DAPI (blue) in the regenerating TA muscle of C57BL/6 five days after CTX injection. Scale bar: 50 μm.

2.3. Effect of Dlk1-Depletion in Mesenchymal Progenitors during Regeneration

Next, we examined the importance of Dlk1 in mesenchymal progenitors during muscle regeneration using $Pdgfra^{CreERT2/+}$ and $Dlk1^{flox/flox}$ mice (Figure 4A). First, we confirmed the successful depletion of Dlk1 in Pa-cKO mice (Figure 4B). Efficient recombination (about 80%) by $Pdgfra^{CreERT2/+}$ with Tm was also confirmed using Rosa-YFP reporter mice. Using these mice, we injected CTX into Pa-cKO or Pa-control mice, which were sacrificed at 14 days after injection. Unexpectedly, the histology of Pa-cKO mice was comparable to that of control mice (Figure 4C). Although Dlk1 inhibits adipogenic differentiation and mesenchymal progenitors have adipogenic differentiation ability, we observed no apparent abnormalities, including the appearance of adipocytes, in Pa-cKO mice compared to in Pa-control mice using Hematoxylin-Eosin staining (Figure 4C) or Oil-red O staining. The diameter of regenerated myofibers in Pa-cKO was also similar to that in control mice, indicating normal muscle regeneration in both Pa-cKO and Pa-control mice (Figure 4D,E). Collectively, these results indicate that Dlk1 expression is remarkably induced in mesenchymal progenitors during muscle regeneration, but also that Dlk1 is dispensable for CTX-induced muscle regeneration.

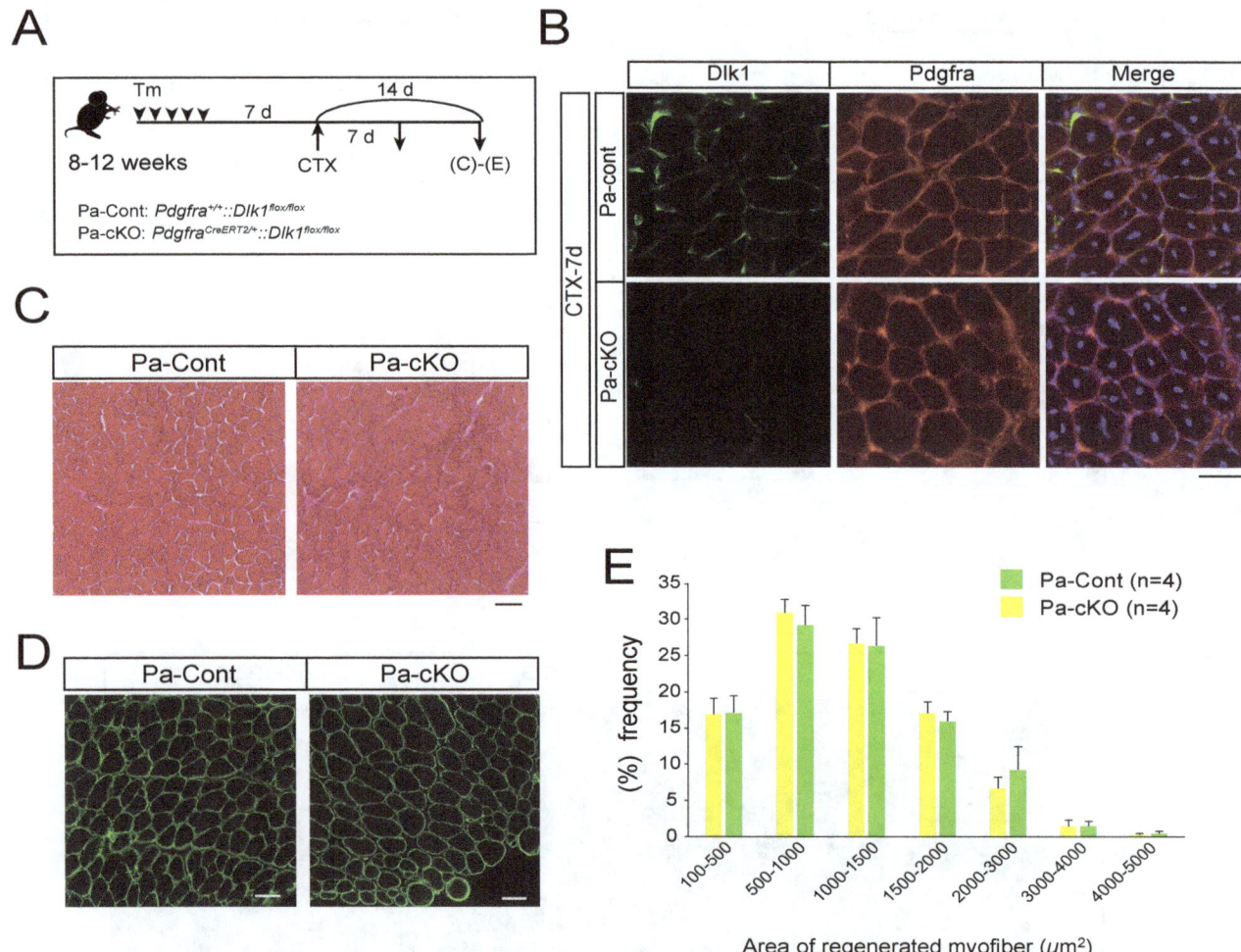

Figure 4. Depletion of Dlk1 in mesenchymal progenitors. (**A**) Cardiotoxin (CTX) and tamoxifen (Tm) time scheme for analysis of the regenerative potential in Pa-control and Pa-cKO mice. (**B**) Immunostaining of Dlk1 (green), Pdgfrα (red), and DAPI (blue) in the regenerating TA muscle of Pa-control and Pa-cKO seven days after CTX injection. Scale bar: 50 μm. (**C**) TA muscle sections of Pa-control and Pa-cKO mice were examined by H&E staining two weeks after CTX injection. Scale bar: 50 μm. (**D**) Immunostaining of laminin α2 (green) in Pa-control and Pa-cKO regenerated TA muscle 14 days after CTX injection. Scale bar: 50 μm. (**E**) Graphs indicate the quantitative analyses of the myofiber areas in Pa-control (green bar) and Pa-cKO (yellow bar) mice. The y-axis shows the percentage of each size of myofibers. The x-axis shows the size of myofibers. Data show the average of four mice per group from two independent experiments with SD.

3. Discussion

3.1. Dlk1 Expression in Mesenchymal Progenitors

In this study, we observed cell type and time-specific expression of Dlk1 during muscle regeneration processes. Because Dlk1 expression is detected in proliferative hepatoblasts from the fetal liver [21,22] and in cancer cells [23,24], Dlk1 expression may also reflect the proliferative ability of mesenchymal progenitors. However, we observed that suppression of Dlk1 in mesenchymal progenitors did not affect the process of muscle regeneration. Considering the timing of the peak cell number (three days after

CTX injection) and the important roles of mesenchymal progenitors during muscle regeneration [25], these results indicate that Dlk1 is dispensable for the function of mesenchymal progenitors.

In agreement with previous reports on knife-cut lesion model [7], Dlk1 expression is rarely observed in myogenic lineage cells of adult regenerating muscle of CTX-injury model. Previously, we reported that doublecortin is expressed specifically in myogenic cells during the middle stage of regenerating muscle [26]. In the middle stage of regeneration, new nascent myofibers become mature myofibers and the environment clearly differs from that in the early stage of regeneration [27]. Presumably, this difference in environment affects the middle stage-specific expression of Dlk1 in mesenchymal progenitors, and Dlk1$^+$ mesenchymal progenitors have some roles that differ from Dlk1$^-$ mesenchymal progenitor in the early stage of muscle regeneration, although Dlk1 itself has no impact on muscle regeneration process.

3.2. Dlk1 and Adipogenic Differentiation

Mesenchymal progenitors are defined by their ability to differentiate into adipocytes [17,18], and ectopic adipocyte accumulation in the skeletal muscle is detected in patients with muscular dystrophy. In contrast, mesenchymal progenitors also promote the process of muscle regeneration [25]. The origin of this duality is currently unclear. Because Dlk1 has anti-adipogenesis effects [28], Dlk1 is a candidate as the regulator of this duality. However, we found that fat accumulation was not accelerated by the loss of Dlk1 in regenerated muscle. Additional studies are necessary to determine the molecular mechanism directing this duality, which may lead to the development of therapeutic agents for muscular dystrophy.

3.3. Function of Dlk1 in Myogenic Cells

Inheritance of the *callipyge* sheep phenotype is known as an unusual mode of inheritance known as the *callipyge* phenotype. This phenotype is observed when a mutated allele is passed on only by the father. Thus, double mutated allele sheep exhibit a wild-type phenotype. Gao et al. proposed that a mutation in the maternal allele induces expression of the *miR−379/miR−544* cluster, which suppresses Dlk1 expression, as deletion of the maternal *miR−379/miR−544* cluster led to muscle hypertrophy following Dlk1 up-regulation [29]. Additionally, transgenic mice expressing ovine *Dlk1* under the muscle specific murine Myosin light chain 3F promoter and 2E enhancer (*Mlc 3F/2E*) exhibited muscular hypertrophy [4], indicating that Dlk1 derived from myogenic cells is functionally important for muscle hypertrophy. However, the expression of Dlk1 is rarely detected in normal and regenerating adult skeletal muscle cells including myofibers and satellite cells. In contrast, developmental myogenic cells express high levels of Dlk1 [8,30]. Considering our result and those observed in *Myf5-Dlk1* cKO and *Dlk1*-null mice, the expression pattern and function of Dlk1 is completely different during the developmental and regenerative processes in the skeletal muscle, and Dlk1 is dispensable for myogenic cells in adult intact and regenerating muscle.

4. Materials and Methods

4.1. Mice

Pax7$^{CreERT2/+}$ (Stock No: 012476) [31], *Dlk1 $^{flox/flox}$* (Stock No: 019074) [32], and *Pdgfra$^{CreERT2/+}$* (Stock No: 018280) [33] mice were obtained from Jackson Laboratories (Bar Harbor, ME, USA). Relocation of *Rosa26$^{EYFP/+}$* (Stock No: 006148) [34] from the the Experimental Animal Care and Use Committee at Osaka University (Approval No. 25-9-3, 25 June 2017; 30-1-1, 8 May 2019). To generate *Pax7$^{CreERT2/+}$::Dlk1 $^{flox/flox}$* or *Pdgfra$^{CreERT2/+}$::Dlk1 $^{flox/flox}$* mice, male *Pax7$^{CreERT2/+}$::Dlk1 $^{flox/+}$* or *Pdgfra$^{CreERT2/+}$::Dlk1 $^{flox/+}$* mice and female *Dlk1 $^{flox/+}$* were crossed. Mice were injected twice (*Pax7$^{CreERT2/+}$*) or five times (*Pdgfra$^{CreERT2/+}$*) (24 h apart) intraperitoneally with 200–300 µL tamoxifen (20 mg/mL; #T5648, Sigma-Aldrich, St. Louis, MO, USA) dissolved in sunflower seed oil (#S5007, Sigma-Aldrich) containing 5% ethanol. Three animals were housed in one cage designed for six mice and maintained in a controlled environment (temperature of 24 ± 2 °C, humidity of $50 \pm 10\%$) with a 12:12 h light/dark cycle. The mice received sterilized standard chow (DC−8, Nihon Clea, Tokyo, Japan) and water ad libitum. All procedures involving experimental animals were approved by the Experimental Animal Care and Use Committee at Osaka University. Primer pairs for genotyping are as follows: 5′- ACT AGG CTC CAC TCT GTC CTT C and 5′- GCA GAT GTA GGG ACA TTC CAG TG for $Pax7^{CreERT2/+}$; 5′- TCA GCC TTA AGC TGG GAC AT and 5′- ATG TTT AGC TGG CCC AAA TG for $Pdgfra^{CreERT2/+}$; 5′- AGA TTC CCC CAC CTC CAA C and 5′- TTC CCA AAC TGG ACA TGA GC for $Dlk1^{flox/flox}$; 5′- AAA GTC GCT CTG AGT TGT TAT, 5′- AAG ACC GCG AAG AGT TTG TC, and 5′-GGA GCG GGA GAA ATG GAT AT G for $Rosa26^{EYFP/+}$.

4.2. Muscle Injury

Muscles were injured by injecting cardiotoxin from *Naja pallida* (10 μM in saline)(Latoxan, Valence, France) into the hindlimb muscles (tibialis anterior (TA), gastrocnemius (GC), and quadriceps muscle (Qu)) [35].

4.3. Preparation and FACS Analyses of Skeletal Muscle-Derived Mononuclear Cells

Mononuclear cells from injured limb muscles (TA, GC, Qu) were prepared using 0.2% collagenase type II (Worthington Biochemical Corp., Lakewood, NJ, USA) as previously described [36]. Lympholyte (Cedarlane Laboratories, Ltd., Burlington, ON, Canada) was used to remove debris according to the manufacturer's instructions [37].

Mononuclear cells derived from the skeletal muscles were stained with fluorescein isothiocyanate-conjugated anti-CD31, and CD45, phycoerythrin-conjugated anti-Sca−1, and biotinylated-SM/C−2.6 [38] antibodies. Cells were then incubated with streptavidin-labeled allophycocyanin (BD Biosciences, Franklin Lakes, NJ, USA) on ice for 30 min and resuspended in phosphate-buffered saline containing 2% fetal calf serum and 2 μg/mL propidium iodide. Cell sorting was performed using an FACS Aria II™ flow cytometer (BD Immunocytometry Systems, Mountain View, CA, USA). Debris and dead cells were excluded by forward scatter, side scatter, and propidium iodide gating. Data were collected using FACSDiva™ software (BD Biosciences).

4.4. Real-Time PCR

Total RNA was extracted from sorted cells using Trizol LS reagent (Thermo Fisher Scientific, Waltham, MA, USA) and a QIAGEN RNeasy Micro Kit according to the manufacturer's instructions (Hilden, Germany). Total RNA was extracted from uninjured and injured TA muscles using Qiagen Tissue Ruptor Disposable Probes (Nonsterile) (#990890), Qiagen Tissue Ruptor (#9001271), and a Qiagen RNeasy Fibrous Tissue Mini Kit (#74704) according to the manufacturer's instructions. The isolated total RNA was reverse-transcribed into cDNA using a QuantiTect Reverse Transcription Kit (QIAGEN). Real-time PCR was performed using SYBR Green Universal Mix (#13608700, Roche Diagnostics, Mannheim, Germany) and StepOnePlus Real-Time PCR System (Applied Biosystems, Foster City, CA, USA). Specific forward and reverse primers for optimal amplification in real-time PCR of reverse transcribed cDNAs were as follows: 5′-AAG CAT CCG AGA CAC ACA CA and 5′-GGC AAG ACA TAC CAG GGA GA for mouse F4/80; 5′-GAC GAG TGT CCT TCG CCA AAG TG and 5′-CAA AAT CCG ACC AAG CAC GAG G for mouse Pdgfra; 5′-GTC TGG TTC AGT AAC CGG CGT G and 5′-GGT TAG CTC CTG CCT GCT TA for mouse Pax7; 5′-AGA TTC CCC CAC CTC CAA C and 5′-TTC CCA AAC TGG ACA TGA GC for mouse Dlk1; 5′-CAA CTG CTC TGA TGG CAT GAT G and 5′-AGA TGC GCT CCA CTA TGC TG for mouse MyoD; 5′-TCC CAA CCC AGG AGA TCA TTT G and 5′-ACA ATC TCA GTT GGG CAT GG for mouse myogenin; 5′-TGT CAA GCT CAT TTC CTG G and 5′-TTG GGG GCC GAG TTG GGA TA for mouse Gapdh. Quantitative gene expression data are often normalized to the expression levels of Gapdh.

4.5. Immunohistochemistry

For immunohistological analyses, transverse cryosections (6–8 μm) were fixed with 4% paraformaldehyde for 10 min. Anti-embryonic myosin heavy chain (eMyHC) or anti-laminin α2 antibodies were purchased from the Developmental Studies Hybridoma Bank (clone F1.652, Iowa City, IA, USA) or Enzo Life Sciences (clone 4H8–2, Plymouth Meeting, PA, USA), respectively. Goat anti-YFP or goat anti-Pdgfrα antibodies were purchased from R&D Systems (Minneapolis, MN, USA) or SICGEN-Research and Development in Biotechnology Ltd. (#AB0020–200, Carcavelos, Portugal), respectively. Rabbit anti-Dlk1 antibody used in this study was reported previously [7]. For staining with mouse anti-eMyHC antibody, transverse cryosections were fixed in cooled acetone for 10 min, and a MOM kit (Vector Laboratories, Burlingame, CA, USA) was used to block endogenous mouse IgG before the reaction with primary antibodies. The signals were recorded photographically using a BZ-X700 fluorescence microscope, and eMyHC-positive areas and myofiber-diameters were quantified with Hybrid Cell Count software (Keyence, Osaka, Japan). For the quantification, all the area of one section was used.

4.6. Statistics

Values were expressed as the means ± SD. Statistical significance was assessed by Student's t test. In comparisons of more than two groups, non-repeated measures analysis of variance followed by the Bonferroni test (vs. control) or Student-Newman-Keuls test (multiple comparisons) were used. A probability of less than 5% ($p < 0.05$) or 1% ($p < 0.01$) was considered statistically significant.

5. Conclusions

During muscle regeneration, mesenchymal progenitors almost exclusively express Dlk1 during the middle stage of regeneration processes, but Dlk1 is nonetheless dispensable for muscle regeneration processes. These results suggest the limited importance of Dlk1 in post-developmental processes.

Author Contributions: L.Z. performed most of the experimental work in the study; T.K. assisted L.Z. in some experiments; A.U., D.C.A. and C.H.J. provided critical materials for the study; L.Z., A.U., K.T. and S.-i.F. designed experiments; L.Z., A.U. and S.-i.F. interpreted experimental data; S.-i.F. conceived and supervised the study, and mounted figures. D.C.A., C.H.J. and S.-i.F. wrote the manuscript.

References

1. Wust, S.; Drose, S.; Heidler, J.; Wittig, I.; Klockner, I.; Franko, A.; Bonke, E.; Gunther, S.; Gartner, U.; Boettger, T.; et al. Metabolic Maturation during Muscle Stem Cell Differentiation Is Achieved by miR−1/133a-Mediated Inhibition of the Dlk1-Dio3 Mega Gene Cluster. *Cell Metab.* **2018**, *27*, 1026–1039.e6. [CrossRef] [PubMed]

2. Qian, P.; He, X.C.; Paulson, A.; Li, Z.; Tao, F.; Perry, J.M.; Guo, F.; Zhao, M.; Zhi, L.; Venkatraman, A.; et al. The Dlk1-Gtl2 Locus Preserves LT-HSC Function by Inhibiting the PI3K-mTOR Pathway to Restrict Mitochondrial Metabolism. *Cell Stem Cell* **2016**, *18*, 214–228. [CrossRef] [PubMed]

3. Carpenter, C.E.; Rice, O.D.; Cockett, N.E.; Snowder, G.D. Histology and composition of muscles from normal and callipyge lambs. *J. Anim. Sci.* **1996**, *74*, 388–393. [CrossRef] [PubMed]

4. Davis, E.; Jensen, C.H.; Schroder, H.D.; Farnir, F.; Shay-Hadfield, T.; Kliem, A.; Cockett, N.; Georges, M.; Charlier, C. Ectopic expression of DLK1 protein in skeletal muscle of padumnal heterozygotes causes the callipyge phenotype. *Curr. Biol.* **2004**, *14*, 1858–1862. [CrossRef] [PubMed]

5. Waddell, J.N.; Zhang, P.; Wen, Y.; Gupta, S.K.; Yevtodiyenko, A.; Schmidt, J.V.; Bidwell, C.A.; Kumar, A.; Kuang, S. Dlk1 is necessary for proper skeletal muscle development and regeneration. *PLoS ONE* **2010**, *5*, e15055. [CrossRef] [PubMed]

6. Moon, Y.S.; Smas, C.M.; Lee, K.; Villena, J.A.; Kim, K.H.; Yun, E.J.; Sul, H.S. Mice lacking paternally expressed Pref−1/Dlk1 display growth retardation and accelerated adiposity. *Mol. Cell Biol.* **2002**, *22*, 5585–5592. [CrossRef] [PubMed]

7.   Andersen, D.C.; Laborda, J.; Baladron, V.; Kassem, M.; Sheikh, S.P.; Jensen, C.H. Dual role of delta-like 1 homolog (DLK1) in skeletal muscle development and adult muscle regeneration. *Development* **2013**, *140*, 3743–3753. [CrossRef] [PubMed]

8.   Andersen, D.C.; Petersson, S.J.; Jorgensen, L.H.; Bollen, P.; Jensen, P.B.; Teisner, B.; Schroeder, H.D.; Jensen, C.H. Characterization of DLK1+ cells emerging during skeletal muscle remodeling in response to myositis, myopathies, and acute injury. *Stem Cells* **2009**, *27*, 898–908. [CrossRef] [PubMed]

9.   Seale, P.; Sabourin, L.A.; Girgis-Gabardo, A.; Mansouri, A.; Gruss, P.; Rudnicki, M.A. Pax7 is required for the specification of myogenic satellite cells. *Cell* **2000**, *102*, 777–786. [CrossRef]

10. Fukada, S.I. The roles of muscle stem cells in muscle injury, atrophy and hypertrophy. *J. Biochem.* **2018**, *163*, 353–358. [CrossRef] [PubMed]

11. Wang, Y.X.; Rudnicki, M.A. Satellite cells, the engines of muscle repair. *Nat. Rev. Mol. Cell Biol.* **2011**, *13*, 127–133. [CrossRef] [PubMed]

12. Relaix, F.; Zammit, P.S. Satellite cells are essential for skeletal muscle regeneration: The cell on the edge returns centre stage. *Development* **2012**, *139*, 2845–2856. [CrossRef] [PubMed]

13. Mauro, A. Satellite cell of skeletal muscle fibers. *J. Biophys Biochem Cytol.* **1961**, *9*, 493–495. [CrossRef] [PubMed]

14. Sabourin, L.A.; Rudnicki, M.A. The molecular regulation of myogenesis. *Clin. Genet.* **2000**, *57*, 16–25. [CrossRef] [PubMed]

15. Buckingham, M.; Bajard, L.; Chang, T.; Daubas, P.; Hadchouel, J.; Meilhac, S.; Montarras, D.; Rocancourt, D.; Relaix, F. The formation of skeletal muscle: From somite to limb. *J. Anat.* **2003**, *202*, 59–68. [CrossRef] [PubMed]

16. Smas, C.M.; Sul, H.S. Pref−1, a protein containing EGF-like repeats, inhibits adipocyte differentiation. *Cell* **1993**, *73*, 725–734. [CrossRef]

17. Uezumi, A.; Fukada, S.; Yamamoto, N.; Takeda, S.; Tsuchida, K. Mesenchymal progenitors distinct from satellite cells contribute to ectopic fat cell formation in skeletal muscle. *Nat. Cell Biol.* **2010**, *12*, 143–152. [CrossRef]

18. Joe, A.W.; Yi, L.; Natarajan, A.; Le Grand, F.; So, L.; Wang, J.; Rudnicki, M.A.; Rossi, F.M. Muscle injury activates resident fibro/adipogenic progenitors that facilitate myogenesis. *Nat. Cell Biol.* **2010**, *12*, 153–163. [CrossRef]

19. Uezumi, A.; Fukada, S.; Yamamoto, N.; Ikemoto-Uezumi, M.; Nakatani, M.; Morita, M.; Yamaguchi, A.; Yamada, H.; Nishino, I.; Hamada, Y.; et al. Identification and characterization of PDGFRalpha(+) mesenchymal progenitors in human skeletal muscle. *Cell Death Dis.* **2014**, *5*, e1186. [CrossRef]

20. Yamaguchi, M.; Watanabe, Y.; Ohtani, T.; Uezumi, A.; Mikami, N.; Nakamura, M.; Sato, T.; Ikawa, M.; Hoshino, M.; Tsuchida, K.; et al. Calcitonin Receptor Signaling Inhibits Muscle Stem Cells from Escaping the Quiescent State and the Niche. *Cell Rep.* **2015**, *13*, 302–314. [CrossRef]

21. Kubota, H.; Reid, L.M. Clonogenic hepatoblasts, common precursors for hepatocytic and biliary lineages, are lacking classical major histocompatibility complex class I antigen. *Proc. Natl. Acad. Sci. USA* **2000**, *97*, 12132–12137. [CrossRef] [PubMed]

22. Tanimizu, N.; Nishikawa, M.; Saito, H.; Tsujimura, T.; Miyajima, A. Isolation of hepatoblasts based on the expression of Dlk/Pref−1. *J. Cell Sci.* **2003**, *116*, 1775–1786. [CrossRef] [PubMed]

23. Yanai, H.; Nakamura, K.; Hijioka, S.; Kamei, A.; Ikari, T.; Ishikawa, Y.; Shinozaki, E.; Mizunuma, N.; Hatake, K.; Miyajima, A. Dlk−1, a cell surface antigen on foetal hepatic stem/progenitor cells, is expressed in hepatocellular, colon, pancreas and breast carcinomas at a high frequency. *J. Biochem.* **2010**, *148*, 85–92. [CrossRef] [PubMed]

24. Traustadottir, G.A.; Lagoni, L.V.; Ankerstjerne, L.B.S.; Bisgaard, H.C.; Jensen, C.H.; Andersen, D.C. The imprinted gene Delta like non-canonical Notch ligand 1 (Dlk1) is conserved in mammals, and serves a growth modulatory role during tissue development and regeneration through Notch dependent and independent mechanisms. *Cytokine Growth Factor Rev.* **2019**, *46*, 17–27. [CrossRef] [PubMed]

25. Wosczyna, M.N.; Konishi, C.T.; Perez Carbajal, E.E.; Wang, T.T.; Walsh, R.A.; Gan, Q.; Wagner, M.W.; Rando, T.A. Mesenchymal Stromal Cells Are Required for Regeneration and Homeostatic Maintenance of Skeletal Muscle. *Cell Rep.* **2019**, *27*, 2029–2035. [CrossRef]

26. Ogawa, R.; Ma, Y.; Yamaguchi, M.; Ito, T.; Watanabe, Y.; Ohtani, T.; Murakami, S.; Uchida, S.; De Gaspari, P.; Uezumi, A.; et al. Doublecortin marks a new population of transiently amplifying muscle progenitor cells and is required for myofiber maturation during skeletal muscle regeneration. *Development* **2015**, *142*, 51–61. [CrossRef]

27. Bentzinger, C.F.; Wang, Y.X.; von Maltzahn, J.; Soleimani, V.D.; Yin, H.; Rudnicki, M.A. Fibronectin regulates Wnt7a signaling and satellite cell expansion. *Cell Stem Cell* **2013**, *12*, 75–87. [CrossRef]

28. Lee, K.; Villena, J.A.; Moon, Y.S.; Kim, K.H.; Lee, S.; Kang, C.; Sul, H.S. Inhibition of adipogenesis and development of glucose intolerance by soluble preadipocyte factor−1 (Pref−1). *J. Clin. Investig.* **2003**, *111*, 453–461. [CrossRef]

29. Gao, Y.Q.; Chen, X.; Wang, P.; Lu, L.; Zhao, W.; Chen, C.; Chen, C.P.; Tao, T.; Sun, J.; Zheng, Y.Y.; et al. Regulation of DLK1 by the maternally expressed miR−379/miR−544 cluster may underlie callipyge polar overdominance inheritance. *Proc. Natl. Acad. Sci. USA* **2015**, *112*, 13627–13632. [CrossRef]

30. Floridon, C.; Jensen, C.H.; Thorsen, P.; Nielsen, O.; Sunde, L.; Westergaard, J.G.; Thomsen, S.G.; Teisner, B. Does fetal antigen 1 (FA1) identify cells with regenerative, endocrine and neuroendocrine potentials? A study of FA1 in embryonic, fetal, and placental tissue and in maternal circulation. *Differentiation* **2000**, *66*, 49–59. [CrossRef]

31. Lepper, C.; Conway, S.J.; Fan, C.M. Adult satellite cells and embryonic muscle progenitors have distinct genetic requirements. *Nature* **2009**, *460*, 627–631. [CrossRef] [PubMed]

32. Appelbe, O.K.; Yevtodiyenko, A.; Muniz-Talavera, H.; Schmidt, J.V. Conditional deletions refine the embryonic requirement for Dlk1. *Mech. Dev.* **2013**, *130*, 143–159. [CrossRef] [PubMed]

33. Kang, S.H.; Fukaya, M.; Yang, J.K.; Rothstein, J.D.; Bergles, D.E. NG2 + CNS glial progenitors remain committed to the oligodendrocyte lineage in postnatal life and following neurodegeneration. *Neuron* **2010**, *68*, 668–681. [CrossRef] [PubMed]

34. Srinivas, S.; Watanabe, T.; Lin, C.S.; William, C.M.; Tanabe, Y.; Jessell, T.M.; Costantini, F. Cre reporter strains produced by targeted insertion of EYFP and ECFP into the ROSA26 locus. *BMC Dev. Biol.* **2001**, *1*, 4. [CrossRef]

35. Takemoto, Y.; Inaba, S.; Zhang, L.; Tsujikawa, K.; Uezumi, A.; Fukada, S.I. Implication of basal lamina dependency in survival of Nrf2-null muscle stem cells via an antioxidative-independent mechanism. *J. Cell Physiol.* **2019**, *234*, 1689–1698. [CrossRef] [PubMed]

36. Uezumi, A.; Ojima, K.; Fukada, S.; Ikemoto, M.; Masuda, S.; Miyagoe-Suzuki, Y.; Takeda, S. Functional heterogeneity of side population cells in skeletal muscle. *Biochem. Biophys. Res. Commun.* **2006**, *341*, 864–873. [CrossRef]

37. Segawa, M.; Fukada, S.; Yamamoto, Y.; Yahagi, H.; Kanematsu, M.; Sato, M.; Ito, T.; Uezumi, A.; Hayashi, S.; Miyagoe-Suzuki, Y.; et al. Suppression of macrophage functions impairs skeletal muscle regeneration with severe fibrosis. *Exp. Cell Res.* **2008**, *314*, 3232–3244. [CrossRef]

38. Fukada, S.; Higuchi, S.; Segawa, M.; Koda, K.; Yamamoto, Y.; Tsujikawa, K.; Kohama, Y.; Uezumi, A.; Imamura, M.; Miyagoe-Suzuki, Y.; et al. Purification and cell-surface marker characterization of quiescent satellite cells from murine skeletal muscle by a novel monoclonal antibody. *Exp. Cell Res.* **2004**, *296*, 245–255. [CrossRef]

2

Conditional Deletion of Dicer in Adult Mice Impairs Skeletal Muscle Regeneration

Satoshi Oikawa[ID], **Minjung Lee and Takayuki Akimoto** *

Faculty of Sport Sciences, Waseda University, Saitama 359-1192, Japan; s-oikawa@aoni.waseda.jp (S.O.);
namoonyousun@gmail.com (M.L.)
* Correspondence: axi@waseda.jp;

Abstract: Skeletal muscle has a remarkable regenerative capacity, which is orchestrated by multiple processes, including the proliferation, fusion, and differentiation of the resident stem cells in muscle. MicroRNAs (miRNAs) are small noncoding RNAs that mediate the translational repression or degradation of mRNA to regulate diverse biological functions. Previous studies have suggested that several miRNAs play important roles in myoblast proliferation and differentiation in vitro. However, their potential roles in skeletal muscle regeneration in vivo have not been fully established. In this study, we generated a mouse in which the *Dicer* gene, which encodes an enzyme essential in miRNA processing, was knocked out in a tamoxifen-inducible way (iDicer KO mouse) and determined its regenerative potential after cardiotoxin-induced acute muscle injury. *Dicer* mRNA expression was significantly reduced in the tibialis anterior muscle of the iDicer KO mice, whereas the expression of muscle-enriched miRNAs was only slightly reduced in the Dicer-deficient muscles. After cardiotoxin injection, the iDicer KO mice showed impaired muscle regeneration. We also demonstrated that the number of PAX7$^+$ cells, cell proliferation, and the myogenic differentiation capacity of the primary myoblasts did not differ between the wild-type and the iDicer KO mice. Taken together, these data demonstrate that Dicer is a critical factor for muscle regeneration in vivo.

Keywords: Dicer; microRNA; skeletal muscle; muscle regeneration

1. Introduction

Adult skeletal muscle has a remarkable regenerative capacity. After muscle injury, the resident muscle stem cells leave their quiescent state and begin to proliferate. These cells ultimately differentiate into multinucleated myotubes, which fuse with existing damaged myofibers [1]. Muscle regeneration is impaired by treatment with a mitosis inhibitor, colchicine, which inhibits cellular proliferation during regeneration [2]. Primary satellite cells (SCs) derived from mutant mice lacking PAX7, a marker of SCs, showed reduced proliferation and fewer myosin heavy chain (MyHC)-positive myotubes [3,4]. The adult *Pax7*-mutant mice also showed impaired injury-induced muscle regeneration [3]. These findings indicate that the proliferation and myogenic differentiation of resident muscle stem cells are necessary for muscle regeneration.

MicroRNAs (miRNAs) are small noncoding RNAs that repress the expression of their target genes at the posttranscriptional level to control diverse biological functions [5]. These small RNAs can bind to a complementary site, called "seed sequences", in the 3′ untranslated region (UTR) of a target mRNA, resulting in the degradation or translational repression of that mRNA [5]. miRNAs are transcribed as long primary transcripts, called "primary miRNAs", by an RNA polymerase II. The transcripts are cleaved by a nuclear ribonuclease III, Drosha, and then exported to the cytoplasm and further cleaved by a cytoplasmic ribonuclease III, Dicer, into double-stranded RNA. This miRNA duplex is loaded onto an Argonaute protein to form a ribonucleoprotein complex called the "RNA-induced silencing complex" [6].

Growing evidence indicates that miRNA-mediated gene silencing plays an important role in skeletal muscle cell growth and myogenic differentiation [7–11]. Mutant mice in which Dicer is inactivated during embryonic myogenesis show a variety of abnormal muscle phenotypes, suggesting that Dicer-mediated miRNA processing plays an essential role in muscle development [12]. An expression profiling analysis showed that three miRNAs, miR-1, miR-133, and miR-206, are abundantly expressed in skeletal muscles [13]. These three miRNAs are transcriptionally regulated by myogenic regulatory factors, which are master transcriptional factors for skeletal muscle cell-fate determination and development, and are upregulated during muscle differentiation [14–17]. It has been shown that miR-1 and miR-206, which have identical seed sequences, promote myogenesis in vitro, whereas miR-133 promotes myoblast proliferation [7,8]. A previous study also demonstrated that miR-1 and miR-206 regulate apoptosis by repressing *Pax3* gene expression in *Myod*-KO myoblasts [18]. Although these data indicate that miRNAs are important regulators of the proliferation and differentiation of muscle cells in vitro, their potential roles in muscle regeneration in vivo have not been fully established.

In this study, we generated a tamoxifen-inducible conditional *Dicer*-KO (iDicer KO) mouse to deplete all mature miRNAs and analyzed its regenerative capacity during cardiotoxin-induced muscle regeneration. Our data suggest that Dicer-mediated miRNA processing is necessary for skeletal muscle regeneration in vivo.

2. Results

2.1. Expression of Dicer and miRNAs in iDicer KO Mice

To investigate the role of miRNAs in muscle regeneration, we first generated a mutant mouse with the tamoxifen-inducible disruption of the *Dicer* gene (iDicer KO). Consistent with our previous data [19], a real-time PCR analysis confirmed the significant reduction in *Dicer* mRNA expression in the tibialis anterior (TA) muscles of the iDicer KO mice (Figure 1A), whereas the expression levels of the muscle-enriched miRNAs miR-1, miR-133a and miR-26a, and other miRNAs (miR-15b, miR-20a, miR-199a-3p, miR-214, miR-146a, miR-21 and miR-24) were modestly reduced in the iDicer KO mice (Figure 1B).

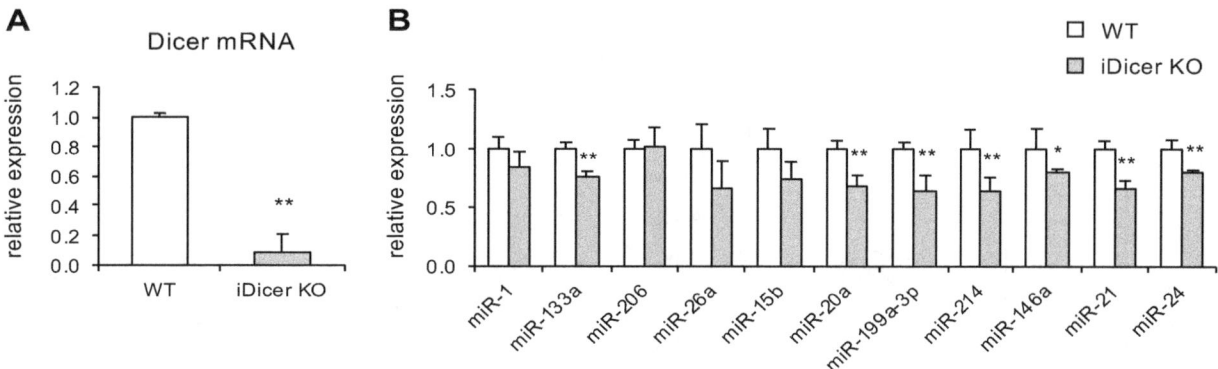

Figure 1. Expression levels of *Dicer* mRNA and muscle-enriched miRNAs in tibialis anterior (TA) muscles of tamoxifen-induced *Dicer* knock-out (iDicer KO) mice. (**A**) Tamoxifen induced a large reduction in *Dicer* mRNA expression in the iDicer KO mice ($n = 5$). (**B**) Expression levels of muscle-enriched miR-1, miR-133a and miR-26a and other miRNAs (miR-15b, miR-20a, miR-199a-3p, miR-214, miR-146a, miR-21 and miR-24) were slightly reduced in TA muscle of the iDicer KO mice by tamoxifen injection ($n = 3–5$). Data are means ± SE, * $p < 0.05$, ** $p < 0.01$.

2.2. Skeletal Muscle Regeneration Is Impaired in iDicer KO Mice

We next determined the regenerative potential of the iDicer KO mice during skeletal muscle regeneration. Wild-type (WT) and iDicer KO mice were injected intramuscularly with cardiotoxin (CTX) to induce muscle injury, and the cross-sectional area (CSA) of the regenerating myofibers was analyzed with hematoxylin–eosin (H&E) staining. Fourteen days after CTX injection, the mean CSA of the regenerating myofibers with central nuclei in the iDicer KO mice was smaller than that in the WT mice (Figure 2A–C).

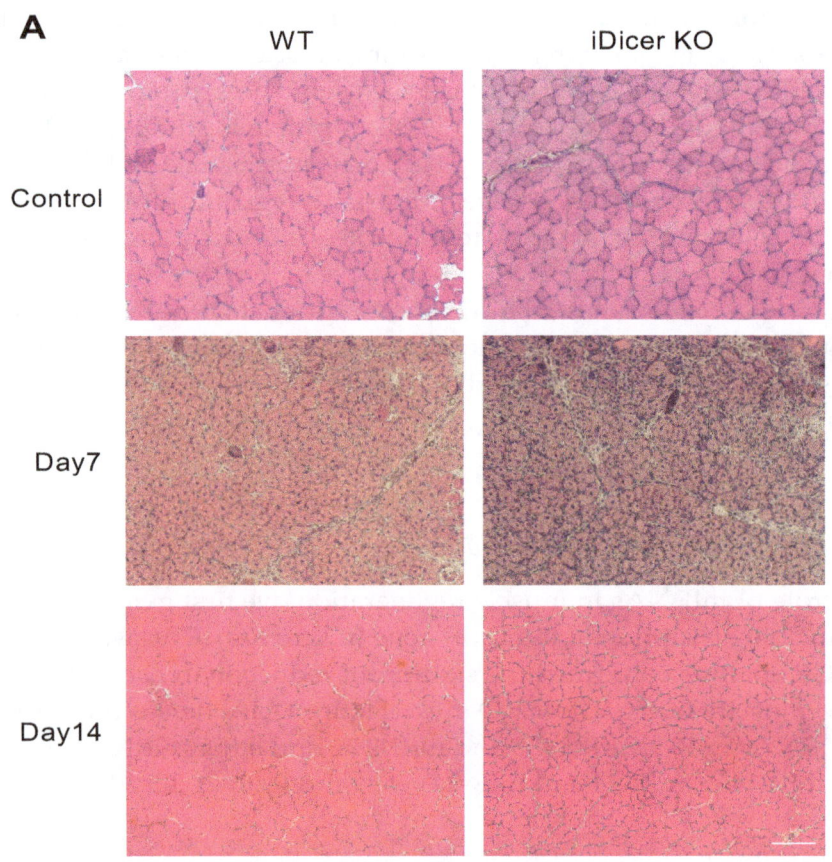

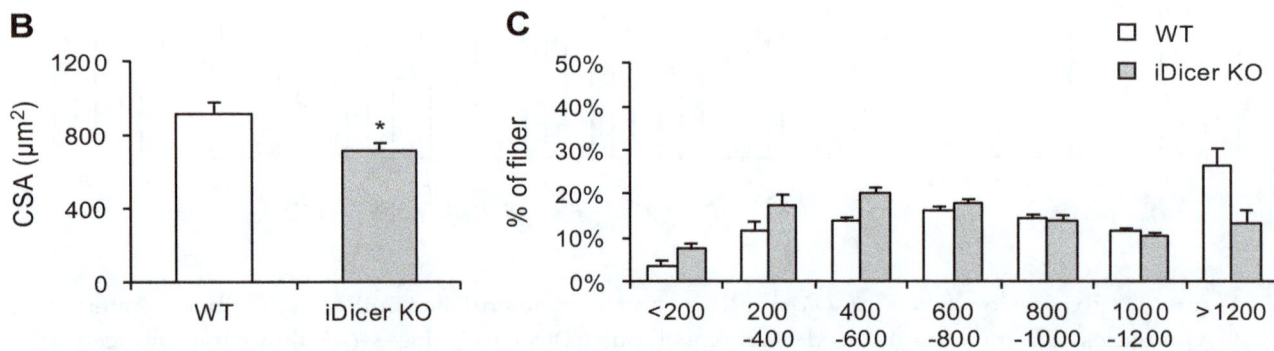

Figure 2. Skeletal muscle regeneration in the iDicer KO mice. (**A**) Representative image of sections of TA muscle stained with hematoxylin–eosin (H&E). Scale bar = 100 μm. (**B,C**) Mean cross-sectional area (CSA) of regenerating muscle fibers with central nuclei in the iDicer KO mice was significantly smaller than that in the WT mice ($n = 7$). Data are means ± SE, * $p < 0.05$.

2.3. Inducible Knockout of Dicer Does Not Affect Cell Proliferation or Differentiation of Primary Myoblasts

Because the regenerative capacity of adult skeletal muscle largely depends on the functions of the resident muscle stem cells, such as muscle SCs, we investigated their numbers and the myogenic differentiation potential of primary myoblasts isolated from iDicer KO mice. Fourteen days after CTX injection, the number of PAX7$^+$ cells on the cryosections did not differ in the WT and iDicer KO mice (Figure 3A,B). Furthermore, the cell viability and fusion index of the primary myoblasts isolated from the iDicer KO mice with tamoxifen injection were similar to those of the WT mice (Figure 3C–E).

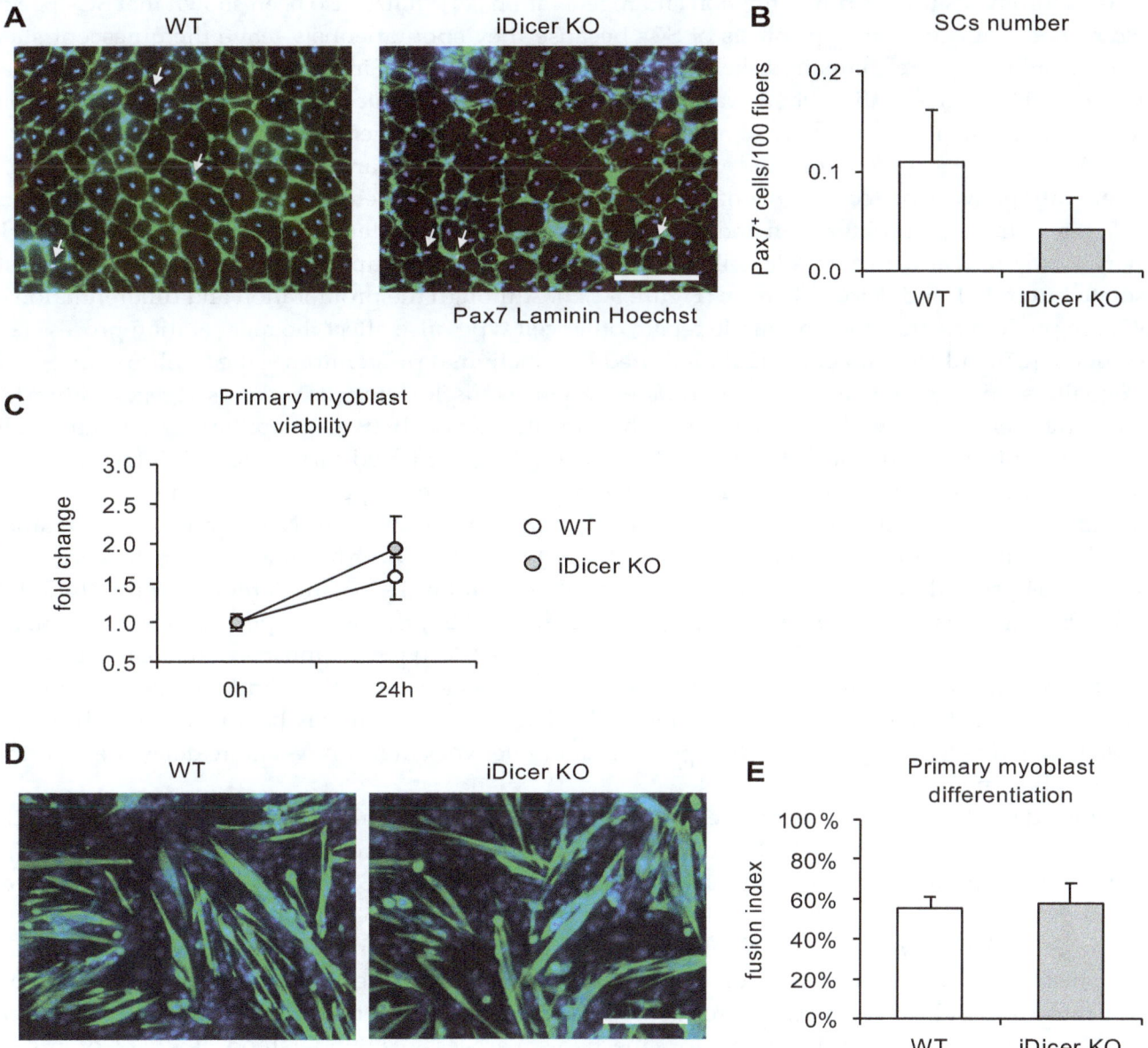

Figure 3. Satellite cell (SC) numbers and myogenic differentiation potential in primary myoblasts isolated from WT and iDicer KO mice (**A,B**). Immunofluorescence analysis revealed that the number of PAX7$^+$ SCs in the iDicer KO mice was similar to that in the WT mice (n = 6–8) (**C–E**). There was no difference in the cell viability of the primary myoblasts (**C**) or their fusion indices (**D,E**) in the WT and iDicer KO mice (n = 3–4). Data are means ± SE. Scale bar = 100 μm.

3. Discussion

The tamoxifen-inducible knockout of Dicer in adult mice impaired the skeletal muscle regeneration that occurred in response to CTX injury (Figure 2). However, we found no reductions in the PAX7$^+$ cell numbers, cell viability, or the myogenic differentiation potential of the primary myoblasts isolated from the iDicer KO mice (Figure 3). These data suggest that Dicer plays a prominent role in skeletal muscle regeneration in vivo. However, the molecular mechanism by which Dicer regulates skeletal muscle regeneration in this model is still unclear.

Recent studies have demonstrated that multiple miRNAs act as key regulators of skeletal muscle regeneration in adult mice [20–24]. For example, miR-26a, which is specifically expressed in skeletal muscle, is upregulated during muscle differentiation in vitro and muscle regeneration in vivo [10,21]. The inhibition of miR-26a with a miRNA decoy in vivo delayed muscle regeneration, indicating that miR-26a promotes muscle differentiation and regeneration [21]. It has also been shown that SC-specific *Dicer* knockout causes the apoptosis of SCs because they spontaneously leave the quiescent state, which results in severely impaired skeletal muscle regeneration after injury [25]. We also demonstrated that the CSA of regenerating fibers was reduced in the iDicer KO mice (Figure 2). Taken together, our data demonstrate the importance of miRNAs in skeletal muscle regeneration in mice.

Because the proliferation and differentiation of myoblasts are essential for skeletal muscle regeneration, we isolated the primary myoblasts from the skeletal muscles of iDicer KO mice, and determined the proliferation and myogenic differentiation potential of these cells. Surprisingly, there were no clear differences in cell viability or differentiation capacity of the primary myoblasts isolated from WT and iDicer KO mice (Figure 3C,D). Although the proliferation and differentiation of SCs are predominant factors in muscle repair, other cell types also affect the regeneration process [26]. Joe et al., [27] and Uezumi et al., [28] identified mesenchymal progenitors, called "fibro-adipogenic progenitors", that enhance the myogenic differentiation of muscle stem cells and muscle regeneration [27, 29]. Another recent work demonstrated that an interaction between capillary endothelial cells and SCs controls SC functions through a Notch-signaling-mediated direct cell–cell interaction [30]. Future research with mice in which individual miRNAs are cell-type-specifically knocked out may provide greater insight into the functions and regulatory mechanisms of miRNAs in muscle regeneration.

We found that muscle regeneration was disrupted in the iDicer KO mice, whereas expressions of muscle-enriched miRNAs (miR-1, miR-133a, miR-206 and miR-26a) and other miRNAs (miR-15b, miR-20a, miR-119a-3p, miR-214, miR-146a, miR-21 and miR-24) that were reported to be upregulated during muscle regeneration [31], were reduced only ~20–40% in the TA muscle of the iDicer KO mice compared with those in the WT mice (Figure 1B). It is not clear how the slight changes in miRNAs could contribute to the delayed regeneration in the iDicer KO mice. It may be possible that the global reduction in miRNAs is enough to disrupt a regulatory network of miRNAs and to delay the myofiber regeneration in vivo.

Our data showed that the muscle-enriched miRNAs were highly stable in the TA muscle of the iDicer KO mice (Figure 1B), which is consistent with our previous report [19]. Similarly, recent data on tamoxifen-inducible, skeletal muscle-specific Dicer knockout (HSA-MCM; Dicer$^{fl/fl}$) mice showed that the expression levels of miRNAs including miR-1, miR-133a and miR-206 were slightly affected by the Dicer depletion [32]. Several lines of evidence indicate that the mature miRNAs expressed in liver, heart, and neuron are also stable in vivo [33–35]. A pulse-chase approach and high-throughput sequencing of miRNAs revealed the production and turnover rates of miRNAs in vitro [36,37], whereas miRNA turnover in vivo and its regulatory mechanism are less well understood. It will be of interest in future works to investigate how miRNA turnover is regulated in vivo.

4. Materials and Methods

4.1. Animal Experiments

All mice were maintained in temperature-controlled quarters (21 °C) under a 12 h light–dark cycle and provided with a standard chow diet. The generation of tamoxifen-inducible Dicer knockout (CAG-Cre^{ERT2}, Dicer$^{fl/fl}$) mice has been described previously [19]. The mice were maintained in a B6 background and intraperitoneally injected with 1 mg of tamoxifen at 8 weeks old for 5 consecutive days.

The tibialis anterior (TA) muscles of 9-week-old wild-type (WT) and iDicer KO mice were injected with cardiotoxin (CTX) from *Naja pallida* (Latoxan, Portes-lès-Valence, France) with a 27-gauge needle. The TA muscles were harvested 7 and 14 days after CTX injury, frozen in liquid nitrogen, and stored at −80 °C. The animal protocols were approved by the Animal Care and Use Committees of Waseda University, Japan (numbers: 2017-A103a, 2018-A122, 2019-108).

4.2. qPCR

Total RNA was extracted with Isogen II (Wako Chemicals, Osaka, Japan), and 1 μg of total RNA was converted to cDNA with ReverTra Ace reverse transcriptase (Toyobo, Osaka, Japan). Real-time PCR was performed with Thunderbird® SYBR® qPCR Mix (Toyobo), with gene-specific primers. The following primers were used for real-time PCR: Dicer, 5′-CACACGCCTCCTACCACTACAACAC-3′ and 5′-CCGTGGGTCTTCATAAAGGT-3′; glyceraldehyde 3-phosphate dehydrogenase (GAPDH), 5′-AAATGGTGAAGGTCGGTGTG-3′ and 5′-TGAAGGGGTCGTTGATGG-3′. For the real-time PCR analysis of mature miRNA expression, the TaqMan® MicroRNA Reverse Transcription Kit and TaqMan® MicroRNA Assays (Applied Biosystems, Foster City, CA, USA) were used, according to the manufacturer's protocols [38,39].

4.3. Histological Analysis

Cross-sections of frozen TA muscle were stained with H&E and immunofluorescence. The cross-sections were incubated with the following antibodies: anti-PAX7 (DSHB; University of Iowa, Iowa City, IA), anti-laminin (10765; Cappel Reseach Reagent, Turnholt, Belgium), and Hoechst 33342 (Invitrogen, Carlsbad, CA). The secondary antibodies were Alexa-Fluor-594-conjugated anti-mouse IgG antibody for PAX7 and Alexa-Fluor-488-conjugated anti-rabbit IgG antibody for laminin (Jackson ImmunoResearch Laboratories, West Grove, PA, USA). The cross-sectional area (CSA) was quantified using ImageJ software (National Institutes of Health, Bethesda, MD, USA).

4.4. Isolation and Culture of Primary Myoblasts

Primary myoblasts were isolated as previously described [40,41]. Briefly, after tamoxifen injection, the gastrocnemius, TA, and quadriceps muscles were collected and digested with 0.2% collagenase type II (Worthington Biochemical Corporation, Freehold, NJ, USA) at 37 °C for 30 min. After incubation, the muscle slurries were triturated with an 18-gauge needle and then incubated again at 37 °C for 15 min. The muscle mixtures were filtered sequentially through 100 μm and 40 μm filters (Falcon, Sunnyvale, CA, USA), and then centrifuged at 200× g for 5 min. The cells were resuspended in growth medium containing Ham's F-10 Nutrient Mix (Thermo Fisher Scientific, Waltham, MA, USA) supplemented with 20% fetal bovine serum, 1% penicillin–streptomycin, and 2.5 ng/mL basic fibroblast growth factor (G5071; Promega, Madison, WI, USA), and seeded in gelatin-coated dishes. To evaluate cell viability, 3000 cells/well were seeded in 96-well plates and a CellTiter-Glo® 2.0 Cell Viability Assay (Promega) was performed, according to the manufacturer's protocol. To induce cell differentiation, the myoblasts in the 96-well plate at 80–90% confluence were switched to differentiation medium (DM; DMEM supplemented with 2% horse serum). The DM was changed daily for 5 days. After differentiation, the cells were immunofluorescently stained with Hoechst 33342 and anti-α-actinin antibody (A7732; Sigma-Aldrich, St Louis, MO, USA) to identify nuclei and differentiated myotubes, respectively. The secondary antibody for anti-α-actinin was an Alexa-Fluor-488-conjugated goat anti-mouse IgG_1 antibody (Jackson ImmunoResearch Laboratories). The fusion index was calculated manually as the ratio of the number of nuclei within the α-actinin-positive myotubes with more than two nuclei to the total number of nuclei, using ImageJ software (LOCI, University of Wisconsin, Madison, WI, USA).

Author Contributions: S.O. and T.A. conceived and designed the research; S.O. and M.L. performed experiments; S.O. and M.L. analyzed the data; S.O., M.L., and T.A. interpreted the results of the experiments; S.O. prepared the figures; S.O. and T.A. drafted the manuscript.

Acknowledgments: We thank Brian Harfe (University of Florida) for providing the Dicer1-floxed mice.

Abbreviations

SC	Satellite cell
miRNA	microRNA
TA	Tibialis anterior
WT	Wild-type
CSA	Cross-sectional area
CTX	Cardiotoxin

References

1.   Chargé, S.B.; Rudnicki, M.A. Cellular and molecular regulation of muscle regeneration. *Physiol. Rev.* **2004**, *84*, 209–238. [CrossRef] [PubMed]

2.   Pietsch, P. The effects of colchicine on regeneration of mouse skeletal muscle. *Anat. Rec.* **1961**, *139*, 167–172. [CrossRef]

3.   Oustanina, S.; Hause, G.; Braun, T. Pax7 directs postnatal renewal and propagation of myogenic satellite cells but not their specification. *Embo. J.* **2004**, *23*, 3430–3439. [CrossRef] [PubMed]

4.   Seale, P.; Sabourin, L.A.; Girgis-Gabardo, A.; Mansouri, A.; Gruss, P.; Rudnicki, M.A. Pax7 is Required for the Specification of Myogenic Satellite Cells. *Cell* **2000**, *102*, 777–786. [CrossRef]

5.   Bartel, D.P. MicroRNAs Genomics, Biogenesis, Mechanism, and Function. *Cell* **2004**, *116*, 281–297. [CrossRef]

6.   Ha, M.; Kim, N.V. Regulation of microRNA biogenesis. *Nat. Rev. Mol. Cell Biol.* **2014**, *15*, 509–524. [CrossRef]

7.   Chen, J.-F.; Mandel, E.M.; Thomson, M.J.; Wu, Q.; Callis, T.E.; Hammond, S.M.; Conlon, F.L.; Wang, D.-Z. The role of microRNA-1 and microRNA-133 in skeletal muscle proliferation and differentiation. *Nat. Genet.* **2005**, *38*, 228–233. [CrossRef]

8.   Kim, H.; Lee, Y.; Sivaprasad, U.; Malhotra, A.; Dutta, A. Muscle-specific microRNA miR-206 promotes muscle differentiation. *J. Cell Biol.* **2006**, *174*, 677–687. [CrossRef]

9.   Chen, J.-F.; Tao, Y.; Li, J.; Deng, Z.; Yan, Z.; Xiao, X.; Wang, D.-Z. microRNA-1 and microRNA-206 regulate skeletal muscle satellite cell proliferation and differentiation by repressing Pax7. *J. Cell Biol.* **2010**, *190*, 867–879. [CrossRef]

10.   Wong, C.; Tellam, R.L. MicroRNA-26a Targets the Histone Methyltransferase Enhancer of Zeste homolog 2 during Myogenesis. *J. Biol. Chem.* **2008**, *283*, 9836–9843. [CrossRef]

11.   Silva, W.; Graça, F.; Cruz, A.; Silvestre, J.; Labeit, S.; Miyabara, E.; Yan, C.; Wang, D.; Moriscot, A. miR-29c improves skeletal muscle mass and function throughout myocyte proliferation and differentiation and by repressing atrophy-related genes. *Acta Physiol.* **2019**, *226*, e13278. [CrossRef] [PubMed]

12.   O'Rourke, J.; Georges, S.; Seay, H.; Tapscott, S.; McManus, M.; Goldhamer, D.; Swanson, M.; Harfe, B. Essential role for Dicer during skeletal muscle development. *Dev. Biol.* **2007**, *311*, 359–368. [CrossRef] [PubMed]

13.   Sempere, L.F.; Freemantle, S.; Pitha-Rowe, I.; Moss, E.; Dmitrovsky, E.; Ambros, V. Expression profiling of mammalian microRNAs uncovers a subset of brain-expressed microRNAs with possible roles in murine and human neuronal differentiation. *Genome Biol.* **2004**, *5*, R13. [CrossRef] [PubMed]

14.   Liu, N.; Williams, A.H.; Kim, Y.; McAnally, J.; Bezprozvannaya, S.; Sutherland, L.B.; Richardson, J.A.; Bassel-Duby, R.; Olson, E.N. An intragenic MEF2-dependent enhancer directs muscle-specific expression of microRNAs 1 and 133. *Proc. Natl. Acad. Sci. USA* **2007**, *104*, 20844–20849. [CrossRef]

15.   Rao, P.K.; Kumar, R.M.; Farkhondeh, M.; Baskerville, S.; Lodish, H.F. Myogenic factors that regulate expression of muscle-specific microRNAs. *Proc. Natl. Acad. Sci. USA* **2006**, *103*, 8721–8726. [CrossRef]

16.   Sweetman, D.; Goljanek, K.; Rathjen, T.; Oustanina, S.; Braun, T.; Dalmay, T.; Munsterberg, A. Specific requirements of MRFs for the expression of muscle specific microRNAs, miR-1, miR-206 and miR-133. *Dev. Biol.* **2008**, *321*, 491–499. [CrossRef]

17. Koutsoulidou, A.; Mastroyiannopoulos, N.P.; Furling, D.; Uney, J.B.; Phylactou, L.A. Expression of miR-1, miR-133a, miR-133b and miR-206 increases during development of human skeletal muscle. *BMC Dev. Biol.* **2011**, *11*, 34. [CrossRef]

18. Hirai, H.; Verma, M.; Watanabe, S.; Tastad, C.; Asakura, Y.; Asakura, A. MyoD regulates apoptosis of myoblasts through microRNA-mediated down-regulation of Pax3. *J. Cell Biol.* **2010**, *191*, 347–365. [CrossRef]

19. Oikawa, S.; Lee, M.; Motohashi, N.; Maeda, S.; Akimoto, T. An inducible knockout of Dicer in adult mice does not affect endurance exercise-induced muscle adaptation. *Am. J. Physiol. Cell Physiol.* **2019**, *316*, C285–C292. [CrossRef]

20. Snyder, C.M.; Rice, A.L.; Estrella, N.L.; Held, A.; Kandarian, S.C.; Naya, F.J. MEF2A regulates the Gtl2-Dio3 microRNA mega-cluster to modulate WNT signaling in skeletal muscle regeneration. *Development* **2013**, *140*, 31–42. [CrossRef]

21. Dey, B.K.; Gagan, J.; Yan, Z.; Dutta, A. miR-26a is required for skeletal muscle differentiation and regeneration in mice. *Genes Dev.* **2012**, *26*, 2180–2191. [CrossRef] [PubMed]

22. Lee, K.-P.; Shin, Y.; Panda, A.C.; Abdelmohsen, K.; Kim, J.; Lee, S.-M.; Bahn, Y.; Choi, J.; Kwon, E.-S.; Baek, S.-J.; et al. miR-431 promotes differentiation and regeneration of old skeletal muscle by targeting Smad4. *Genes Dev.* **2015**, *29*, 1605–1617. [CrossRef] [PubMed]

23. Bronisz-Budzyńska, I.; Chwalenia, K.; Mucha, O.; Podkalicka, P.; Karolina, B.-S.; Józkowicz, A.; Łoboda, A.; Kozakowska, M.; Dulak, J. miR-146a deficiency does not aggravate muscular dystrophy in mdx mice. *Skelet. Muscle* **2019**, *9*, 22. [CrossRef] [PubMed]

24. Qiu, H.; Liu, N.; Luo, L.; Zhong, J.; Tang, Z.; Kang, K.; Qu, J.; Peng, W.; Liu, L.; Li, L.; et al. MicroRNA-17-92 regulates myoblast proliferation and differentiation by targeting the ENH1/Id1 signaling axis. *Cell Death Differ.* **2016**, *23*, 1658–1669. [CrossRef] [PubMed]

25. Cheung, T.H.; Quach, N.L.; Charville, G.W.; Liu, L.; Park, L.; Edalati, A.; Yoo, B.; Hoang, P.; Rando, T.A. Maintenance of muscle stem-cell quiescence by microRNA-489. *Nature* **2012**, *482*, 524–528. [CrossRef] [PubMed]

26. Baghdadi, M.B.; Tajbakhsh, S. Regulation and phylogeny of skeletal muscle regeneration. *Dev. Biol.* **2018**, *433*, 200–209. [CrossRef]

27. Joe, A.W.; Yi, L.; Natarajan, A.; Grand, F.; So, L.; Wang, J.; Rudnicki, M.A.; Rossi, F.M. Muscle injury activates resident fibro/adipogenic progenitors that facilitate myogenesis. *Nat. Cell Biol.* **2010**, *12*, 153–163. [CrossRef]

28. Uezumi, A.; Fukada, S.; Yamamoto, N.; Takeda, S.; Tsuchida, K. Mesenchymal progenitors distinct from satellite cells contribute to ectopic fat cell formation in skeletal muscle. *Nat. Cell Biol.* **2010**, *12*, 143–152. [CrossRef]

29. Wosczyna, M.N.; Konishi, C.T.; Carbajal, E.E.; Wang, T.T.; Walsh, R.A.; Gan, Q.; Wagner, M.W.; Rando, T.A. Mesenchymal Stromal Cells Are Required for Regeneration and Homeostatic Maintenance of Skeletal Muscle. *Cell Rep.* **2019**, *27*, 2029–2035. [CrossRef]

30. Verma, M.; Asakura, Y.; Murakonda, B.; Pengo, T.; Latroche, C.; Chazaud, B.; McLoon, L.K.; Asakura, A. Muscle Satellite Cell Cross-Talk with a Vascular Niche Maintains Quiescence via VEGF and Notch Signaling. *Cell Stem Cell* **2018**, *23*, 530–543. [CrossRef]

31. Liu, N.; Williams, A.H.; Maxeiner, J.M.; Bezprozvannaya, S.; elton, J.; Richardson, J.A.; Bassel-Duby, R.; Olson, E.N. microRNA-206 promotes skeletal muscle regeneration and delays progression of Duchenne muscular dystrophy in mice. *J. Clin. Investig.* **2012**, *122*, 2054–2065. [CrossRef] [PubMed]

32. Vechetti, I.J.; Wen, Y.; Chaillou, T.; Murach, K.A.; Alimov, A.P.; Figueiredo, V.C.; Dal-Pai-Silva, M.; McCarthy, J.J. Life-long reduction in myomiR expression does not adversely affect skeletal muscle morphology. *Sci. Rep. UK* **2019**, *9*, 5483. [CrossRef] [PubMed]

33. Gatfield, D.; Martelot, L.G.; Vejnar, C.; Gerlach, D.; Schaad, O.; Fleury-Olela, F.; Ruskeepaa, A.; Oresic, M.; Esau, C.; Zdobnov, E.; et al. Integration of microRNA miR-122 in hepatic circadian gene expression. *Genes Dev.* **2009**, *23*, 1313–1326. [CrossRef] [PubMed]

34. Van Rooij, E.; Sutherland, L.; Qi, X.; Richardson, J.; Hill, J.; Olson, E. Control of stress-dependent cardiac growth and gene expression by a microRNA. *Science* **2007**, *316*, 575–579. [CrossRef] [PubMed]

35. Schaefer, A.; O'Carroll, D.; Tan, C.; Hillman, D.; Sugimori, M.; Llinas, R.; Greengard, P. Cerebellar neurodegeneration in the absence of microRNAs. *J. Exp. Med.* **2007**, *204*, 1553–1558. [CrossRef]

36. Reichholf, B.; Herzog, V.A.; Fasching, N.; Manzenreither, R.A.; Sowemimo, I.; Ameres, S.L. Time-Resolved Small RNA Sequencing Unravels the Molecular Principles of MicroRNA Homeostasis. *Mol. Cell* **2019**, *75*, 756–768. [CrossRef]

37. Marzi, M.J.; Ghini, F.; Cerruti, B.; de Pretis, S.; Bonetti, P.; Giacomelli, C.; Gorski, M.M.; Kress, T.; Pelizzola, M.; Muller, H.; et al. Degradation dynamics of microRNAs revealed by a novel pulse-chase approach. *Genome Res.* **2016**, *26*, 554–565. [CrossRef]

38. Oikawa, S.; Wada, S.; Lee, M.; Maeda, S.; Akimoto, T. Role of endothelial microRNA-23 clusters in angiogenesis in vivo. *Am. J. Physiol. Heart C* **2018**, *315*, H838–H846. [CrossRef]

39. Wada, S.; Kato, Y.; Okutsu, M.; Miyaki, S.; Suzuki, K.; Yan, Z.; Schiaffino, S.; Asahara, H.; Ushida, T.; Akimoto, T. Translational suppression of atrophic regulators by microRNA-23a integrates resistance to skeletal muscle atrophy. *J. Biol. Chem.* **2011**, *286*, 38456–38465. [CrossRef]

40. Rando, T.; Blau, H. Primary mouse myoblast purification, characterization, and transplantation for cell-mediated gene therapy. *J. Cell Biol.* **1994**, *125*, 1275–1287. [CrossRef]

41. Hindi, L.; McMillan, J.; Afroze, D.; Hindi, S.; Kumar, A. Isolation, Culturing, and Differentiation of Primary Myoblasts from Skeletal Muscle of Adult Mice. *Bio. Protoc.* **2017**, *7*, 7. [CrossRef] [PubMed]

3

Effect of Ishophloroglucin A, a Component of *Ishige okamurae*, on Glucose Homeostasis in the Pancreas and Muscle of High Fat Diet-Fed Mice

Hye-Won Yang [1,†], Myeongjoo Son [2,3,†] (ID), Junwon Choi [2,3], Seyeon Oh [3], You-Jin Jeon [1,4] (ID), Kyunghee Byun [2,3,*] and BoMi Ryu [1,4,*]

[1]   Department of Marine Life Science, School of Marine Biomedical Sciences, Jeju National University, 1 Ara 1-dong, Jejudaehak-ro, Jeju 63243, Korea; koty221@naver.com (H.-W.Y.); youjinj@jejunu.ac.kr (Y.-J.J.)
[2]   Department of Anatomy & Cell Biology, Gachon University College of Medicine, Incheon 21936, Korea; mjson@gachon.ac.kr (M.S.); choijw88@gc.gachon.ac.kr (J.C.)
[3]   Functional Cellular Networks Laboratory, College of Medicine, Department of Medicine, Graduate School and Lee Gil Ya Cancer and Diabetes Institute, Gachon University, Incheon 21999, Korea; seyeon8965@gachon.ac.kr
[4]   Marine Science Institute, Jeju National University, Jeju 63333, Korea
*   Correspondence: khbyun1@gachon.ac.kr (K.B.); bmryu@jejunu.ac.kr (B.R.);
†   These authors contributed equally to this work.

Abstract: Ishophloroglucin A (IPA), a component of *Ishige okamurae* (IO), was previously evaluated to standardize the antidiabetic potency of IO. However, the potential of IPA as a functional food for diabetes prevention has not yet been evaluated. Here, we investigated if 1.35 mg/kg IPA, which is the equivalent content of IPA in 75 mg/kg IO, improved glucose homeostasis in high-fat diet (HFD)-induced diabetes after 12 weeks of treatment. IPA significantly ameliorated glucose intolerance, reducing fasting glucose levels as well as 2 h glucose levels in HFD mice. In addition, IPA exerted a protective effect on the pancreatic function in HFD mice via pancreatic β-cells and C-peptide. The level of glucose transporter 4 (GLUT4) in the muscles of HFD mice was stimulated by IPA intake. Our results suggested that IPA, which is a component of IO, can improve glucose homeostasis via GLUT4 in the muscles of HFD mice. IO may be used as a functional food for the prevention of diabetes.

Keywords: functional food; diabetes; *Ishige okamurae*; Ishophloroglucin A

1. Introduction

Seaweeds contain bioactive substances, such as polysaccharides, proteins, lipids, and polyphenols, and have been reported to have nutraceutical and pharmaceutical potential in functional foods [1,2]. *Ishige okamurae* (IO), an edible seaweed, possesses bioactive substances, such as ishophloroglucin A (IPA), diphlorethohydroxycarmalol (DPHC), and fucoxanthin, as well as other secondary metabolites [3]. In our previous study, we suggested that IPA could be used to standardize the antidiabetic activity potency of IO extract in vitro [4]. However, the use of IPA in functional foods for diabetes prevention in vivo, in high-fat diet (HFD)-fed mice, has not yet been determined.

Diabetes mellitus is a chronic metabolic disorder caused by the inadequate balance of glucose homeostasis [5]. Glucose homeostasis is maintained by the tight regulation of blood glucose by insulin and glucagon [6]. In particular, glucose transporters (GLUT), with substrate specificities that dictate their functional roles, regulate glucose level both outside and inside of the cell [7]. Most of the current drugs for the treatment of diabetes aim to improve insulin production and metabolic regulation. Furthermore, previous studies have focused on the prevention of diabetes for both type 1 and type 2 diabetes [8,9]. In addition, the improper balance of glucose homeostasis can be prevented or reduced by functional foods. Therefore, there has recently been much interest in the use of natural products as a source of stronger and safer antidiabetic therapies [10–12].

Previous studies have reported that complementary and alternative natural products, such as herbal therapies, have been used for the prevention and/or treatment of diseases, such as diabetes, hypertension, and cardiovascular disease [13,14]. Increased intake of high-calorie and high-fat diets and decreased physical activity have led to a high rate of chronic diseases, such as heart diseases, diabetes, and hypertension [15]. Health is recognized by many as an important personal and social value; consumers have become increasingly interested in the benefits of food that can help achieve or maintain a healthy lifestyle [16,17]. Previous studies have reported that adequate nutrition is an essential aspect of diet and chronic diseases, as well as influencing a person's health status [18,19]. In addition, the studies have shown that health is an important motivation for nutraceutical consumption [20].

Therefore, this study evaluated the effect of IPA on glucose transporters, such as GLUT2 and GLUT4, which are involved in glucose homeostasis. In addition, we examined if their related transcription factors in the pancreas and muscle could regulate the blood glucose level in HFD mice. The data from this study address the effect of IPA on glucose homeostasis in the pancreas and muscle of HFD mice, and shed further light on the strategic potential of IPA as a functional food for the improvement of diabetes in the future.

2. Results

2.1. Improvement in Glucose Tolerance by IPA in HFD Mice

To assess whether the increased metabolic disorders in HFD mice were improved by IPA, we investigated the body weight, food intake, and fasting and feeding glucose levels in HFD mice. The concentration of IPA used in this experiment was the equivalent content of IPA (1.35 mg/kg) in IO extract (75 mg/kg). As shown in Figure 1A, the body weight of HFD mice was not different at the beginning of the study between groups. After 4 weeks of the HFD/IO treatment, we fed mice IO extract (50 and 75 mg/kg, HFD/IO), IPA (1.35 mg/kg, HFD/IPA), and guava (75 mg/kg, HFD/Guava), used as positive control for blood glucose level control in diabetes [21], for 12 weeks. After 12 weeks, the HFD group gained more body weight at each time point compared with the NFD group. However, the HFD/IPA (1.35 mg/kg) group showed a significantly lower increased in body weight compared with the HFD group. In addition, the amount of HFD consumed is required to maintain a constant energy intake [22]. A previous study has reported that HFD may be overconsumed in an attempt to derive the necessary levels of energy [23]. The HFD group had a higher food intake than the NFD group (Figure 1B). The increased food intake of mice fed the HFD was significantly decreased by IO (50 and 75 mg/kg), IPA (1.35 mg/kg), and guava (75 mg/kg).

To investigate the effect of IPA on glucose tolerance, oral glucose tolerance tests (OGTTs) were conducted at different time points (30, 60, 90, and 120 min) after 12 weeks of HFD/IO, HFD/IPA, and HFD/Guava treatment. As shown in Figure 1C, HFD groups showed a lower glucose tolerance, with higher glucose level after 120 min, compared with the NFD group. However, the increased glucose levels were significantly reversed by HFD/IO (50 and 75 mg/kg), HFD/IPA (1.35 mg/kg), and HFD/Guava (75 mg/kg). To evaluate the degree of the glucose tolerance impairment, we calculated the area under the glucose curve (AUC) in the OGTT in each group. In Figure 1D, the AUC of OGTT in the HFD group was significantly increased compared with that in the NFD group. The AUC of OGTT in the HFD/IO, HFD/IPA and HFD/Guava groups was significantly decreased compared with that in the HFD group. Fasting glucose and 2 h glucose levels play a role in maintaining glucose homeostasis in diabetes. As shown in Figure 1D,E, fasting and 2 h glucose levels were significantly increased in the HFD group compared with that in the NFD group. Increased fasting and 2 h glucose levels were significantly decreased by HFD/IO (50 and 75 mg/kg), HFD/IPA (1.35 mg/kg), and HFD/Guava (75 mg/kg) treatments. These data suggested that IPA and IO containing IPA can improve glucose tolerance in HFD mice. We further evaluated the maintenance of glucose homeostasis in the blood of HFD mice as a means to control blood glucose level.

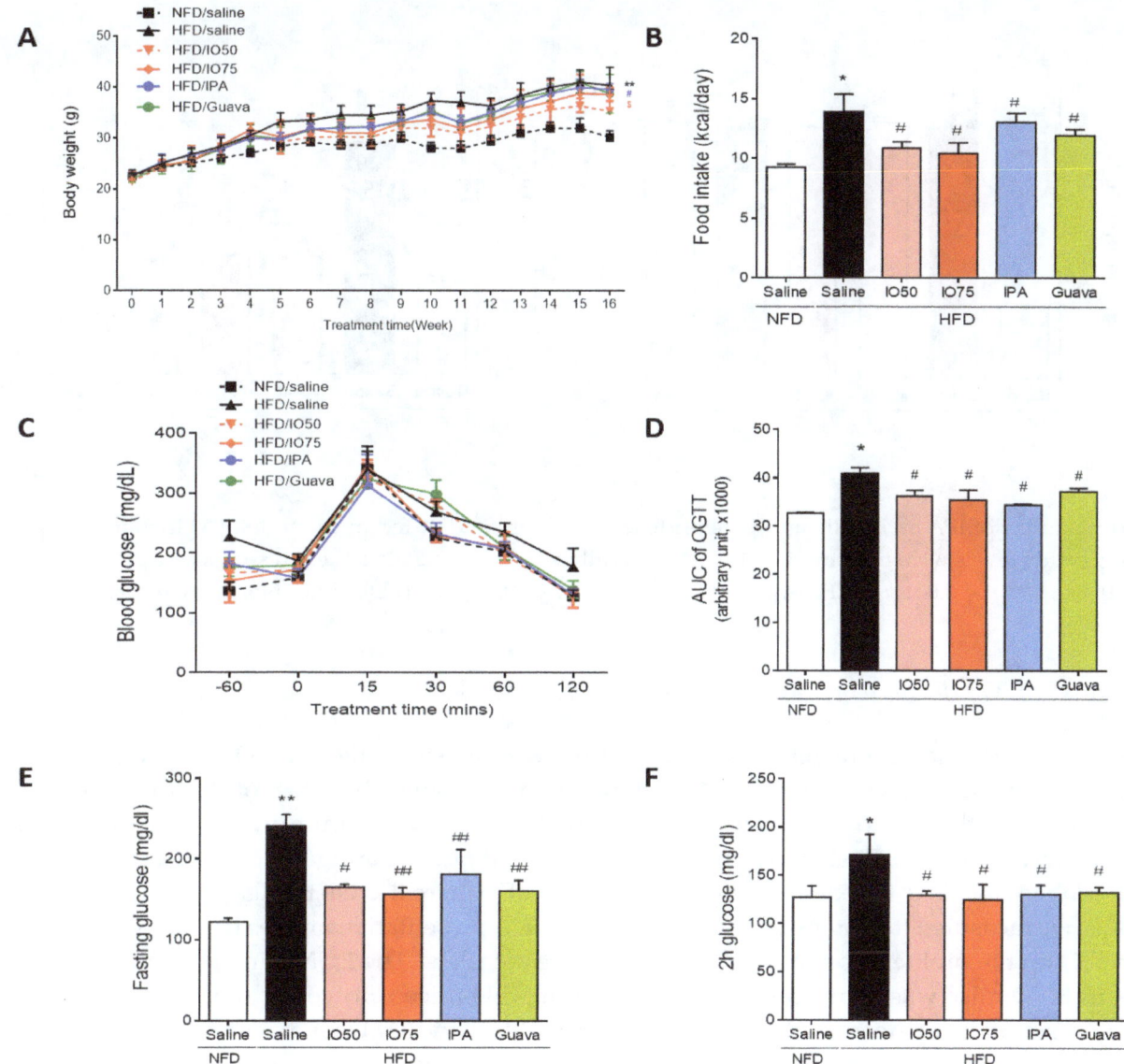

Figure 1. Effect of Ishophloroglucin A (IPA) on serum glucose level in high fat diet-fed mice model. The mice receiving 45% high fat diet for 8 weeks exhibit improved glucose tolerance but, IPA oral administration reduced glucose tolerance. (**A**) Body weight and (**B**) food intake were measured weekly during 14 weeks on different diets/treatments. (**C,D**) Oral glucose tolerance tests (OGTT) were measured and calculated area under the curve (AUC) from the GTT in all mice groups. (**E**) Fasting and (**F**) feeding glucose levels were in all mice group. Data are expressed as mean ± S.D. * $p < 0.05$ or ** $p < 0.01$ vs. NFD/saline; # $p < 0.05$, ## $p < 0.01$ vs. HFD/saline; $ $p < 0.05$ vs. HFD/Guava.

2.2. Regulation of Glucose Homeostatic Imbalance by IPA in HFD Mice

Next, we assessed whether the activation of the insulin and C-peptide level in the blood of HFD mice was regulated by HFD/IPA to control glucose metabolism. As shown in Figure 2A, the insulin level was significantly higher in HFD mice than in NFD mice, indicating that insulin resistance was induced in HFD mice. However, the insulin level was significantly lower in the HFD/IO (75 mg/kg) and HFD/IPA (1.35 mg/kg) groups than in HFD mice. As shown in Figure 2B, the C-peptide level was significantly higher in HFD mice than in NFD mice, indicating that the pancreas produced insulin to regulate glucose homeostasis. In contrast, the increase in C-peptide level was markedly decreased by HFD/IO (50 and 75 mg/kg), HFD/IPA (1.35 mg/kg), and HFD/Guava (75 mg/kg) treatment. These results showed that the decrease in insulin and C-peptide levels by IPA and IO containing IPA could regulate glucose homeostasis in HFD-induced insulin resistance.

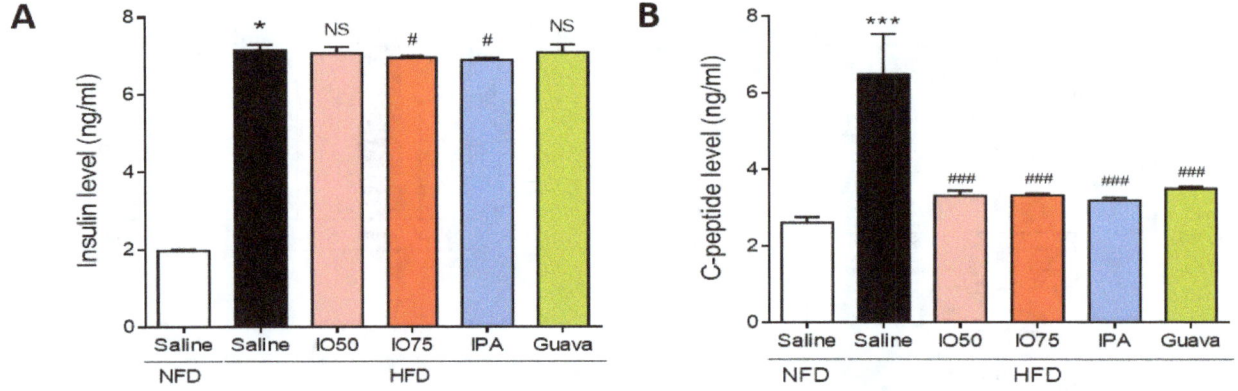

Figure 2. Effect of IPA on insulin and C-peptide level in high fat diet-fed mice model. (**A**) Insulin and (**B**) C-peptide levels were measured by ELISA kit in all mice groups. Data are expressed as mean ± S.D. * $p < 0.05$ or *** $p < 0.001$ vs. NFD/saline; # $p < 0.05$, ### $p < 0.001$ vs. HFD/saline. NS, not significant.

2.3. Protective Effect of IPA on Pancreatic Dysfunction in HFD Mice

To examine whether the increased number of pancreatic islet cells in HFD mice was reduced by IPA and IO for the protection of β-cell function, we investigated the effect of IPA on the change in morphology and the area of pancreatic islets in HFD mice by using immunohistochemistry and hematoxylin and eosin (H & E) staining. The proliferating cell nuclear antigen (PCNA), a proliferative cell marker, was detected to examine the proliferation of pancreatic islet cells [24]. As shown in Figure 3A,B, we measured the intensity of PCNA staining in representative images to quantify the effect of IPA and IO on the proliferation of β-cells in the pancreatic islets. The PCNA intensity in pancreatic islet cells in HFD mice was significantly higher than in NFD mice. However, the increased PCNA intensity was significantly decreased in the HFD/IO, HFD/IPA, and HFD/Guava groups. As shown in Figure 3C,D, the size of pancreatic islets from the histological changes in HFD mice was markedly elevated compared with that in NFD mice, whereas the size of pancreatic islets was significantly reduced in the HFD/IO, HFD/IPA, and HFD/Guava groups. These data suggested that IPA and IO containing IPA could protect against pancreatic dysfunction that occurs in HFD-induced diabetes.

Next, we examined Ins2 mRNA expression in the pancreas of HFD mice by using qRT-PCR to evaluate β-cell function by HFD/IPA. As shown in Figure 3E, Ins2 mRNA expression was markedly increased in HFD mice compared with that in NFD mice. However, the Ins2 mRNA expression was significantly decreased in the HFD/IO, HFD/IPA, and HFD/Guava mice. Interestingly, 1.35 mg/kg HFD/IPA, which is the equivalent content of IPA in IO, reduced Ins2 mRNA, as well as 75 mg/kg HFD/IO. These results suggested that the decrease in Ins2 mRNA level induced by IPA was able to regulate the elevated blood glucose level in HFD mice.

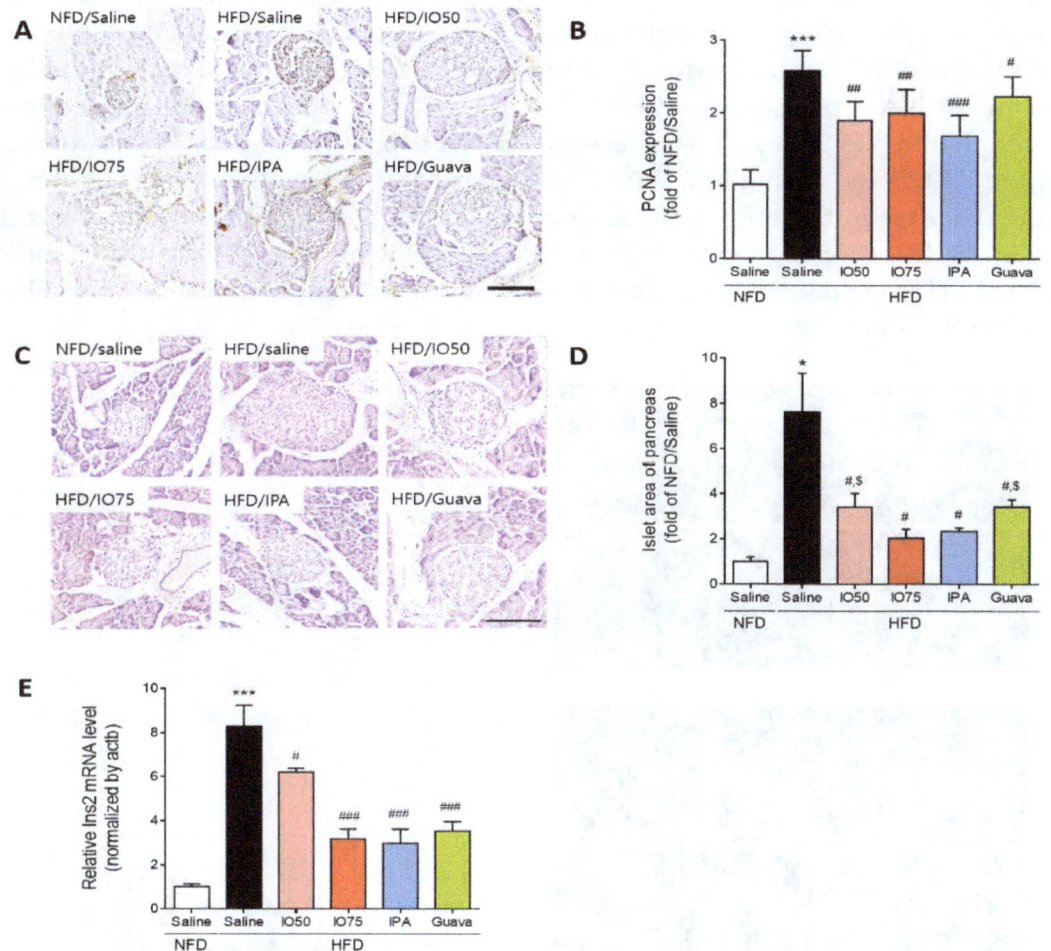

Figure 3. Effect of IPA on the morphology and area of pancreatic islets in high fat diet-fed mice model. (**A**) Proliferative cell marker (Proliferating cell nuclear antigen, PCNA) was detected by immunohistochemistry and (**B**) quantitative graph shows the level of PCNA expression on pancreatic islet from representative images. (**C**) Hematoxylin and eosin (H&E) stained histological images show islets of pancreas (round shape and pale color) and (**D**) pancreatic islet size were measured by image j software from representative images. (**E**) The expression level of Ins2 was measured by qRT-PCR. Scale bar = 100 μm, Data are expressed as mean ± S.D. * $p < 0.05$, or *** $p < 0.001$ vs. NFD/saline; [#] $p < 0.05$, [##] $p < 0.01$, or [###] $p < 0.001$ vs. HFD/saline; [$] $p < 0.05$ vs. HFD/Guava.

2.4. Effect of IPA on Glucose Transport in the Pancreas and Skeletal Muscle of Mice

The glucose transporter 2 (GLUT2) is an essential agent in the induction of glucose-stimulated insulin secretion and glucose tolerance in the β-cells of the pancreas [25]. Thus, we evaluated the effect of IPA on GLUT2 expression in the pancreas of HFD mice by using immunofluorescence, as shown in Figure 4A,B. The intensity of GLUT2 in HFD mice was significantly decreased compared to that in NFD mice. After the treatment with IO (50 and 75 mg/kg), IPA (1.35 mg/kg), and Guava (75 mg/kg), no significant decrease in the intensity of GLUT2 in HFD mice was found compared with that in HFD mice.

Previous studies reported that the defects of glucose transporter 4 (GLUT4) translocation were caused by impairment of glucose metabolism in HFD mice [26]. Thus, we examined the effect of IPA on the translocation of GLUT4 in the membrane of muscles in HFD mice by using immunofluorescence, as shown in Figure 4C,D. HFD/IO mice showed a slight increase in GLUT4 intensity, with a significant increase in the 75 mg/kg HFD/IO group. HFD/IPA and HFD/Guava treatment resulted in significantly increased GLUT4 translocation. These results showed that the increase in GLUT4 by IPA could improve glucose metabolism in the skeletal muscle of HFD mice.

Interestingly, the transcription of GLUT2 and GLUT4 is known to regulate glucose sensing and glucose transporters [27]. We measured the mRNA expression of GLUT2 and GLUT4 in the pancreas and skeletal muscle of HFD mice by qRT-PCR to evaluate glucose metabolism by IPA. As shown in Figure 4E,F, the mRNA expression of GLUT2 and GLUT4 was significantly decreased in HFD mice compared with that in NFD mice. The decrease in mRNA expression of GLUT2 was not significantly different in the IO (25 and 75 mg/kg), IPA (1.35 mg/kg), and Guava (75 mg/kg) treatment groups. However, the decrease in the mRNA expression of GLUT4 was significantly increased by the IO (25 and 75 mg/kg), IPA (1.35 mg/kg), and Guava (75 mg/kg) treatments. These results indicated that the increase in GLUT4 expression by IPA can improve glucose transport, thereby controlling glucose homeostasis, in HFD mice.

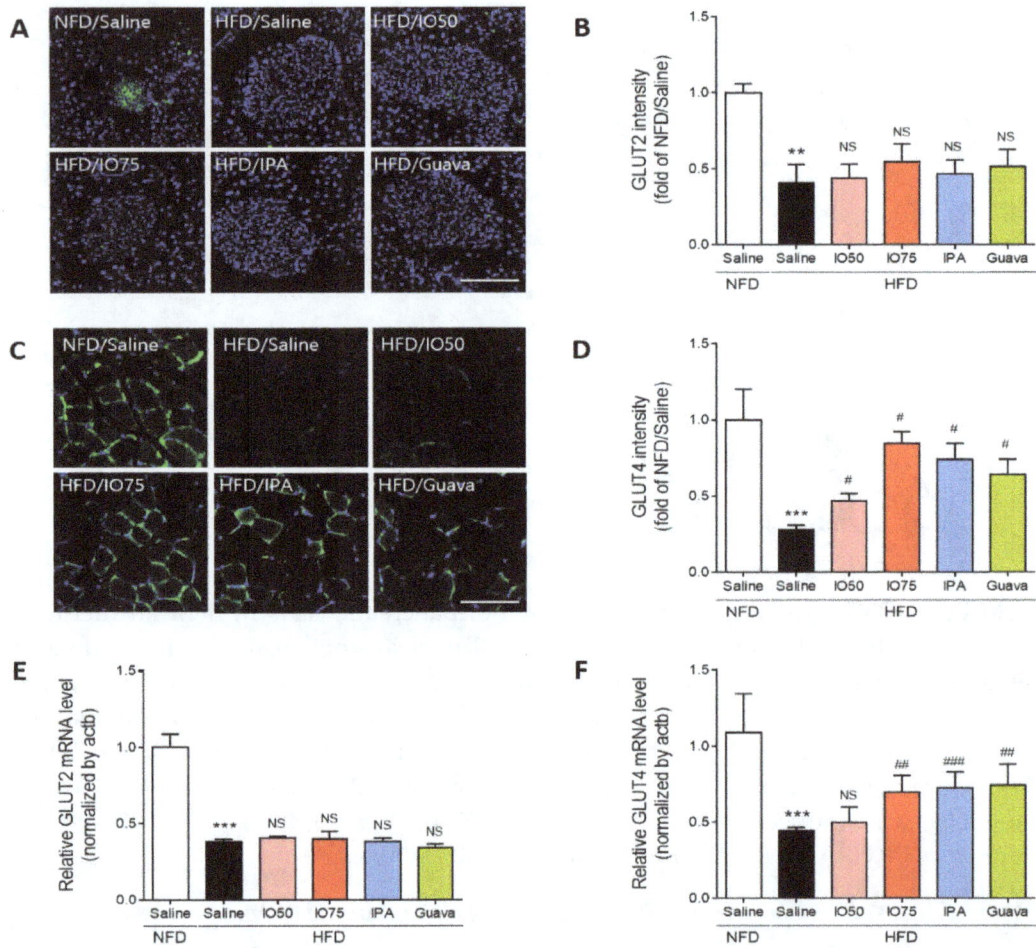

Figure 4. Effect of IPA on GLUT2 and GLUT4 expression increase of pancreas and skeletal muscle in high fat diet-fed mice model. (**A**) Confocal microscopic images show GLUT2 expression and GLUT2 (green) and nuclei (blue; DAPI) were detected of pancreas tissue of mice. (**B**) Quantitative graph was show level of GLUT2 expression from representative images and Zen 2012 software was used for measurement. (**C**) Confocal microscopic images show GLUT4 expression and GLUT4 (green) and nuclei (blue; DAPI) were detected of skeletal muscle tissue of mice. (**D**) Quantitative graph was show level of GLUT4 expression from representative images and Zen 2012 software was used for measurement. (**E,F**) The expression levels of GLUT2 and GLUT4 were measured by qRT-PCR. Scale bar = 100 μm, Data are expressed as mean ± S.D. ** $p < 0.01$, or *** $p < 0.001$ vs. NFD/saline; # $p < 0.05$, ## $p < 0.01$, or ### $p < 0.001$ vs. HFD/saline. NS, nor significant.

3. Discussion

A previous study reported that IPA isolated from IO and the equivalent content of IPA in IO extract showed an antidiabetic activity similar to that of IO extract [4]. However, the effect of IO, including IPA, as an agent for diabetes prevention has not yet been assessed on glucose homeostasis in the pancreas and muscles of HFD mice. In this study, our data suggest that IPA can improve glucose homeostasis in the pancreas and muscle, resulting in the regulation of blood glucose level in HFD-induced diabetes.

The HFD mouse is a robust and efficient model for type 2 diabetes and can be used for mechanistic studies [28]. Type 2 diabetes is a metabolic disorder characterized by insulin resistance and pancreatic β-cell dysfunction [29]. Insulin and C-peptide are present in the pancreas at equivalent concentrations [30]. C-peptide promotes the activation of the insulin receptor and increases glycogen synthesis via the insulin signaling pathway, but it does not affect glucose lowering [31,32]. It is also suggested that C-peptide may have a suppressive effect on insulin action in type 2 diabetes [31]. IPA significantly decreased the insulin and C-peptide levels in the plasma of HFD mice, suggesting the protective action of IPA against pancreatic dysfunction in HFD-induced diabetes.

The maintenance of glucose homeostasis is regulated by insulin secretion from pancreatic β-cells and hepatic glucose production, as well as glucose disposal into the muscle and adipose tissue [33]. The failure of β-cell function in pancreas is associated with HFD-induced diabetes [34]. Previous studies reported that the decrease in pancreatic β-cell mass was a common characteristic of subjects with diabetes [35,36]. In addition, in HFD mice, type 2 diabetes occurs when β-cells in the pancreas fail to secrete sufficient amounts of insulin to meet the metabolic demand [33]. The response of the elevated glucose levels in pancreatic β-cells was regulated by an increase in insulin hormone production and secretion. However, the prolonged stimulation of pancreatic β-cells by increased blood glucose levels results in β-cell function failure and insulin release reduction [37,38]. We confirmed that IPA treatment reduced β-cell function failure in HFD mice.

Hyperglycemia and glucose intolerance were improved by glucose transporters such as GLUT2 and GLUT4; their function is to regulate glucose level both outside and inside the cell [7,39]. In addition, glucose transport occurs in pancreatic β-cells, muscles, adipose tissue, and the brain to maintain glucose homeostasis and metabolic harmony [40]. GLUT4 plays a key role in the skeletal muscle, suppressing glucose intolerance and insulin resistance. The skeletal muscle is a major organ in insulin-mediated GLUT4 translocation for glucose metabolism [41]. The GLUT2 level in the pancreas was not changed by IPA treatment, whereas the GLUT4 level in the muscle was increased by IPA treatment in HFD mice. This indicated that IPA improved glucose homeostasis in HFD-induced diabetes via GLUT4 translation.

4. Materials and Methods

4.1. Preparation of IO and IPA

A 50% ethanol extract of IO was provided by Shinwoo Co. Ltd. (Lot No. SW9E29SA, Gyeonggi-do, Korea). Briefly, the IO used in this study was standardized on the assumption of diphlorethohydroxycarmalol (DPHC, 2.37%) by an HPLC analysis method [4] with a slight modification. IPA was purified on a pure C-850 FlashPrep chromatography system equipped with a PDA detector or an ELSD detector (all from Buchi, Flawil, Switzerland), equipped with an YMC Pack ODS-A (20 mm × 250 mm, 5 μm). The mobile phase consisted of (A) 0.1% formic acid in water and (B) ACN containing 0.1% formic acid. The HPLC elution was conducted as follows: 20%–40% B for 25 min, followed by a 10 min re-equilibration period of the column. The flow rate was maintained at 9 mL/min and the injection volume was 2 mL. IPA was verified by using quadrupole time-of-flight liquid chromatography-mass spectrometry (Q-TOF LC-MS/MS) using an electrospray ionization (ESI) source (maXis-HD, Bruker Daltonics, Breman, Germany) at the Korea Basic Science Institute (KBSI; Ochang, South Korea), targeted at the m/z 1986.26 fragment.

4.2. Animals

Six-week-old C57BL/6N male mice were used in this research. Animals were acclimated for 1 week. After acclimation, the mice were fed a 45% high-fat diet (HFD; Research Diets, Inc., New Brunswick, NJ, USA) for 8 weeks, except for the control group. After 4 weeks, the mice were allocated into six treatment groups: NFD/Saline, HFD/Saline, HFD/IO50, HFD/IO75, HFD/IPA, HFD/Guava. Each group was orally administrated saline and IO50 (50 mg/kg/day), IO75 (75 mg/kg/day), IPA (1.35 mg/kg/day) for 4 weeks after the separation. During the 8 weeks, the body weight, fasting glucose test, and feeding glucose test was measured once every week. An oral glucose tolerance test (OGTT) was performed once before the animals were sacrificed and the data were analyzed through the calculation of the area under curve (AUC). The animal protocol for the experiments was approved by the Animal Center of Lee Gil Ya Cancer and the Diabetes Institute of Gachon University. All experiments conformed to the AAALAC international guidelines and veterinary advice. The number of this study is LCDI-2018-0112.

4.3. Insulin Measurement

The rat/mouse insulin ELISA Kit (Millipore, Burlington, MA, USA) was used to measure the concentration of insulin in the blood. The blood serum was collected before the animals were sacrificed and then centrifuged at 2,000 g for 10 min. The supernatant and serum were transferred to the new tube and used for this study. The absolute concentration of insulin (Abcam, San Francisco, CA, USA) was measured by using an ELISA kit. The absorbance of the solution at 450 nm was measured by using an ELISA plate reader (Molecular Devices, San Jose, CA, USA).

4.4. C-peptide Measurement

A mouse C-peptide ELISA kit (KAMIYA Biomedical Company, Tukwila, WA, USA) was used to measure the absolute concentration of C-peptide in the blood. The absorbance of the solution at 450 nm was measured by using an ELISA plate reader (Molecular Devices, Suunyvale, CA, USA).

4.5. Sample Preparation

4.5.1. RNA Isolation and cDNA Synthesis

Visceral fat tissues were homogenized by the protocol innated in MACS (Miltenyi Biotec, Bergisch Gladbach, Germany) machine with 500 µL of RNisol (TAKARA, Tokyo, Japan). The supernatant of the tissue lysates was transferred to the new tube and 100 µL of chloroform was added. After vortex mixing for 3 s and incubation on ice for 10 min, the lysates were centrifuged at 12,000 g for 15 min at 4 °C. Remove the supernatant gently. RNA pellets were washed in 70% ethanol (EtOH), then centrifuged at 12,000 g for 15 min at 4 °C. The RNA pellet was dissolved in 40 µL of diethyl pyrocarbonate water (DEPC), and 1 µg of RNA was synthesized into complimentary DNA by using Prime Script 1st-strand cDNA Synthesis Kit (TAKARA, Shiga, Japan).

4.5.2. Tissue Preparation

Visceral fat tissue was fixed in 4% paraformaldehyde (PFA) solution to fix for 1 week. The fixed tissue was washed for 10 min in running water. To prepare a paraffin block, the tissues were incubated in the tissue processor machine (Shandon Citadel, Ramsey, MN, USA) for 14 h. Subsequently, after the machine process was finished, the tissues were embedded in the cassette with the paraffin. Blocks were stored at room temperature.

4.6. Quantitative Real Time Polymerase Chain Reaction (qRT-PCR)

To validate the gene expression of each factor, 1 µg of cDNA was used with the primers (Supplementary Table S1.) and distilled water. The solution was added 10 µL of cyber green solution (CYBG, TAKARA, Mountain View, CA, USA). The mixed solution was distributed in a 384-well plate (Bio-RAD, Hercules, CA, USA). CFX386 touch (Bio-Rad, Hercules, California, USA) was used to perform the qRT-PCR. The reaction efficiency and the number of cycles were determined by innate software.

4.7. Immunohistochemistry: 3, 3 -Diaminobenzidine (DAB) Staining

Paraffin-sectioned slides were deparaffinized with xylene for 5 min twice times. And then, the slides were incubated in antigen-retrieval solution for 5 min in the microwave. The slides were washed in running water for 5 min, and blocking solution was added to the tissue, depending on the host, for 1 h. After three washes in PBS, for 5 min each, the slides were incubated with the primary antibody (Supplementary Table S2.) overnight. Proliferating cell nuclear antigen (PCNA, Abcam) primary antibody was diluted to 1:100 with blocking solution. The slides were washed three times with PBS solution, for 5 min each, and secondary antibody was added to the slides. Biotinylated secondary antibody were diluted to 1:200 with PBS for 2 h. To amplify the signal, ABC kit (Vector Laboratories Inc, Burlingame, CA, USA) was used for 30 min (dilution 1:50 in PBS). The slides were washed three times in PBS, for 5 min each, and then developed by the application of DAB solution until signal was visible. After development, the slides were washed with running water for 10 min and mounted with DPX solution (Sigma-Aldrich, St. Louis, MO, USA). Images were taken by light microscopy (Olympus, Tokyo, Japan). To measure the intensity of DAB staining, ImageJ software (NIH, Bethesda, MD, USA) was used.

4.8. Immunohistochemistry: Fluorescence Staining

Paraffin-sectioned slides were deparaffinized twice with xylene for 5 min. After serial incubation in EtOH, the slides were incubated in antigen-retrieval solution for 5 min in the microwave. The slides were washed in running water for 5 min and then incubated in blocking solution, depending on the host, for 1 h. After three washes in PBS, for 5 min each, the slides were incubated with the primary antibody overnight. Glut2 (Santa Cruz Biotechnology Inc, Santa Cruz, CA, USA) and Glut4 (Santa Cruz) primary antibody were diluted to 1:100 with blocking solution. The slides were washed with 0.1% Triton X-100 in PBS (TPBS), and then incubated with 488-fluorescent anti-mouse secondary antibody (Abcam) solution 2 h. The secondary antibody was diluted 1:200. After incubation for 2 h in the dark at room temperature, the slides were washed three times with TPBS for 10 min. The slides were mounted by using with Vectashield (Vector Laboratories Inc, Burlingame, CA, USA) and images were taken by using a confocal laser microscope (LSM 710, Carl Zeiss, Oberkochen, Germany). To measure the intensity of the immunofluorescence staining, ImageJ software (NIH) was used.

4.9. Histology: Hematoxylin and Eosin Staining

Paraffin-sectioned slides were deparaffinized twice with xylene for 5 min. After serial incubation in EtOH and running water to rehydrate, the slides were stained with hematoxylin (DAKO, Carpinteria, CA, USA) for 2 min at room temperature. The slides were washed with running water for 5 min, stained with eosin (Sigma-Aldrich) for 7 s, and washed with running water for 5 min. The slides were mounted by using DPX (Sigma-Aldrich) solution and viewed by light microscopy. The size of visceral fat was measured by using ImageJ (NIH).

4.10. Statistics

The Kruskal–Wallis test and the Mann–Whitney U post-hoc test were used to compare the statistical differences between the groups, computed by using SPSS version 22 (IBM Corporation, Armonk, NY, USA). The results were presented as the mean ± standard deviation (SD). Differences were considered significant at * $p < 0.05$ vs. NFD/Saline; ** $p < 0.01$ vs. NFD/Saline, *** $p < 0.001$ vs. NFD/Saline; # $p < 0.05$ vs. HFD/Saline; ## $p < 0.01$ vs. HFD/Saline; ### $p < 0.001$ vs. HFD/Saline.

5. Conclusions

Collectively, we demonstrated the effect of IPA on glucose homeostasis in the pancreas and muscles of mice with HFD-induced diabetes and determined potential strategies to ameliorate metabolic disorders in patients with diabetes in the future. IO, containing IPA, may be used to develop functional foods for diabetes prevention.

Author Contributions: H.-W.Y.; Provide the substance and draft preparation; M.S. and S.O.; Data Assembly and interpretation; S.O. and J.C.; Formal analysis and data collection; Y.-J.J. and K.B.; Study conceptualization and methodology; K.B. and B.R.; Supervision and provision of funding acquisition.

Acknowledgments: All authors thank Dong-Min Chung and Shinwoo Co. Ltd. (Korea) for assistance in preparing IO extract.

References

1. Holdt, S.L.; Kraan, S. Bioactive compounds in seaweed: Functional food applications and legislation. *J. Appl. Phycol.* **2011**, *23*, 543–597. [CrossRef]
2. Kiuru, P.; D'Auria, M.V.; Muller, C.D.; Tammela, P.; Vuorela, H.; Yli-Kauhaluoma, J. Exploring marine resources for bioactive compounds. *Planta Med.* **2014**, *80*, 1234–1246. [CrossRef] [PubMed]
3. Sanjeewa, K.A.; Lee, W.W.; Kim, J.-I.; Jeon, Y.-J. Exploiting biological activities of brown seaweed *Ishige okamurae* Yendo for potential industrial applications: A review. *J. Appl. Phycol.* **2017**, *29*, 3109–3119. [CrossRef]
4. Ryu, B.; Jiang, Y.; Kim, H.-S.; Hyun, J.-M.; Lim, S.-B.; Li, Y.; Jeon, Y.-J. Ishophloroglucin A, a novel phlorotannin for standardizing the anti-α-glucosidase activity of *Ishige okamurae*. *Mar. Drugs* **2018**, *16*, 436. [CrossRef]
5. Rudkowska, I. Functional foods for health: Focus on diabetes. *Maturitas* **2009**, *62*, 263–269. [CrossRef]
6. Koolman, J.; Röhm, K.-H.; Wirth, J.; Robertson, M. *Color Atlas of Biochemistry*; Thieme: Stuttgart, Germany, 2005; Volume 2.
7. Shepherd, P.R.; Kahn, B.B. Glucose transporters and insulin action—Implications for insulin resistance and diabetes mellitus. *N. Engl. J. Med.* **1999**, *341*, 248–257. [CrossRef]
8. Cohen, N.; Shaw, J. Diabetes: Advances in treatment. *Intern. Med. J.* **2007**, *37*, 383–388. [CrossRef]
9. Nathan, D.M. Diabetes: Advances in diagnosis and treatment. *JAMA* **2015**, *314*, 1052–1062. [CrossRef]
10. Kazeem, M.I.; Davies, T.C. Anti-diabetic functional foods as sources of insulin secreting, insulin sensitizing and insulin mimetic agents. *J. Funct. Foods* **2016**, *20*, 122–138. [CrossRef]
11. Xing, X.-H.; Zhang, Z.-M.; Hu, X.-Z.; Wu, R.-Q.; Xu, C. Antidiabetic effects of *Artemisia sphaerocephala* Krasch. gum, a novel food additive in China, on streptozotocin-induced type 2 diabetic rats. *J. Ethnopharmacol.* **2009**, *125*, 410–416. [CrossRef]
12. Latha, R.C.R.; Daisy, P. Insulin-secretagogue, antihyperlipidemic and other protective effects of gallic acid isolated from *Terminalia bellerica* Roxb. in streptozotocin-induced diabetic rats. *Chem. Biol. Interact.* **2011**, *189*, 112–118. [CrossRef] [PubMed]
13. Egede, L.E.; Ye, X.; Zheng, D.; Silverstein, M.D. The prevalence and pattern of complementary and alternative medicine use in individuals with diabetes. *Diabetes Care* **2002**, *25*, 324–329. [CrossRef] [PubMed]
14. Tindle, H.A.; Davis, R.B.; Phillips, R.S.; Eisenberg, D.M. Trends in use of complementary and alternative medicine by US adults: 1997–2002. *Altern. Ther. Health Med.* **2005**, *11*, 42. [PubMed]
15. Buettner, R.; Parhofer, K.; Woenckhaus, M.; Wrede, C.; Kunz-Schughart, L.; Scholmerich, J.; Bollheimer, L. Defining high-fat-diet rat models: Metabolic and molecular effects of different fat types. *J. Mol. Endocrinol.* **2006**, *36*, 485–501. [CrossRef] [PubMed]
16. Chrysochou, P. Food health branding: The role of marketing mix elements and public discourse in conveying a healthy brand image. *J. Mark. Commun.* **2010**, *16*, 69–85. [CrossRef]
17. Goetzke, B.; Nitzko, S.; Spiller, A. Consumption of organic and functional food. A matter of well-being and health? *Appetite* **2014**, *77*, 96–105. [CrossRef]
18. Altgeld, T.; Gene, R.; Glaeske, G.; Koli, P.; Rosenbrock, R.; Trojan, A. Prevention and Health Promotion. In *A Program for Improved Health and Social Policy*; Bonner Universitaet Sdruckerei: Bonn, Germany, 2006.
19. Ballali, S.; Lanciai, F. Functional food and diabetes: A natural way in diabetes prevention? *Int. J. Food Sci. Nutr.* **2012**, *63*, 51–61. [CrossRef]

20. Bech-Larsen, T.; Grunert, K.G. The perceived healthiness of functional foods: A conjoint study of Danish, Finnish and American consumers' *perception* of functional foods. *Appetite* **2003**, *40*, 9–14. [CrossRef]

21. Deguchi, Y.; Miyazaki, K. Anti-hyperglycemic and anti-hyperlipidemic effects of guava leaf extract. *Nutr. Metab.* **2010**, *7*, 9. [CrossRef]

22. Rolls, B.J.; Shide, D.J. The influence of dietary fat on food intake and body weight. *Nutr. Rev.* **1992**, *50*, 283–290. [CrossRef]

23. Tremblay, A.; Lavallee, N.; Alméras, N.; Allard, L.; Després, J.-P.; Bouchard, C. Nutritional determinants of the increase in energy intake associated with a high-fat diet. *Am. J. Clin. Nutr.* **1991**, *53*, 1134–1137. [CrossRef] [PubMed]

24. Bringhenti, I.; Moraes-Teixeira, J.A.; Cunha, M.R.; Ornellas, F.; Mandarim-de-Lacerda, C.A.; Aguila, M.B. Maternal obesity during the preconception and early life periods alters pancreatic development in early and adult life in male mouse offspring. *PLoS ONE* **2013**, *8*, e55711. [CrossRef] [PubMed]

25. Bonny, C.; Roduit, R.; Gremlich, S.; Nicod, P.; Thorens, B.; Waeber, G. The loss of GLUT2 expression in the pancreatic β-cells of diabetic db/db mice is associated with an impaired DNA-binding activity of islet-specific trans-acting factors. *Mol. Cell. Endocrinol.* **1997**, *135*, 59–65. [CrossRef]

26. Tremblay, F.; Lavigne, C.; Jacques, H.; Marette, A. Defective insulin-induced GLUT4 translocation in skeletal muscle of high fat–fed rats is associated with alterations in both Akt/protein kinase B and atypical protein kinase C (ζ/λ) activities. *Diabetes* **2001**, *50*, 1901–1910. [CrossRef] [PubMed]

27. Chung, M.J.; Cho, S.-Y.; Bhuiyan, M.J.H.; Kim, K.H.; Lee, S.-J. Anti-diabetic effects of lemon balm (*Melissa officinalis*) essential oil on glucose-and lipid-regulating enzymes in type 2 diabetic mice. *Br. J. Nutr.* **2010**, *104*, 180–188. [CrossRef]

28. Winzell, M.S.; Ahrén, B. The high-fat diet–fed mouse: A model for studying mechanisms and treatment of impaired glucose tolerance and type 2 diabetes. *Diabetes* **2004**, *53*, S215–S219. [CrossRef]

29. Srinivasan, K.; Viswanad, B.; Asrat, L.; Kaul, C.; Ramarao, P. Combination of high-fat diet-fed and low-dose streptozotocin-treated rat: A model for type 2 diabetes and pharmacological screening. *Pharmacol. Res.* **2005**, *52*, 313–320. [CrossRef]

30. Heding, L.G.; Larsen, U.; Markussen, J.; Jørgensen, K.; Hallund, O. Radioimmunoassays for human, pork and ox C-peptides and related substances. In *Radioimmunoassays for Insulin, C-Peptide and Proinsulin*; Springer: Berlin/Heidelberg, Germany, 1988; pp. 43–47.

31. Sima, A.A.; Kamiya, H.; Li, Z.G. Insulin, C-peptide, hyperglycemia, and central nervous system complications in diabetes. *Eur. J. Pharmacol.* **2004**, *490*, 187–197. [CrossRef]

32. Grunberger, G.; Sima, A.A. The C-peptide signaling. *J. Diabetes Res.* **2004**, *5*, 25–36. [CrossRef]

33. Kasuga, M. Insulin resistance and pancreatic β cell failure. *J. Clin. Investig.* **2006**, *116*, 1756–1760. [CrossRef]

34. Matveyenko, A.V.; Gurlo, T.; Daval, M.; Butler, A.E.; Butler, P.C. Successful versus failed adaptation to high-fat diet–induced insulin resistance: The role of IAPP-induced β-cell endoplasmic reticulum stress. *Diabetes* **2009**, *58*, 906–916. [CrossRef] [PubMed]

35. Butler, A.E.; Janson, J.; Soeller, W.C.; Butler, P.C. Increased β-cell apoptosis prevents adaptive increase in β-cell mass in mouse model of type 2 diabetes: Evidence for role of islet amyloid formation rather than direct action of amyloid. *Diabetes* **2003**, *52*, 2304–2314. [CrossRef] [PubMed]

36. Rahier, J.; Guiot, Y.; Goebbels, R.; Sempoux, C.; Henquin, J.-C. Pancreatic β-cell mass in European subjects with type 2 diabetes. *Diabetes Obes. Metab.* **2008**, *10*, 32–42. [CrossRef] [PubMed]

37. Poitout, V.; Robertson, R.P. An integrated view of β-cell dysfunction in type-II diabetes. *Annu. Rev. Med.* **1996**, *47*, 69–83. [CrossRef]

38. Durning, S.P.; Flanagan-Steet, H.; Prasad, N.; Wells, L. O-linked β-N-acetylglucosamine (O-GlcNAc) acts as a glucose sensor to epigenetically regulate the insulin gene in pancreatic beta cells. *J. Biol. Chem.* **2016**, *291*, 2107–2118. [CrossRef]

39. Nishiumi, S.; Bessyo, H.; Kubo, M.; Aoki, Y.; Tanaka, A.; Yoshida, K.-I.; Ashida, H. Green and black tea suppress hyperglycemia and insulin resistance by retaining the expression of glucose transporter 4 in muscle of high-fat diet-fed C57BL/6J mice. *J. Agric. Food Chem.* **2010**, *58*, 12916–12923. [CrossRef]

40. Herman, M.A.; Kahn, B.B. Glucose transport and sensing in the maintenance of glucose homeostasis and metabolic harmony. *J. Clin. Investig.* **2006**, *116*, 1767–1775. [CrossRef]

41. Shan, W.-F.; Chen, B.-Q.; Zhu, S.-J.; Jiang, L.; Zhou, Y.-F. Effects of GLUT4 expression on insulin resistance in patients with advanced liver cirrhosis. *J. Zhejiang Univ. Sci. B* **2011**, *12*, 677. [CrossRef]

4

Platelet-Rich Plasma Modulates Gap Junction Functionality and Connexin 43 and 26 Expression During TGF-β1–Induced Fibroblast to Myofibroblast Transition: Clues for Counteracting Fibrosis

Roberta Squecco [1,†], **Flaminia Chellini** [2,†], **Eglantina Idrizaj** [1], **Alessia Tani** [2,†], **Rachele Garella** [1], **Sofia Pancani** [2], **Paola Pavan** [3], **Franco Bambi** [3], **Sandra Zecchi-Orlandini** [2] and **Chiara Sassoli** [2,*,†]

1   Department of Experimental and Clinical Medicine, Section of Physiological Sciences, University of Florence, 50134 Florence, Italy; roberta.squecco@unifi.it (R.S.); eglantina.idrizaj@unifi.it (E.I.); rachele.garella@unifi.it (R.G.)

2   Department of Experimental and Clinical Medicine, Section of Anatomy and Histology, University of Florence, 50134 Florence, Italy; flaminia.chellini@unifi.it (F.C.); alessia.tani@unifi.it (A.T.); sofia.pancani@stud.unifi.it (S.P.); sandra.zecchi@unifi.it (S.Z.-O.)

3   Transfusion Medicine and Cell Therapy Unit, "A. Meyer" University Children's Hospital, 50134 Florence, Italy; paola.pavan@meyer.it (P.P.); franco.bambi@meyer.it (F.B.)

*   Correspondence: chiara.sassoli@unifi.it;

†   Interuniversity Institute of Myology (IIM) (https://www.coram-iim.it).

Abstract: Skeletal muscle repair/regeneration may benefit by Platelet-Rich Plasma (PRP) treatment owing to PRP pro-myogenic and anti-fibrotic effects. However, PRP anti-fibrotic action remains controversial. Here, we extended our previous researches on the inhibitory effects of PRP on in vitro transforming growth factor (TGF)-β1-induced differentiation of fibroblasts into myofibroblasts, the effector cells of fibrosis, focusing on gap junction (GJ) intercellular communication. The myofibroblastic phenotype was evaluated by cell shape analysis, confocal fluorescence microscopy and Western blotting analyses of α-smooth muscle actin and type-1 collagen expression, and electrophysiological recordings of resting membrane potential, resistance, and capacitance. PRP negatively regulated myofibroblast differentiation by modifying all the assessed parameters. Notably, myofibroblast pairs showed an increase of voltage-dependent GJ functionality paralleled by connexin (Cx) 43 expression increase. TGF-β1-treated cells, when exposed to a GJ blocker, or silenced for Cx43 expression, failed to differentiate towards myofibroblasts. Although a minority, myofibroblast pairs also showed not-voltage-dependent GJ currents and coherently Cx26 expression. PRP abolished the TGF-β1-induced voltage-dependent GJ current appearance while preventing Cx43 increase and promoting Cx26 expression. This study adds insights into molecular and functional mechanisms regulating fibroblast-myofibroblast transition and supports the anti-fibrotic potential of PRP, demonstrating the ability of this product to hamper myofibroblast generation targeting GJs.

Keywords: α-smooth muscle actin; confocal microscopy; connexin 43; connexin 26; fibrosis; gap junctions; myofibroblasts; Platelet-Rich Plasma; skeletal muscle; transforming growth factor (TGF)-β1

1. Introduction

Adult skeletal muscle can efficiently repair/regenerate after focal damages [1]. Several studies showed that many different cell types endowed with inducible myogenic potential, residing within the muscle tissue or recruited via the blood, might contribute to the formation of nascent contractile myofibers [2–6]. Nevertheless, muscle resident satellite cells are widely recognized as the main players in the repair/regenerative processes [7,8]. After focal injuries, satellite cells undergo activation to essentially recapitulate the steps of embryonic and fetal myogenesis forming new myofibers or fusing with injured myofibers to repair the damage [1,9]. To accomplish their task, satellite cells (but even the myogenic non-satellite cells), require the establishment of a suitable and conductive surrounding microenvironment. This essentially includes pro-myogenic factors, biochemical and physical pro-myogenic signals, juxtacrine, and paracrine interaction with different interstitial nursing cells and a spatially and temporally limited reparative fibrotic response [1,10–15].

1.1. Fibrotic Response in Skeletal Muscle

The activation of fibrogenic pathways represents an adaptive physiological response of tissues, including skeletal muscle, to damage. A crucial process in such a fibrotic response is represented by the differentiation of fibroblasts resident in the extracellular matrix (ECM) towards myofibroblasts [16]. This is essentially promoted by the combined action of pro-fibrogenic agents, such as transforming growth factor (TGF)-β1, mainly released by infiltrating inflammatory cells (particularly macrophages) at the site of the injury and by the fibroblasts/myofibroblasts itself, and mechanical stimuli coming from the damaged microenvironment [16,17]. Myofibroblasts are characterized by a prominent rough endoplasmic reticulum, typical of collagen-synthetically active fibroblasts, by the de novo expression of α-smooth muscle actin (α-sma) within well-assembled stress fibers that confers contractile properties to the cells. Stress fibers are anchored to fibronexus, a specialized focal adhesion complex on the myofibroblast surface, to link intracellular actin filaments with extracellular fibronectin fibrils. Through fibronexus, the force generated by stress fibers can be transmitted to the surrounding ECM, and vice-versa the ECM mechanical signals can be transduced via this mechano-transduction system into intracellular signals [18]. Moreover, even if myofibroblasts are not regarded as electrically excitable cells, they show peculiar biophysical properties and trans-membrane ion currents typical of smooth muscle cells. In this regard, it has been reported that human atrial myofibroblasts can express a Na$^+$ current (I_{Na}) and biophysical properties that could give rise to regenerative action potentials [19,20]. In addition, myofibroblasts typically show the inward-rectifier K$^+$ current (I_{kir}), which especially increases under TGF-β1-treatment [21–24]. In physiological conditions, the permanence and function of myofibroblasts after muscle damage are temporally and spatially limited. Indeed, they are responsible for the deposition of ECM components to form a transient contractile scar essentially required to rapidly restore tissue integrity and preserve muscle function, to support activated SCs and the nascent myofibers mechanically. Once the tissue regeneration has taken place, the scar will be degraded thanks to the balanced and finely tuned activity of proteolytic enzymes selectively digesting individual components of ECM, namely matrix metalloproteinases (MMPs), and of their specific tissue inhibitors (TIMPs), that are mainly secreted by different cells including, among others, fibroblasts and inflammatory cells [25]. Myofibroblasts progressively disappear, undergoing apoptosis and/or senescence or reverting to a quiescent state [26,27]. By contrast, the persistence of myofibroblasts in an activated state has been associated with an aberrant maladaptive reparative response to chronic or extended damage leading to the formation of a permanent scar replacing the normal functional tissue and hampering the endogenous cell mediated-mechanism of muscle regeneration [10,16,17,28,29]. Therefore, therapies aimed to limit myofibroblast generation and functionality may result strategical and effective for preventing tissue fibrosis development and thus promoting the regeneration of damaged muscles.

1.2. PRP as an Anti-fibrotic Agent

In this regard, Platelet-Rich Plasma (PRP)—defined as a plasma fraction with a concentration of platelets above baseline levels and representing a source of numerous biologically active molecules—may offer promising perspectives [30]. Indeed, many in vitro and in vivo studies have demonstrated the anti-fibrotic potential of this blood product in different tissues [31–38], including skeletal muscle [30,39–46], and have indicated the fibroblast-myofibroblast transition as the cell process target of its action [31–33,36,38,44,47,48]. Furthermore, the positive contribution of PRP to skeletal muscle regeneration has been demonstrated either in vivo or in vitro, thanks to its capability to promote the myogenic program [30]. Nevertheless, the anti-fibrotic potential of PRP needs to be investigated more in-depth, and the molecular targets of the action of this plasma product need to be clearly identified.

1.3. Gap Junction Intercellular Communication (GJIC)

The gap junction (GJ) channels are dynamic membrane domains built of two docking hemichannels called connexons assembled in the plasma membranes of two adjacent cells. Each connexon is a hexameric structure consisting of six transmembrane proteins named connexins (Cxs) that may have different molecular weights [49] and form an aqueous pore. The opening of these channels allows the flow of ions and small molecules (less than 1000 MW molecular weight size fractions) such as sugars, amino acids, oxygen, as well as second messengers such as cAMP, inositol phosphates, and calcium directly from one cell to another. The type of molecules (second messengers) passing through GJs can be influenced by the Cx isoform composition of the GJ channels. When the Cx isoforms are of the same type within a hemichannel, the resulting structure is called homomeric, whereas it is called heteromeric if more than one Cx isoform is present. The GJ channels composed of two identical hemichannels are named homotypic, and those consisting of two different hemichannels are named heterotypic. These two types of GJ channels exhibit peculiar and different gating properties influencing their voltage sensitivity [50]. GJIC is proposed to play a role in regulating the fibroblasts transition towards myofibroblasts as well as to be involved in the functional coupling of myofibroblasts to coordinate their activity [18,51–54]; however, GJ channel functionality and Cx composition during the phenotypic progression of fibroblasts into the myofibroblasts have not been fully elucidated yet and deserve more attention.

In the present in vitro study, by combining morphological, biomolecular, biochemical, and electrophysiological analyses, we extended our previous researches further exploring the potential molecular targets of the inhibitory action of PRP on myofibroblast generation. In particular, we focused the attention on the GJIC. The experimental model to evaluate fibroblast to myofibroblast transition has been previously validated [23,24,48,55–57] and consists in the culture of the cells in low serum conditions in the presence of TGF-β1. The treatment with PRP was also conducted as previously reported [48,57,58].

Here, while confirming the anti-fibrotic potential of PRP we provide the first experimental evidence that voltage-dependent GJ functionality and the expression of Cx43, a typical Cx forming voltage-dependent connexons, are important mechanisms by which TGF-β1 endorses fibroblasts differentiation towards myofibroblasts, and that PRP treatment hampers this effect. Moreover, we also demonstrated the involvement of not-voltage dependent GJs and Cx26, a typical Cx type forming not (or at least, scarcely) voltage-dependent connexons.

2. Materials and Methods

2.1. Platelet-Rich Plasma (PRP) Preparation

For the present experiments, thawed ready-to-use activated PRP aliquots classified as not suitable for transfusion-infusion purposes previously prepared and stored at −80 °C were used [48]. Briefly, PRP was collected from the blood of healthy adult donors subjected to plasma-platelet apheresis (Haemonetics MCS®, Haemonetics, Milan, Italy) as previously reported in detail [57]. The final platelet concentration in each PRP (without leukocytes) aliquot was 2×10^6 platelets/μL. Platelet activation was induced by the addition of a calcium digluconate solution (10%). The donors gave their written informed consent to allow the use of PRP for in vitro experimentations for which the Ethical Committee's approval is not required. PRP treatment was performed as previously reported [48,57].

2.2. Cell Culture and Treatments

Murine NIH/3T3 fibroblastic cells were obtained from American Type Culture Collection (ATCC, Manassas, VA, USA). The cells were grown in proliferation medium (PM), consisting of Dulbecco's Modified Eagle's Medium (DMEM; Sigma, Milan, Italy) containing 4.5 g/L glucose supplemented with 10% fetal bovine serum (FBS) and 1% penicillin/streptomycin (Sigma), at 37 °C in a humidified atmosphere of 5% CO_2. Fibroblastic cells were induced to differentiate into myofibroblasts by shifting them in differentiation medium (DM) consisting of DMEM supplemented with 2% FBS and 2 ng/mL TGF-β1 (PeproTech, Inc., Rocky Hill, NJ, USA) for 48 h and 72 h, as previously reported [48]. In parallel experiments, to estimate the influence of PRP on fibroblast-myofibroblast transition, PRP was added to DM (1:50) [48,57]. In some experiments, the cells were cultured in PM, DM, or DM + PRP in the presence of 1 mM heptanol (Sigma), a specific GJ blocker, to evaluate the involvement of GJs in myofibroblastic differentiation.

2.3. Electrophysiological Records

Cell pairs were analyzed by the dual whole-cell patch-clamp technique, as previously reported [59–61]. Both passive membrane properties and GJ functionality were investigated. To this aim, cells were plated on glass coverslips (50,000 cells on each glass coverslips) to be located in the recording chamber and continuously superfused at a rate of 1.8 ml/min by a Pump 33 (Harvard Apparatus) with a physiological bath solution containing (mM) 140 NaCl, 5.4 KCl, 1.8 $CaCl_2$, 1.2 $MgCl_2$, 10 D-glucose, and 5 HEPES (pH set at 7.4 with NaOH). The patch electrodes, pulled from borosilicate glass (GC 150–15; Clark, Reading, UK), were filled with the following solution (mM): 130 KCl, 10 NaH_2PO_4, 0.2 $CaCl_2$, 1 EGTA, 5 MgATP, and 10 HEPES (pH was set to 7.2 with KOH). When filled, the pipette resistance ranged between 1.5 to 3.0 MΩ. Experiments were achieved at room temperature (22 °C). The set up for electrophysiological measurements was as previously reported [61] and consisted of the Axopatch 200 B amplifier (Axon Instruments, Union City, CA), an analog-to-digital/digital-to-analog interface (Digidata 1200; Axon Instruments), and pClamp 6 software (Axon Instruments). Currents were low-pass filtered at 1 kHz with a Bessel filter. The passive membrane properties, membrane resistance (R_m), and membrane linear capacitance (C_m) were consistently estimated in voltage-clamp starting from a holding potential (HP) of -70 mV and applying a 10-mV positive and negative step pulse. In brief, R_m was calculated using the relation: $R_m = (\Delta V - I_m R_a)/I_m$, where ΔV is the command voltage step amplitude, I_m is the steady-state membrane current, and R_a the access resistance [23,62]. C_m was calculated from $C_m = \Delta Q(R_m + R_a)/R_m \Delta V$, corrected according to a previous report [63]. To properly compare the currents recorded from different cells, their values were normalized to C_m, assuming that the specific C_m was constant at 1 μF/cm^2. The ratio I/C_m was intended as current density (in pA/pF). The junction potential of the electrode was estimated before making the patch (about −10 mV) and then was subtracted from the recorded membrane potential. The resting membrane potential (RMP) was recorded in current-clamp mode with a stimulus waveform: I = 0 pA. The protocol of stimulation used to record the currents flowing through GJs in voltage clamp and the recording procedure have been previously reported [61,64,65]. In brief, cell 1 of the pair was stepped from a holding potential (HP) of 0 mV, using a bipolar 5 s pulse protocol starting at trans-junctional voltage $V_j = \pm 10$ mV and ongoing at 20 mV increments up to ± 150 mV. The transjunctional current flowing through GJs is indicated as I_j. Precisely, the amplitude of I_j determined at the peak was named $I_{j,inst}$ (instantaneous transjunctional current), whereas that measured at the end of each pulse is indicated as $I_{j,ss}$ (steady-state transjunctional current). These values were used to calculate the related gap junctional conductances, $G_{j,inst}$ and $G_{j,ss}$, by the ratios: $G_{j,inst} = I_{j,inst}/V_j$ and $G_{j,ss} = I_{j,ss}/V_j$, respectively. The mean values of $G_{j,ss}$ were normalized to those of $G_{j,inst}$, plotted as a function of V_j and fitted, when possible, with a Boltzmann function using the equation: $G_j = (G_{max} - G_{min})/(1 + \exp(-A(V_j - V_0))) + G_{min}$. In a set of experiments, heptanol (1 mM) was acutely applied to the bath solution to block gap junctional currents.

2.4. Silencing of Cx43 Expression by Short Interfering RNA

To inhibit the expression of Cx43, the cells were cultured either in a 6-wells/plate or on sterile glass coverslips put on the bottom of a 6-wells/plate in PM till a confluence of 80% and then transfected with a mix of short interfering RNA duplexes (siRNA; Santa Cruz Biotechnology, Santa Cruz, CA) corresponding to 3 distinct regions of the DNA sequence of mouse Cx43 gene (NM_010288): 5'CCCAACUGAACCUUAAGAA3', 5'CCUCACCAAAUGAUUUCUA3', and 5'CCUACCAGUUUCUUCAAGU3' and/or with a non-specific scrambled (SCR)-siRNA (Santa Cruz Biotechnology) used as control. The siRNA transfections were performed according to manufacturer's instructions (Santa Cruz Biotechnology) and as previously reported [59]. Briefly, the cells were transfected with Cx43-siRNA duplexes or SCR-siRNA (20 nM) for 24 h and then shifted in fresh PM for additional 5 h. Thereafter, the transfected cells were cultured in DM with the addition or not of PRP for 48 h before being processed for Western blotting or immunofluorescence analysis of Cx43 and α-sma.

2.5. Reverse Transcription - Polymerase Chain Reaction (RT-PCR)

Cellular expression levels of Cx43 were evaluated by RT-PCR, as previously reported [48]. Briefly, according to manufacturer's instructions, total RNA was extracted from the cells cultured in the different experimental conditions on the wells of 6-wells/plates, by using TRIzol Reagent (Invitrogen, Life Technologies, Grand Island, NY, USA). One μg of total extracted RNA was reverse transcribed and amplified by using SuperScript One-Step RT-PCR System (Invitrogen, Life Technologies). cDNA synthesis was performed at 55 °C for 30 min; the samples were pre-denatured at 94 °C for 2 min and then subjected to 40 cycles of PCR performed at 94 °C for 15 s, alternating with 55 °C for 30 s and 72 °C for 1 min; the final extension step was performed at 72 °C for 5 min. The mouse gene-specific primers used were as follow: Cx43 (X61576.1), forward 5'-AACAGTCTGCCTTTCGCTGT-3' and reverse 5'-ATCTTCACCTTGCCGTGTTC-3'; β-actin (NM_007393), forward 5'-ACTGGGACGACATGGAGAAG-3' and reverse 5'-ACCAGAGGCATACAGGGACA-3'. β-actin mRNA was used as an internal standard. Blank controls, consisting of no template (water), were performed in each run. The amplified samples were electrophoresed on 1.8% agarose gel containing ethidium bromide staining, and the intensity of the related bands was quantified by densitometric analysis by using ImageJ 1.49v software (NIH, https://imagej.nih.gov/ij/). Each band intensity was normalized to the relative β-actin.

2.6. Confocal Laser Scanning Microscopy

Cells grown on sterile glass coverslips in the different experimental conditions were fixed with paraformaldehyde (PFA) 0.5% diluted in PBS for 10 min at room temperature. Fixed cells were washed and permeabilized with cold acetone for 3 min, incubated with a blocking solution containing 0.5% bovine serum albumin (BSA, Sigma) and 3% glycerol in PBS for 20 min and thereafter incubated overnight at 4 °C with the following antibodies: mouse monoclonal anti-α-sma (1:100; Abcam, Cambridge, UK), rabbit polyclonal anti-Cx43 (1:250; Chemicon, Temecula, CA, USA), rabbit polyclonal anti-type-1 collagen (1:50; Santa Cruz Biotechnology), or mouse monoclonal anti-Cx26 (1:50; Sigma). The immunoreactions were revealed by specific anti-mouse Alexa Fluor 488- or 568 conjugated IgG or anti-rabbit Alexa Fluor 488- conjugated IgG (1:200; Molecular Probes, Eugene, OR, USA). In some experiments the fixed cells were incubated with Alexa Fluor 488-conjugated wheat germ agglutinin (WGA, 1:100; Molecular Probes) for 10 min at room temperature, which binds glycoconjugates present on cell membranes, or counterstained with propidium iodide (PI, 1:30 for 30 s; Molecular Probes), to detect nuclei. Negative controls were carried out by replacing the primary antibodies with non-immune serum, while cross-reactivity of the secondary antibodies was evaluated in control experiments in which primary antibodies were omitted. The immunolabeled samples were washed and mounted with an antifade mounting medium (Biomeda Gel mount, Electron Microscopy Sciences,

Foster City, CA, USA) to allow the observation under a confocal Leica TCS SP5 microscope equipped with a HeNe/Ar laser source for fluorescence measurements and differential interference contrast (DIC) optics (Leica Microsystems, Mannheim, Germany). Observations were performed by means of a Leica Plan Apo 63×/1.43NA oil immersion objective. A series of optical sections (1024×1024 pixels each; pixel size 204.3 nm) 0.4 µm in thickness were taken throughout the depth of the cells preparations at intervals of 0.4 µm, and the images were projected onto a single 'extended focus' image. Densitometric analyses of the intensity of α-sma, type-1 collagen, Cx43 and Cx26 fluorescence signals were performed on digitized images using ImageJ 1.49v software (NIH, https://imagej.nih.gov/ij/) in 20 regions of interest (ROI) of 100 μm^2 for each confocal stack (at least 10).

2.7. Western Blotting

Total proteins extracted from the cells in the different experimental conditions were quantified, as reported previously [48]. Forty µg of total proteins were subjected to electrophoresis on NuPAGE®4%–12% Bis-Tris Gel (Invitrogen, Life Technologies; 200 V, 40 min) and blotted onto polyvinylidene difluoride (PVDF) membranes (Invitrogen, Life Technologies; 30 V, 1 h). The membranes were incubated with mouse monoclonal anti-α-sma (1:1000; Abcam), rabbit polyclonal anti-Cx43 (1:2500; Chemicon), and mouse monoclonal anti-Cx26 (1:500; Sigma) overnight at 4 °C. Immunodetection was performed according to the Western Breeze®Chromogenic Western Blot Immunodetection Kit protocol (Invitrogen, Life Technologies). The same membranes were subjected to the immunodetection of the expression of α-tubulin (rabbit polyclonal anti α-tubulin, 1:1000; Merck, Milan, Italy), assumed as control invariant protein. Densitometric analysis of the bands was performed using ImageJ 1.49v software (NIH, https://imagej.nih.gov/ij/), and the values normalized to control.

2.8. Statistical Analysis

Data were expressed as means ± standard error of the mean (S.E.M.) as a result of at least 3 independent experiments performed in triplicate. A 95% confidence level was used, assuming a normal distribution of values. Unpaired Student's t-test was used to compare the means of two conditions for independent data, statistically. The one-way analysis of variance (ANOVA) for any single independent variable was used to compare the differences between more than 2 groups and was followed by Tukey HSD or Bonferroni's post hoc adjustment. In electrophysiological experiments, 'n' indicates the number of cells analyzed. Values of $p < 0.05$ were considered statistically significant. Calculations were performed using GraphPad Prism software program (GraphPad, San Diego, CA, USA) and Microsoft Office Excel 2013 (Microsoft Corporation, Redmond, WA, USA).

3. Results

3.1. PRP Prevented TGF-β1- Induced Fibroblast to Myofibroblast Transition

Successful in vitro differentiation of NIH/3T3 fibroblasts towards myofibroblasts induced by the well-known pro-fibrotic factor TGF-β1 and the ability of PRP to prevent this transition were confirmed by morphological, biochemical and electrophysiological evaluations. Fibroblasts induced to differentiate by culturing in DM exhibited the typical features of myofibroblastic phenotype. Indeed, as judged by Western blotting analysis, they showed a significant increase of the expression of α-sma ($p < 0.05$), the most reliable marker of myofibroblasts, after 48 h and even more after 72 h of culture, as compared to control undifferentiated cells in PM (Figure 1A,B). Moreover, the immunocytochemical analysis at confocal microscopy, performed after 72 h of culture, confirmed the data of Western blotting and showed that this protein was well organized along filamentous structures (Figure 1C,D,I).

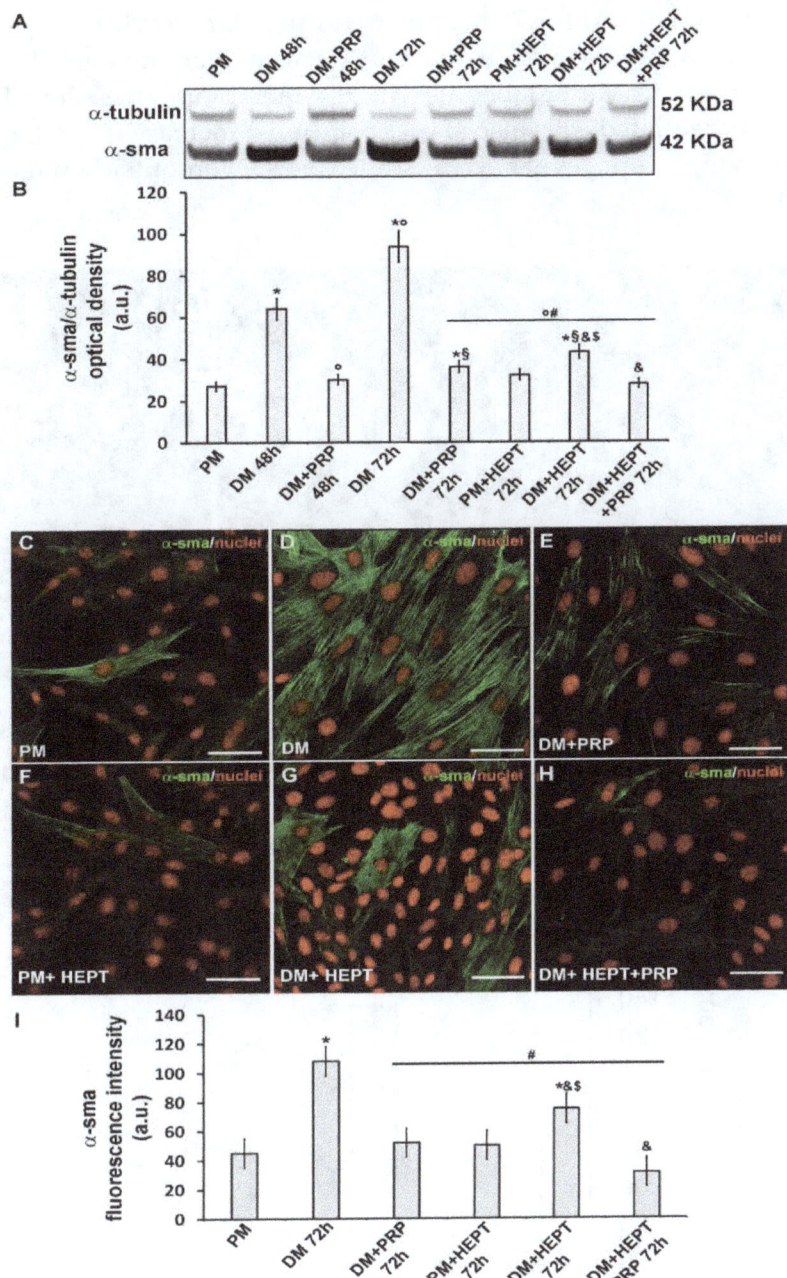

Figure 1. Evaluation of the effects PRP on fibroblast to myofibroblast transition and of the involvement of GJs: α-sma expression. Fibroblasts were induced to differentiate into myofibroblasts by culturing in differentiation medium (DM) in the presence or absence of PRP for 48 h and 72 h. Cells cultured in proliferation medium (PM) served as control undifferentiated cells. In parallel experiments, fibroblasts were cultured in PM or in DM in the presence of heptanol (HEPT), a common GJ channel blocker, in the presence or absence of PRP for 72 h. (**A,B**) Western Blotting analysis of α-sma expression. (**A**) Representative Blot. (**B**) Histogram showing the densitometric analysis of the bands normalized to α-tubulin. (**C–H**) Representative confocal fluorescence images of the cells immunostained with antibodies against α-sma (green) and counterstained with propidium iodide (PI) to detect nuclei. Scale bar: 50 μm. (**I**) Histogram showing the densitometric analysis of the intensity of the α-sma fluorescence signal performed on digitized images in 20 regions of interest (ROI) of 100 μm^2 for each confocal stack (10). Data shown are mean ± S.E.M. and represent the results of at least three independent experiments performed in triplicate. Significance of difference: * $p < 0.05$ versus PM; ° $p < 0.05$ versus DM 48 h; # $p < 0.05$ versus DM 72 h; § $p < 0.05$ versus DM + PRP 48 h; & $p < 0.05$ versus DM + PRP 72 h; $ $p < 0.05$ versus PM + HEPT 72 h (One-way ANOVA followed by the Tukey post hoc test).

Moreover, cells cultured in DM for 72 h, appeared much larger with a more polygonal shape as compared to the cells cultured in PM which, instead, were smaller and spindle-shaped as judged by the confocal fluorescence analysis after labeling with the membrane dye Alexa Fluor 488 conjugated WGA (Figure 2A,B). Differentiated cells also showed a robust increase ($p < 0.05$) in the expression of type-1 collagen at the cytoplasmic level and, in some cases, even outside the cells in a filamentous form (Figure 2D,E,G).

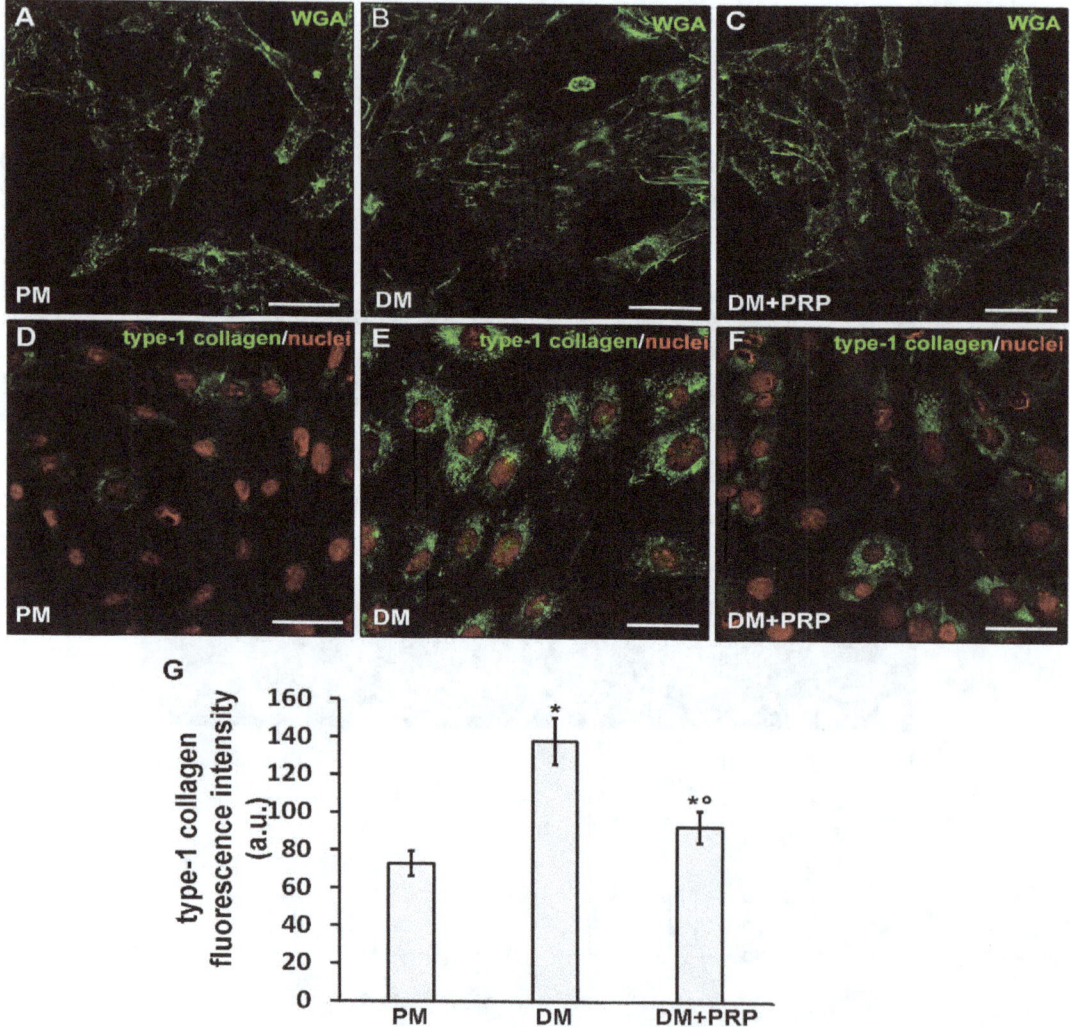

Figure 2. Effects of PRP on fibroblast to myofibroblast transition: Cell morphology and type-1 collagen expression. Fibroblasts were induced to differentiate into myofibroblasts by culturing in differentiation medium (DM) in the presence or absence of PRP for 72 h. The cells cultured in proliferation medium (PM) served as control undifferentiated cells. (**A–F**) Representative confocal fluorescence images of the cells (**A–C**) stained with Alexa Fluor 488-conjugated WGA (green) to reveal the plasma membrane and (**D–F**) immunostained with antibodies against type-1 collagen (green) and counterstained with propidium iodide (PI), to label nuclei. Scale bar: 50 μm. (**G**) Histogram showing the densitometric analysis of the intensity of type-1 collagen fluorescence signal performed on digitized images in 20 regions of interest (ROI) of 100 μm² for each confocal stack (10). Data are reported as mean ± S.E.M. and represent the results of at least three independent experiments performed in triplicate. Significance of difference: * $p < 0.05$ versus PM; ° $p <0.05$ versus DM (One-way ANOVA followed by the Tukey post hoc test).

The electrophysiological analysis of the passive membrane properties achieved by the whole-cell patch-clamp technique confirmed that the cells cultured in DM acquired the myofibroblastic phenotype. First, the resting membrane potential, RMP, was recorded and it was found that the values recorded from the cells cultured in DM for 48 h tended to be more depolarized compared to control undifferentiated fibroblasts in PM, in accordance with previous observations [23,24]. The overall results from all of the experiments done are shown in Figure 3A and Table 1. The statistical analysis of the RMP values between the different conditions was achieved with one–way ANOVA that provided overall results for our data. Despite the observed tendency to depolarization, the differences between the means did not turned out to be statistically significant ($p = 0.26$; $F = 1.45 <$ Fcrit $= 3.15$; df $= 30$).

We then analyzed the cell membrane resistance, R_m, in the voltage-clamp mode of our device. As shown in Figure 3B, R_m increased after 48 h and even more after 72 h of culture in DM. The one-way ANOVA analysis of R_m indicated statistical significance ($p = 0.00010$; $F = 8.99 >$ Fcrit $= 2.83$; df $= 50$). To know which groups were significantly different from another, we used the Bonferroni post-hoc test. The resulting significance is indicated by the symbols depicted in Figure 3B and Table 1.

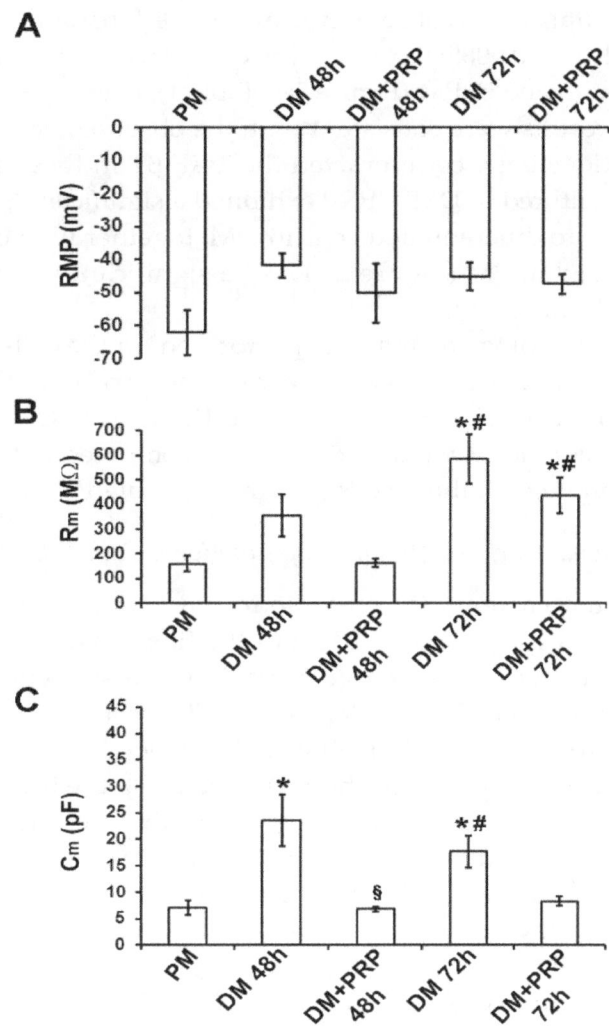

Figure 3. Effects of PRP on fibroblast to myofibroblast transition: Electrophysiological analysis of biophysical properties. (**A**) Resting membrane potential (RMP, in mV) recorded in the different conditions. Myofibroblasts have a tendency to be more depolarized. (**B**) Membrane resistance (R_m, in MΩ) shows higher values in myofibroblasts grown in differentiation medium (DM) compared to fibroblasts grown in proliferation medium (PM). (**C**) Membrane capacitance (C_m, in pF): Myofibroblasts show higher values compared to the undifferentiated cells in PM. All values are reported as mean ± S.E.M. and are listed in Table 1. * $p < 0.05$ versus PM; # $p < 0.05$ versus DM + PRP 48 h; § $p < 0.05$ versus DM 48 h (one-way ANOVA, followed by Bonferroni's post hoc test).

Table 1. Electrophysiological analysis of the membrane passive properties.

	PM	DM 48 h	DM + PRP 48 h	DM 72 h	DM + PRP 72 h
RMP (mV)	-62.0 ± 6.8 ($n = 6$)	-41.7 ± 3.75 ($n = 5$)	-50.2 ± 8.9 ($n = 7$)	-45.16 ± 4.06 ($n = 7$)	-47.37 ± 3.1 ($n = 6$)
R_m (M'Ω)	159.2 ± 31.0 (n = 6)	353.8 ± 85.9 (n = 5)	164.7 ± 17.3 (n = 14)	585.3 ± 100.9 *,# (n=11)	436.2 ± 71.3 *,# (n=15)
C_m (pF)	7.05 ± 1.2 ($n = 6$)	23.5 ± 4.7 * ($n = 9$)	6.82 ± 0.5 § ($n = 9$)	17.6 ± 2.9 *,# ($n = 8$)	8.3 ± 0.9 ($n = 14$)

Data are reported as mean ± S.E.M. * $p < 0.05$ versus PM; # $p < 0.05$ versus DM + PRP 48 h; § $p < 0.05$ versus DM 48 h (one-way ANOVA, followed by Bonferroni's post hoc test). The number of investigated cells is indicated by "n" in brackets for each condition.

Similarly, the cell capacitance, C_m, of cells cultured in DM, usually assumed as an index of cell surface, changed significantly ($p = 0.0085$; F = 4.52 > Fcrit = 2.86; df = 45; one way ANOVA). It tended to increase compared to that estimated in PM (Figure 3C; Table 1), being ($p < 0.05$) higher for cells in DM, especially after 48 h. These results were consistent with the observed cell morphology (Figure 2A,B).

The treatment with PRP actually counteracted the TGF-β1-induced fibroblast to myofibroblast transition. Indeed, the cells cultured in DM + PRP exhibited a significant ($p < 0.05$) reduction of α-sma (Figure 1A,B,E,I) with respect to differentiated cells in DM, together with different morphology, more similar to that of cells cultured in PM (Figure 2C) and a significantly reduced expression of type-1 collagen ($p < 0.05$) (Figure 2F,G).

Of interest, the electrophysiological analyses performed on the cells cultured in DM + PRP for the first time, revealed that R_m values tended to decrease compared to those measured in DM ($p > 0.05$) both after 48 h and 72 h of culture (Figure 3B; Table 1). As well, C_m values evaluated from cells cultured in DM + PRP were significantly reduced ($p < 0.05$) compared to those in DM, consistent with the observed changed morphology of these cells (Figure 3C; Table 1).

3.2. PRP Modifies Transjunctional Currents (I_j) and Gap Junctional Conductance (G_j) in Myofibroblast Pairs

Next, the transjunctional currents (I_j) were analyzed in cell pairs in different experimental conditions by the dual whole-cell technique. Most of the fibroblast pairs cultured in PM exhibited families of I_j current traces with a nearly heterogeneous time course. Typical tracings obtained from a not differentiated cell pair cultured in PM are depicted in Figure 4A.

A minority of the cell pairs cultured in PM (about 20%) showed current records with a symmetrical time course for negative and positive V_j (not shown), indicating the involvement of homotypic GJs. Moreover, they also showed a linear I_j-V_j plot, suggesting the presence of not-voltage-dependent connexons. By contrast, the remaining 80% of the cell pairs investigated showed a non-linear time course. In particular, only 40% of these cells showed a symmetrical voltage dependence for positive and negative V_j, suggesting the involvement of homotypic GJs and voltage-dependent connexons; 60% of the cells showed asymmetrical voltage dependence (Figure 4A). This may suggest the dominant presence of heterotypic GJs in control not differentiating fibroblasts.

We then analyzed the time course of the I_j evoked in myofibroblast pairs. Typical tracings of the I_j evoked in cell pairs cultured in DM for 48 h or 72 h are shown in Figure 4B,C, respectively. About 25% of these cells showed linear not-voltage-dependent I_j. Notably, about 75% of the cell pairs cultured in DM for 48 h exhibited a non-linear time course, suggesting the prevalent expression of voltage-dependent connexons. Only 33% of this kind of cell pairs showed an asymmetrical voltage-dependence suggesting a minor presence of heterotypic voltage-dependent GJs in differentiating myofibroblasts. In contrast, 67% of this kind of response was symmetrical for negative and positive V_j, suggesting that the majority of the GJs involved in this myofibroblastic population were voltage-dependent and homotypic.

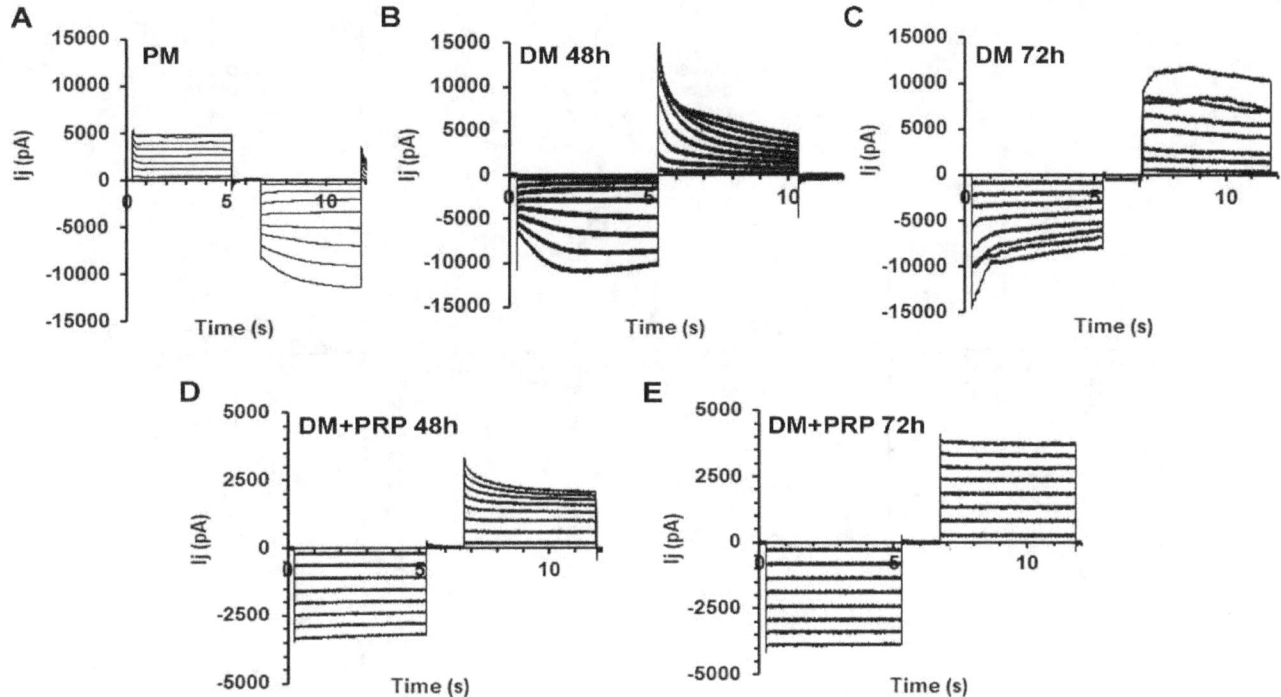

Figure 4. Time course of the transjunctional currents I_j, recorded from fibroblast and myofibroblast pairs in the absence or presence of PRP. (**A**) Representative I_j tracings (in pA) recorded in response to a bipolar pulse protocol applied to a fibroblast pair cultured in proliferation medium (PM). Note the asymmetrical time course between the two voltage polarities with a linear response for positive V_j. (**B,C**) Typical asymmetrical and almost voltage-dependent I_j tracings recorded from (**B**) a myofibroblast pair cultured in differentiation medium (DM) for 48 h and from (**C**) a myofibroblast pair in DM for 72 h. (**D,E**) Representative I_j recorded from a cell pair grown in (**D**) DM with PRP for 48 h (DM + PRP 48 h) and (**E**) for 72 h (DM + PRP 72 h). Note the completely linear and symmetrical responses in the latter condition.

After 72 h of culture in DM, we could observe an increase of the percentage of cell pairs with symmetrical voltage-dependent responses (about 80% in 72 h versus 67% in 48 h), indicating a progressive increase in the number of myofibroblasts exhibiting voltage-dependent and homotypic GJs.

The voltage dependence of I_j was evaluated by plotting the mean values of instantaneous currents, $I_{j,inst}$, (Figure 5A,C,E) and the steady-state currents, $I_{j,ss}$, (Figure 5B,D,F) as a function of V_j (I_j-V_j plot).

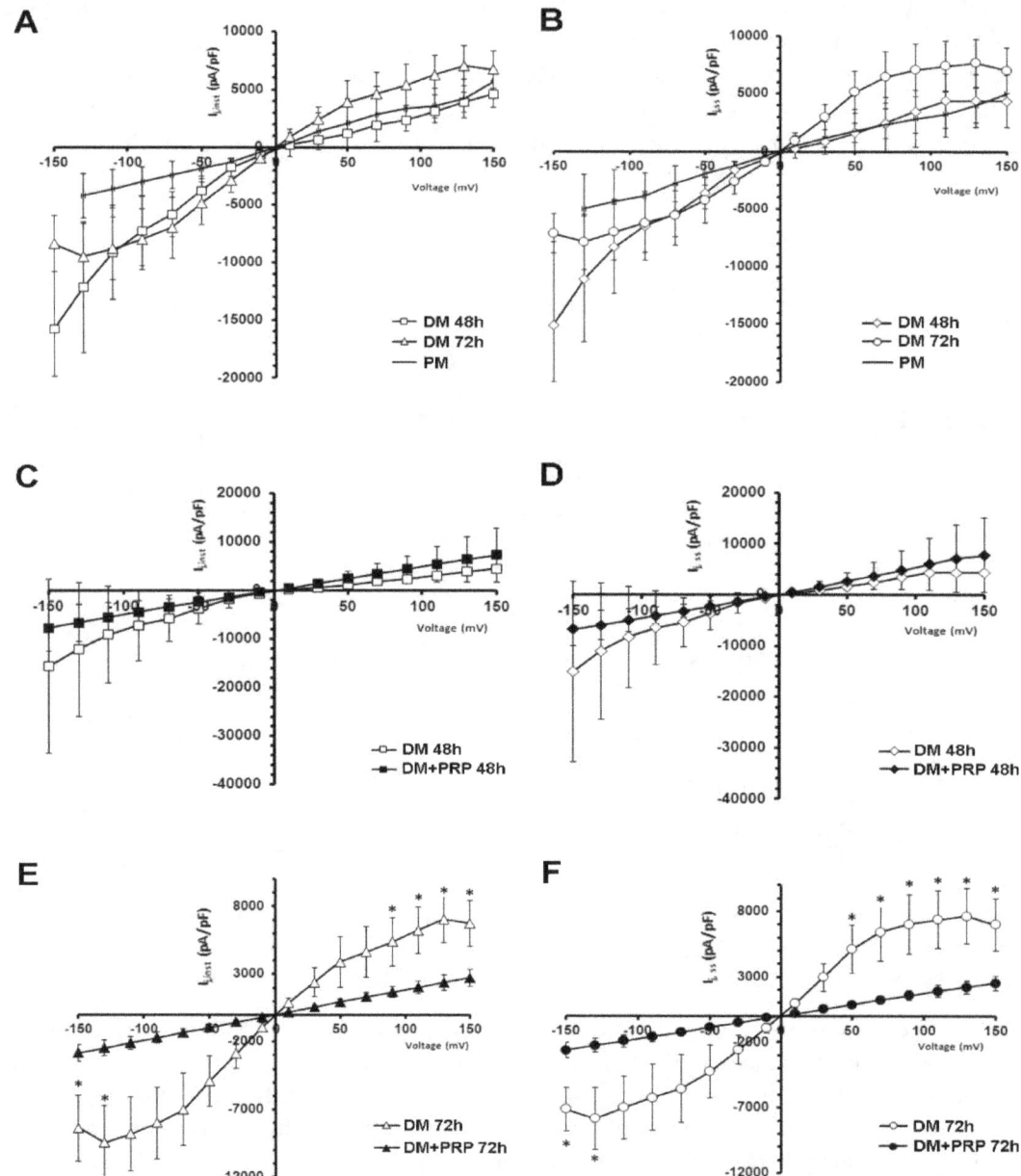

Figure 5. Voltage dependence of the transjunctional currents I_j, recorded from fibroblast and myofibroblast pairs in the absence or presence of PRP. (**A–F**) Transjunctional current values normalized for cell capacitance (in pA/pF), recorded from all of the fibroblast pairs cultured in proliferation medium (PM, continuous line, $n = 6$), and in differentiation medium (DM) for 48 h ($n = 9$) and 72 h ($n = 8$) plotted versus V_j. Panels A, C, and E show the $I_{j,inst}$ values whereas panels B, D, and F show the $I_{j,ss}$ values. Note that the plots related to DM show different slopes. (**C,D**) Comparison between I_j-V_j plot obtained from cell pairs cultured in DM for 48 h (open symbols, $n = 9$) and from cell pairs cultured in DM + PRP for 48 h (filled symbols, $n = 9$). Adding PRP to the culture medium for 48 h, altered the I_j voltage dependence, causing an almost complete linearity with voltage both for $I_{j,inst}$ and $I_{j,ss}$. (**E,F**) I_j-V_j plots related to 72 h treatments. The presence of PRP in DM for 72 h (DM + PRP 72 h, filled symbols, $n = 14$), strongly reduced the mean normalized current amplitude observed in DM 72 h (open symbols, $n = 8$) and altered the I_j voltage dependence, causing an almost complete linearity with voltage both for $I_{j,inst}$ and $I_{j,ss}$. All values represent mean ± S.E.M. * $p < 0.05$ (unpaired Student's t-test).

Notably, from a qualitative point of view, the I_j-V_j plots showed a different shape according to the different culture conditions, namely PM and DM 48 h and 72 h (Figure 5A,B). Ij currents recorded in PM showed the smallest amplitude and a scarce deviation from linearity, especially for negative V_j, showing a similar slope for both the V_j polarities (Figure 5A,B). In contrast, the plot related to DM 48 h was almost linear and smoother for positive V_j (Figure 5A,B). The plot related to DM 72 h showed a kind of shoulder becoming S-shaped (Figure 5A,B). For negative V_j the resulting I_j-V_j plots showed a different steepness compared to that observed for positive V_j, and it was similar at any time in culture in DM for 48 h and 72 h (Figure 5A,B). Again, I_j data showing this asymmetrical V_j -dependence are indicative of heterotypic GJ channels. The I_j evaluated both at the peak ($I_{j,inst}$) and at the steady-state ($I_{j,ss}$) showed a progressively more marked voltage-dependence as the time in culture in DM increased. Based on this observation, we suggest a major involvement of voltage-dependent connexons during the differentiation time. Of note, when cells were cultured in DM + PRP for 48 h, about 75% of the cell pairs showed a linear time course (Figure 4D), even if this kind of response was not perfectly symmetrical for negative and positive V_j for all of the cell pairs investigated. When the mean values of all the $I_{j,inst}$ and $I_{j,ss}$ recorded were plotted versus V_j, the relation resulted approximately linear and symmetrical over the entire voltage range, clearly indicating the prevalence of not voltage-dependent homotypic GJ channels (Figure 5C,D) in this culture condition. On the other hand, the cells cultured in DM + PRP for 72 h exhibited only not-voltage dependent Ij (100%) (Figure 4E). Indeed, they showed a linear response and a perfectly symmetrical time course for positive and negative V_j. Again, the I_j-V_j plot analysis showed the I_j linearity with V_j and a marked symmetry, strongly indicating the presence of not-voltage-dependent homotypic GJ channels (Figure 5E,F). Remarkably, for the largest voltage steps applied, the mean current amplitudes recorded from cells cultured in DM for 72 h were statistically different ($p < 0.05$; multiple unpaired Student's t-test) to those estimated in DM + PRP at the same time. Of note, the comparison of I_j-V_j plots in Figure 5E,F with those in Figure 5C,D indicated that the maximal recorded normalized mean amplitude both of $I_{j,inst}$ and $I_{j,ss}$ resulted smaller in DM + PRP 72 h than in DM + PRP 48 h. For instance, the mean $I_{j,ss}$ value estimated for the +150 mV step pulse was 2508 ± 566 pA/pF in DM + PRP 72 h and 7801 ± 7006 pA/pF in DM + PRP 48 h (Figure 5C,D).

Therefore, the features of I_j observed in the cells cultured in DM + PRP, such as the symmetry of the time course and the linearity of $I_{j,inst}$ and $I_{j,ss}$ versus voltage plots lead us to suggest a lessened contribution of voltage-dependent connexons in this condition.

To test for the current really flowing through GJs, we added heptanol (1 mM), a regularly used GJ channel blocker [59], to the bath solution during the recordings. The I_j was evoked from a cell pair cultured in DM, and then records were acquired from the same cell pair. After that, heptanol was acutely added to the bath solution. The recorded currents were significantly reduced compared to those elicited without heptanol. The mathematical subtraction of these two sets of traces gave the heptanol-sensitive current that is the one flowing through the GJs. In contrast, heptanol added during the recordings to cell pairs cultured in DM in the presence of PRP usually caused only a slight reduction of the current amplitude, suggesting a minor number of functional GJs allowing the current flow. A typical experiment related to cell pairs cultured in DM or in DM + PRP for 72 h is shown in Figure 6A. Only the current amplitude obtained by applying two representative voltage pulses (+130 and −30 mV) is shown as an example. Similar results were systematically observed for the bulk of cell pairs investigated. Since the heptanol sensitive current had a very small value in DM + PRP 72 h, we suggest a very small amount of functional GJs in the cells cultured in this experimental condition (Figure 6B–D).

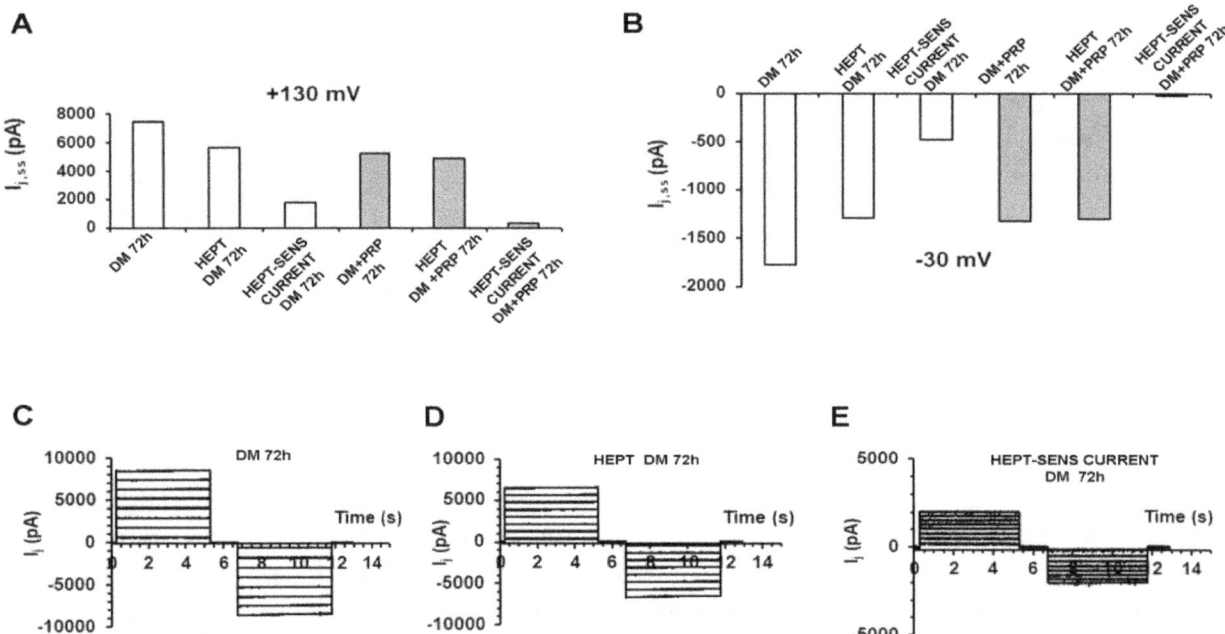

Figure 6. Evaluation of the current flowing through the GJs by acute addition of heptanol under different experimental conditions. (**A,B**) Evaluation of $I_{j,ss}$ (pA) related to a typical cell pair cultured for 72 h in differentiation medium (DM, white bars on the left side of each graph) or to a cell pair cultured for 72 h in DM + PRP (grey bars on the right). For clarity, only the current amplitude values obtained in response to a representative voltage pulse to +130 mV is reported in A, and to −30 mV in B. The current value recorded from the myofibroblast pair (DM 72 h) resulted clearly reduced after the acute addition of heptanol (HEPT, 1 mM) to the bath solution (HEPT DM 72 h). The current flowing through the GJs at the steady-state (HEPT-SENS CURRENT DM 72 h) is obtained by subtracting the current values recorded in the presence of heptanol from those recorded in DM alone. In contrast, the current amplitude recorded from the cell pair cultured in DM + PRP after acute addition of heptanol (HEPT DM + PRP 72 h) showed a slight reduction compared to DM + PRP 72h, having the heptanol-sensitive current a very small value (HEPT-SENS CURRENT DM + PRP 72h). Similar results were systematically observed for any voltage step applied in the bulk of the cell pairs investigated, suggesting a very small amount of functional GJs expressed under PRP treatment. (**C**) Characteristic time course of I_j (pA) recorded from a cell pair cultured in DM (DM 72 h) that exceptionally showed voltage independent features. (**D**) The same current traces recorded after acute heptanol addition (HEPT DM 72 h). (**E**) Resulting current traces (HEPT-SENS CURRENT DM 72 h) obtained by subtracting currents in D from currents in C, and representing the small heptanol-sensitive flux through the GJs. Note the different ordinate scale in E.

Noteworthy, even in those cell pairs cultured in DM for 72 h that exhibited not-voltage-dependent I_j, we could still measure a heptanol-sensitive current, suggesting that also the not-voltage dependent GJ functionality was hampered by the GJ blocker.

Finally, we analyzed the conductive properties of GJs. Intercellular current flow in cell pairs of fibroblasts and myofibroblasts were also used to study the dependency of the gap junctional conductance, G_j, on V_j by means of the G_j-V_j plot analysis. The related results are shown in Figure 7.

Data points obtained from cell pairs cultured in PM (Figure 7A) showed a horizontal distribution for positive V_j, suggesting the involvement of not-voltage-dependent GJs, in contrast to the not-linear distribution observed for negative V_j values. This asymmetrical voltage dependence of the G_j can suggest the prevalence of heterotypic GJs in proliferating fibroblastic cell pairs. These data points obtained from the cell pairs cultured in DM for 48 h (Figure 7B) did not follow a merely symmetrical relationship, being almost linear for negative V_j and more bell-shaped for positive V_j. Again, this may be consistent with the expression of more than one Cx isoform in myofibroblasts (possibly assembling in different combinations compared to those observed in PM) and hence confirms the involvement of heterotypic GJ channels in this cell population. After 72 h in DM, the G_j-V_j plot showed more or less the same shape as 48 h, but the G_j values for positive V_j resulted higher, suggesting a major contribution of the voltage-dependent component. In contrast, G_j-V_j plots related to the cells cultured in DM + PRP both at 48 h and 72 h were symmetrical and linear in any case, suggesting a lack of voltage-dependent GJs. This result suggests the involvement of homotypic GJ channels in this cell population.

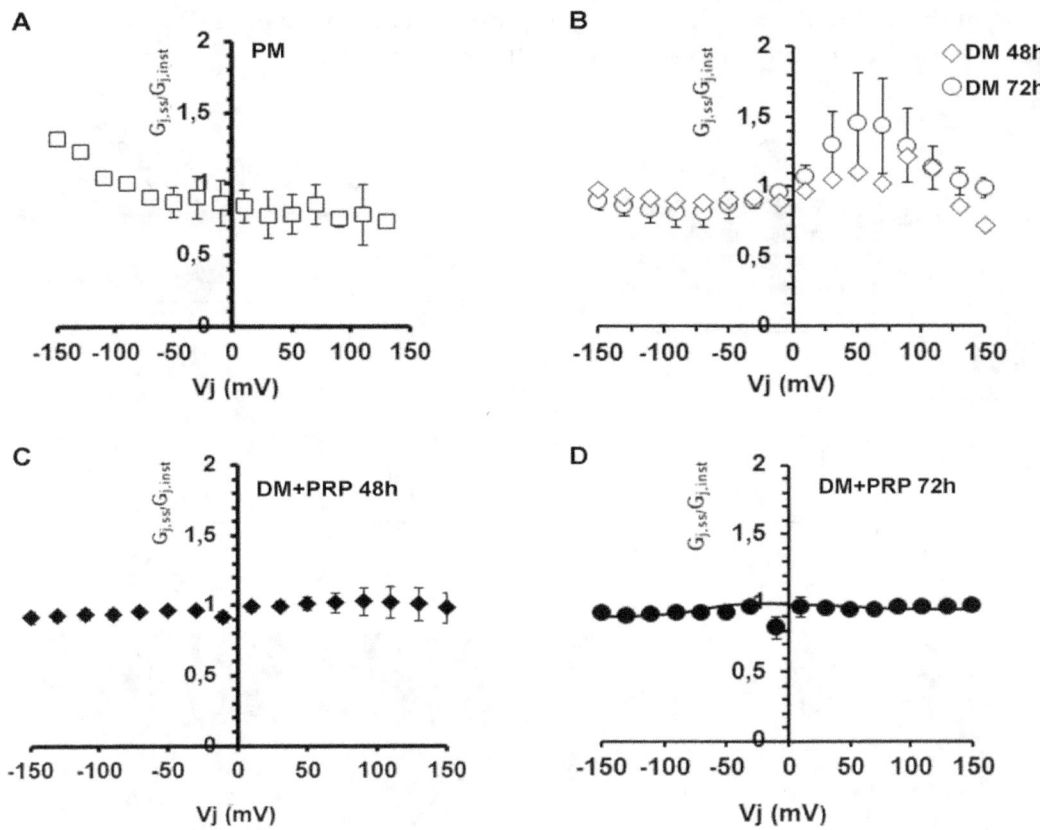

Figure 7. Voltage dependence of the transjunctional conductance G_j. (**A,B**) Voltage dependence of the transjunctional conductance obtained by plotting $G_{j,ss}/G_{j,inst}$ versus V_j related to (**A**) proliferation medium (PM) condition (open squares, $n = 6$), (**B**) differentiation medium (DM) condition at 48 h (open squares, $n = 9$) and 72 h (open circles, $n = 9$). These data obtained in DM show an asymmetrical distribution that becomes more bell-shaped for positive V_j. The treatment for 72 h gave higher values compared to 48 h, although not statistically significant ($p > 0.05$, multiple unpaired Student's t-test). (**C,D**) Symmetrical linear distribution observed under the concomitant treatment in DM + PRP at (**C**) 48 h (filled squares, $n = 9$), and (**D**) 72 h (filled circles, $n = 14$). All values represent mean ± S.E.M. Error bars are visible if they exceed the symbol size.

3.3. PRP Reduces Cx43 Expression and Increases Cx26 Expression in Differentiated Myofibroblasts

Since the electrophysiological experiments showed an increase of I_j and G_j functionality during myo-differentiation of fibroblasts, we cultured the cells in DM in the presence of the GJ channel blocker heptanol (1 mM) for 72 h, to test the effective involvement of GJs in myofibroblast generation. We first analyzed the expression of α-sma in this experimental condition. As assessed by Western blotting and confocal immunofluorescence analyses, the cells exposed to DM + heptanol exhibited a clear reduction of α-sma expression (Figure 1A,B,F,G,I) compared to control differentiated myofibroblasts cultured in DM, supporting a key role of the GJs in the acquisition of myofibroblastic phenotype. Of note, the cells cultured in DM + PRP showed a more robust reduction of α-sma then those cultured in DM + heptanol, likely suggesting that PRP-induced prevention of fibroblast myofibroblast differentiation involves the activation of multiple molecular mechanisms. The cells cultured in DM + heptanol + PRP showed a significantly reduced ($p < 0.05$) expression of α-sma as compared to that observed in the cells exposed to single treatment (i.e., DM + heptanol or DM + PRP).

Then, taking into consideration the increasingly marked voltage dependence of the I_j recorded during differentiation time, we performed experiments aimed to evaluate the expression of the typical Cx types forming voltage- dependent connexins, namely Cx43.

We found that Cx43 expression both at mRNA and protein levels significantly increased ($p <$ 0.05) with time in the cells cultured in DM as compared to control cells in PM as judged by RT-PCR (Figure 8A) and Western blotting analyses (Figure 8B), respectively.

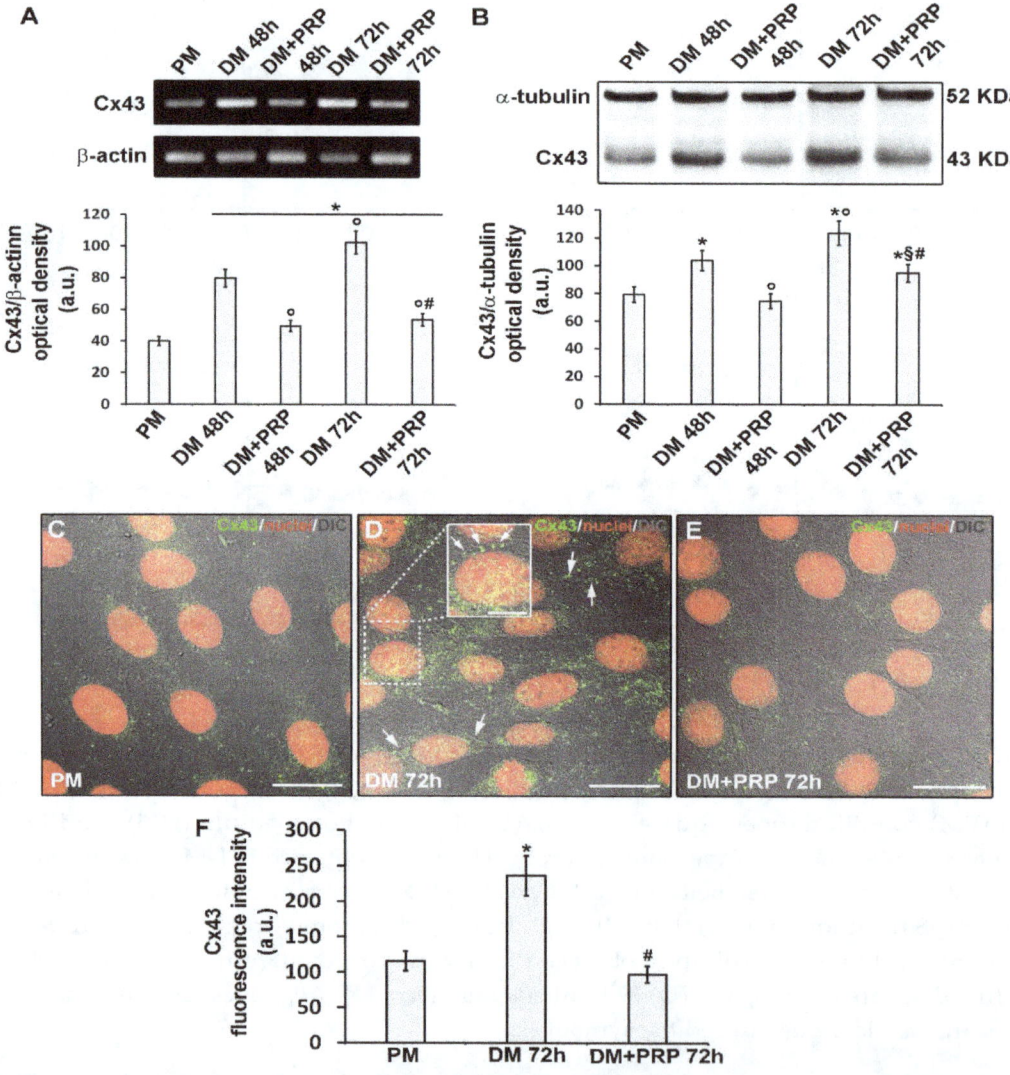

Figure 8. Cx43 expression and localization during fibroblast to myofibroblast transition and related PRP effects. Fibroblasts were induced to differentiate into myofibroblasts by culturing in differentiation medium (DM) in the presence or absence of PRP for 48 h and 72 h. The cells cultured in proliferation medium (PM) were used as control undifferentiated cells. (**A**) RT-PCR analysis of Cx43 expression in the indicated experimental conditions. Representative agarose gel is shown. The densitometric analysis of the bands normalized to β-actin is reported in the histogram. (**B**) Western Blotting analysis of Cx43 expression. Histogram showing the densitometric analysis of the bands normalized to α-tubulin. (**C–E**) Representative superimposed differential interference contrast (DIC, grey) and confocal fluorescence images of the cells immunostained with antibodies against Cx43 (green) and

counterstained with propidium iodide (PI, red) to label nuclei. Scale bar: 30 μm. Scale bar in the inset in D: 15 μm. Arrows indicate the localization of Cx43 at the membrane level of two adjacent cells. **(F)** Histogram showing the densitometric analysis of the intensity of the Cx43 fluorescence signal performed on digitized images in 20 regions of interest (ROI) of 100 μm² for each confocal stack (12). Data shown are mean ± S.E.M. and represent the results of at least three independent experiments performed in triplicate. Significance of difference: * $p < 0.05$ versus PM; ° $p < 0.05$ versus DM 48 h; # $p < 0.05$ versus DM 72 h; § $p < 0.05$ versus DM + PRP 48 h (One-way ANOVA followed by the Tukey post hoc test).

Confocal immunofluorescence analysis confirmed the increase of Cx43 expression in differentiated cells after 48 h (data not shown) and even more after 72 h of culture in DM as compared to control undifferentiated cells in PM (Figure 8C,D,F). Moreover, we demonstrated the protein localization either at the cytoplasmic level or at the cell membrane level of adjacent cells (Figure 8C,D). To confirm the key role of this Cx isoform in fibroblast to myofibroblast transition, we silenced the cells for the expression of Cx43 by specific siRNA before culturing them in DM for 72 h (Figure 9A).

These cells exhibited a significant reduction ($p < 0.05$) of α-sma expression (Figure 9B,C,D,E,I) compared to cell cultured in DM, suggesting that Cx43 was required for the differentiation process. Of note, the cells cultured in DM + PRP concomitantly to reduced α-sma, showed a significant reduction of Cx43 expression (Figure 8A,B,E,F). This outcome was consistent with the electrophysiological data showing the reduction of voltage-dependent responses in these cells. Notably, according to the results of the experiments achieved in cells cultured with heptanol (Figure 1), the cells cultured in DM + PRP showed reduced expression of α-sma with respect to the cells silenced for Cx43 cultured in DM (Figure 9 B–I). Cells silenced for Cx43 expression and exposed to DM + PRP exhibited reduced α-sma expression levels as compared to those observed in the cells exposed to single treatment (i.e., DM + siRNA or DM + PRP) (Figure 9 B–I).

Finally, even the occurrence of a not-voltage-dependent response in myofibroblast pairs (although in a minority) as well as of the increase of this type of response after treatment with PRP, we analyzed the expression of a typical Cx type forming not/scarcely voltage-dependent connexons, namely Cx26. Western blotting (Figure 10A,B) and confocal immunofluorescence (Figure 10C–H) analyses demonstrated that Cx26 expression significantly increased in the cells after culture in DM for 48 h with respect to undifferentiated cells cultured in PM ($p < 0.05$). By contrast, the cells cultured in DM for 72 h exhibited Cx26 expression levels comparable to those of undifferentiated cells. The cells cultured in DM for 48 h in the absence or presence of PRP exhibited comparable levels of Cx26 expression ($p > 0.05$). Of note, the cells cultured in DM + PRP for 72 h exhibited a slight but significant increase ($p > 0.05$) of Cx26 as compared to cells cultured in the absence of PRP (Figure 10A,B,F,G,H).

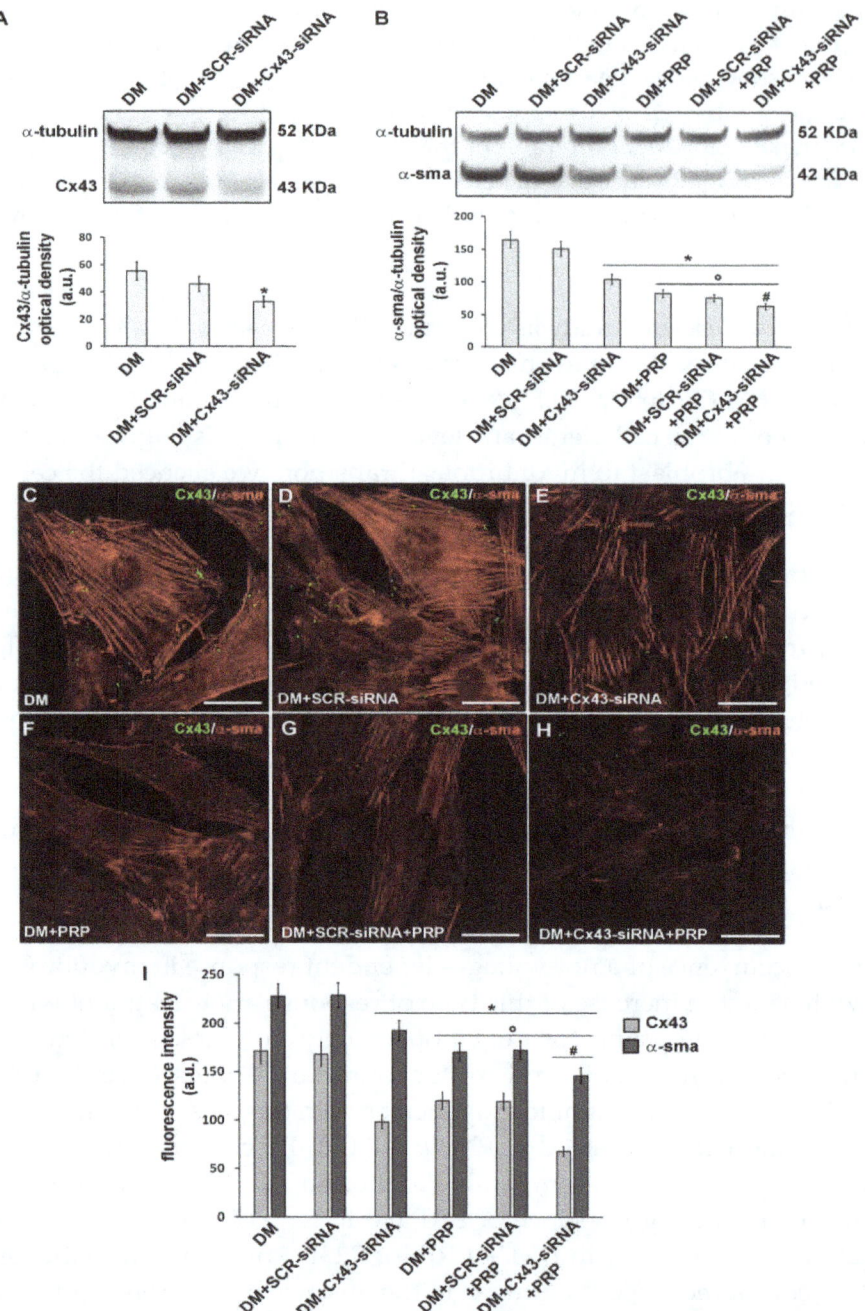

Figure 9. Effect of inhibition of Cx43 expression on fibroblast to myofibroblast transition and related PRP effects. Fibroblasts were silenced by specific Cx43-siRNA duplexes and cultured in differentiation medium (DM) for 48 h in the absence or presence of PRP. SCR-siRNA duplexes were used as an internal control. (**A,B**) Western Blotting analysis of (**A**) Cx43 and (**B**) α-sma expression. The densitometric analysis of the bands normalized to α-tubulin is reported in the histograms. (**C–H**) Representative confocal fluorescence images of the cells double immunostained with antibodies against Cx43 (green) and α-sma (red). Scale bar: 25 μm. (**I**) Histogram showing the densitometric analysis of the intensity of Cx43 and α-sma fluorescence signal performed on digitized images in 20 regions of interest (ROI) of 100 μm^2 for each confocal stack (12). Data shown are mean $\pm$ S.E.M. and represent the results of at least three independent experiments performed in triplicate. Significance of difference: * $p < 0.05$ versus DM; ° $p < 0.05$ versus DM + CX43 − siRNA; # $p < 0.05$ versus DM + PRP (One-way ANOVA followed by the Tukey post hoc test).

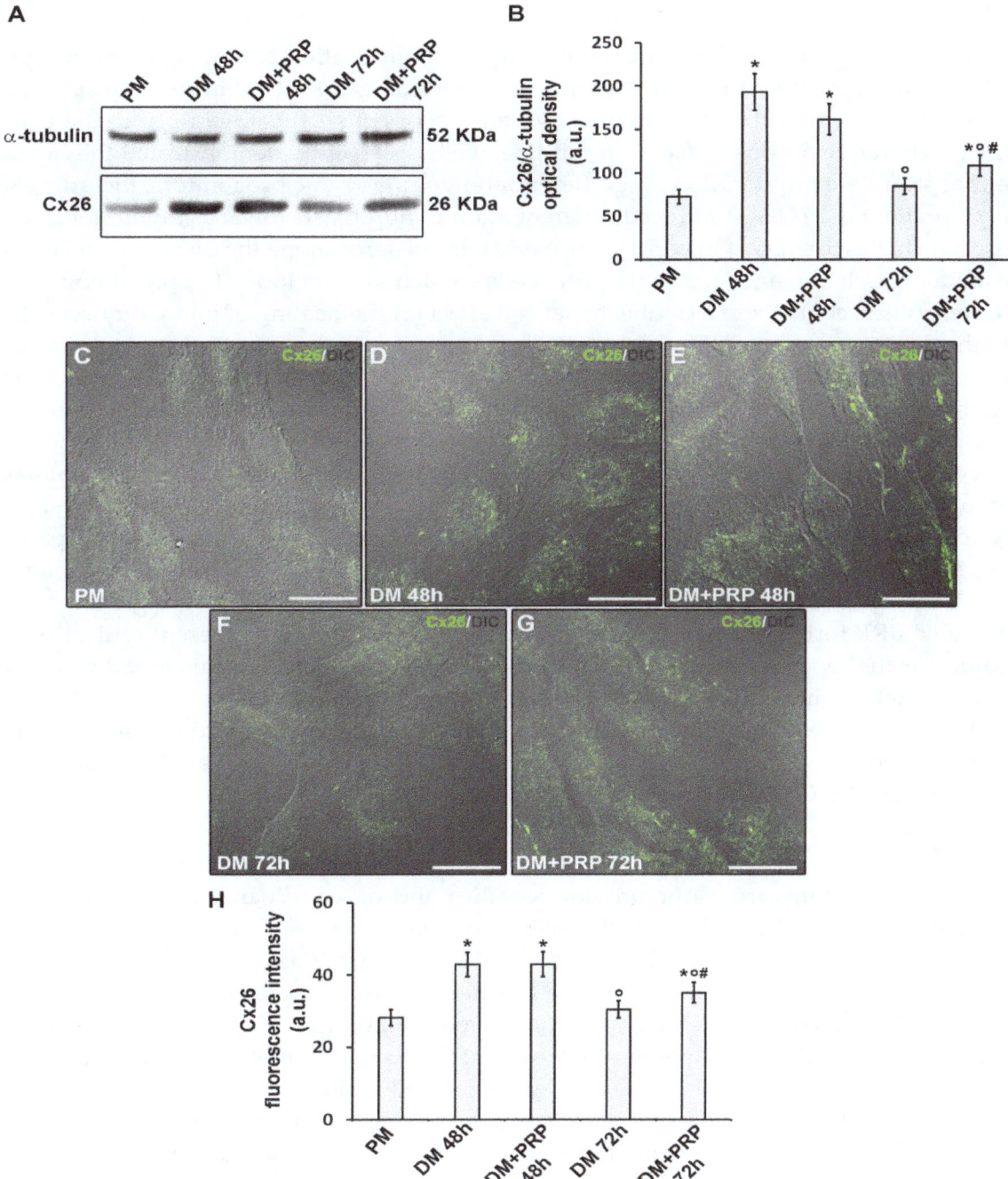

Figure 10. Cx26 expression during fibroblast to myofibroblast transition and related PRP effects. Fibroblasts were induced to differentiate into myofibroblasts by culturing in differentiation medium (DM) in the presence or absence of PRP for 48 h and 72 h. The cells cultured in proliferation medium (PM) served as control undifferentiated cells. (**A,B**) Western Blotting analysis of Cx26 expression. (**A**) Representative blot. (**B**) Histogram showing the densitometric analysis of the bands normalized to α-tubulin. (**C–G**) Representative superimposed differential interference contrast (DIC, grey) and confocal fluorescence images of the cells immunostained with antibodies against Cx26 (green) showing the cellular localization of the protein. Scale bar: 25 μm. (**H**) Histogram showing the densitometric analysis of the intensity of the Cx26 fluorescence signal performed on digitized images in 20 regions of interest (ROI) of 100 μm^2 for each confocal stack (12). Data shown are mean ± S.E.M. and represent the results of at least three independent experiments performed in triplicate. Significance of difference: * $p < 0.05$ versus PM; ° $p < 0.05$ versus DM 48 h; # $p < 0.05$ versus DM 72 h (One-way ANOVA followed by the Tukey post hoc test).

4. Discussion

In recent years, great attention has been paid to the identification of new therapeutic agents and treatments that may promote the repair/regeneration of damaged skeletal muscle. In such a context, several in vitro and in vivo studies provided evidence supporting the advantage of the use of PRP for muscle regenerative purpose [30,66]. In this line, we have recently demonstrated the capability of PRP to either stimulate proliferation and differentiation of myogenic progenitors, including satellite cells [58], or prevent the TGF-β1 induced differentiation of fibroblasts towards myofibroblasts [48,57].

These data led us to suggest that PRP, if properly administered along the cascade of events through which skeletal muscle repair/regeneration proceeds (which also includes the physiological fibrotic reparative response), could exert a double beneficial effect on the healing of injured muscle. This may consist in the direct activation of the resident cells effectors of muscle regeneration, responsible for the formation of new muscle fibers and, in parallel, in the modulation/prevention of an excessive fibrotic response, thus contributing to the recreation of a more hospitable and conducive microenvironment for muscle progenitor functionality and thus the promotion of tissue regeneration. Experiments are ongoing in our lab aimed to assess the effects of PRP on differentiated myofibroblasts, by evaluating the capability of this blood product to modulate their fate. The results should be of interest to support the anti-fibrotic action of PRP. However, the ability of PRP in antagonizing fibrotic signaling pathways is still an issue of debate. Some reports show limited effectiveness or even inefficacy of this blood-derived product in counteracting the skeletal muscle fibrotic response [30,42,44,67–75]. The great heterogeneity of the available PRP formulation, PRP dosage and application timing represent critical points that may account for the reported conflicting results concerning the effects of this blood product in the modulation of skeletal muscle tissue fibrosis.

Based on these considerations, studies aimed to support the anti-fibrotic effect of this blood product are needed, as well as researches focused on the identification of the cellular and molecular target mechanisms of PRP, underpinning its action.

4.1. PRP Counteracts Myofibroblast Generation

According to findings from our previous studies and other research groups [30,47,48,76,77], here we have confirmed the ability of PRP to counteract the core cellular process of the fibrotic response, namely differentiation of fibroblasts towards myofibroblasts induced by the pro-fibrotic agent TGF-β1, based on: i) morphological and biochemical analyses showing that the cells treated with TGF-β1 in the presence of PRP did not acquire a mature myofibroblastic phenotype; indeed they rather appeared more spindle-shaped and showed either a reduction of type-1 collagen expression and a lower expression of α-sma, that was also less organized in filamentous structure as compared to differentiated cells; ii) the novel electrophysiological recordings of the membrane passive properties and gap junctional functionality, showing the ability of PRP to modify such parameters with respect to those recorded in differentiated myofibroblasts. Particularly, in the present experiments we observed that differentiated myofibroblasts tended to have a more positive RMP and PRP treatment counteracted this occurrence. The RMP is always critical for cell function since any small alteration of its value can substantially change cell excitability, contractility, and other properties, such as cell migration [21]. The less positive membrane potential registered in the cells induced to differentiate in the presence of PRP may counteract the depolarization of myofibroblasts and hamper their contractility, leading to an altered functionality. In this regard, it was shown that depolarization causes enhancement of ventricular myofibroblast contractility [21]. In this view, the present findings may suggest that PRP can revert myofibroblast RMP towards a more 'dormant' condition, counteracting their full differentiation.

In addition, PRP action opposed the increase of R_m value observed in differentiating conditions, showing its ability to revert the effect on the resting conductive properties induced by TGF-β1. The R_m parameter, corresponding to the reciprocal value of the membrane conductance, G_m, gives an idea of the total resting ionic fluxes across the membrane; thus, its physiological relevance is strictly linked to cell excitability. Moreover, the C_m value assumed as an index of membrane surface area increased in the cells induced to differentiate as compared to proliferating cells. This observation was in agreement with the morphological analysis showing that the cells tended to increase their size upon TGF-β1-induced differentiation. Both phenomena were counteracted by PRP. Notably, the latter data are in accordance with the electrophysiological results described in our previous report dealing with the anti-fibrotic potential of relaxin [23].

4.2. Role of GJIC and Cx43 in Myofibroblast Generation

The main relevance of our study is the contribution toward defining the molecular and functional mechanisms regulating TGF-β1 induced fibroblast-myofibroblast transition, highlighting the role of GJs in this process as well as the involvement of voltage-dependent connexin isoform, namely Cx43. In particular, we found that the majority of differentiated myofibroblast pairs exhibited an enhancement of I_j amplitude in the course of differentiation, suggesting an increased functionality of GJs, especially of the voltage-dependent ones, with increasing exposure time to TGF-β1. The role of GJs in this differentiation process was confirmed by the use of heptanol, a common GJ blocker. When the cells were induced to differentiate in the presence of heptanol, they actually failed to acquire a myofibroblast phenotype, indicating an essential role of functional GJs in the promotion of fibroblasts differentiation towards myofibroblasts. These data are in good accordance with previous studies showing that the selective blockade of GJs downregulated myofibroblastic phenotype [78,79]. Therefore, it can be stated that GJIC is of crucial importance in our cell model to regulate the fibroblast transformation towards myofibroblast. However, a possible role of such intercellular communications in the functional coupling of mature myofibroblasts to coordinate their activity can also be speculated [18,51–54]. In fact, while it is well accepted that myofibroblasts are responsible for the reparative scar formation and contraction, it is not clear yet whether they act individually or behave synchronically [78]. In this regard, we can propose that myofibroblasts can, at least in part, act as a coordinated functional syncytium, thus that hindering intercellular communication may represent a therapeutic target in diseases characterized by an overabundance of these contractile cells. Another important point is the ability of myofibroblasts to interact, by GJs, with other resident cell types of tissue globally affecting the organ functionality [80–82]. The analysis of the transjunctional conductance, G_j, gave some interesting information. Usually, the higher the G_j, the faster the current flows from a cell to the adjacent one, resulting in faster propagation speed [83]. The estimated G_j is the overall result of the total number of GJ channels docked between cells, the single-channel conductance of each GJ channel, and their functional states (fully open, sub conductance, or closed states). The GJ functional states can be dynamically modulated by chemicals and transjunctional voltage. The transjunctional voltage-dependent gating is an intrinsic property in all characterized GJs. In this study, we found that the G_j in differentiated myofibroblast pairs showed a progressively more marked voltage-dependence, suggesting a prevalent expression of voltage-dependent Cxs in myofibroblasts. From a functional point of view, this may reflect the need for myofibroblasts to be coupled in response to stimuli that cause membrane potential alterations. However, myofibroblasts likely need to express a kind of Cx, such as Cx43, whose trafficking, half-life, and regulation (by phosphorylation) can be maximally modulated during differentiation to myofibroblast [84]. Corroborating this suggestion coming from electrophysiological records, here we found that myofibroblasts showed an increased expression of Cx43. Furthermore, we found that cells silenced for the expression of Cx43 did not exhibit a mature myofibroblastic phenotype when cultured in differentiation condition in the presence of TGF-β1, suggesting the requirement of Cx43 for fibroblast-myofibroblast transition. Collectively these data are in accordance with the findings of our recent study [48] demonstrating an upregulation of mRNA expression of Cx43 in TGF-β1 treated cells (i.e., myofibroblasts). As well they agree with the studies by Asazuma-Nakamura and co-workers (2009) [85] and by Paw and co-workers (2017) [86] showing that Cx43 positively regulated myofibroblastic differentiation of cardiac and bronchial fibroblasts, respectively. In parallel, other studies showed that Cx43 expression is largely modulated during wound repair, and the modulation of Cx43 expression and gap junctional communication can be beneficial to wound healing [87]. This process can be definitely altered by modulating Cx43 expression: wound closure can be delayed when Cx43 is overexpressed or accelerated when the levels of epidermal Cx43 are reduced [88–91]. In line with this, the transient blockade of Cx43 functions has been shown to reduce fibrosis as well as to promote experimental wound healing [89], and the normal GJ functions of Cx43 seems to be important for normal fibroblast function [92]. In this regard, multiple clinical trials are investigating Cx43 modulators and specific peptides targeting the intracellular loop, and the C-terminal tail region of this protein appear promising [93]. Based on our present findings, showing an increase of Cx43 expression in differentiated cells not only at the plasma membrane level but also in the cytoplasm, it is worth mentioning that a GJ independent function of Cx43 during fibroblast to myofibroblast transition cannot be excluded [59,94]. Taking into account the reported channel-independent influence of Cx43 on cytoskeleton remodeling and cell migration, we may speculate a similar role [94] for stress fiber assembly during fibroblast- myofibroblast transition.

4.3. GJs, Cx43, and Cx26 as Molecular Candidate Targets of the Potential Anti-fibrotic Action of PRP

Another main finding of this study is the compelling experimental evidence indicating, for the first time, that GJs and Cx43 are molecular candidate targets of the potential anti-fibrotic action of PRP. Indeed, PRP treatment affected the occurrence of voltage-dependent I_j, which was reduced at 48 h and even abolished after 72 h of culture; concomitantly, it prevented the TGF-β1 induced increase of Cx43 expression. Interestingly, the cells induced to differentiate in the presence of PRP mostly exhibited scarcely/not voltage-dependent I_j along with an observed upregulation of Cx26, especially after 48 h. We may suppose that these events reflect a compensatory mechanism to maintain a sort of cell-to-cell communication, upon PRP treatment. In addition, we may speculate a major role of Cx26 in this condition that may be linked to the ability of this Cx type to form hemichannels rather than highly regulated GJs. We should point out the ability of hemichannels themselves to act as membrane channels able to mediate cell communication with surrounding extracellular environment: recent studies confirm a link between hemichannel-mediated ATP release and the progression and development of fibrosis in different tissue types [95–98]. In this line, the role of Cx26 in forming scarcely voltage-dependent GJs and/or hemichannels and the possible relation with ATP content in our cell model is an interesting topic deserving further investigation.

4.4. Factors Released by PRP Possibly Modulating Cx Expression and GJ Functionality During Myofibroblast Generation

Finally, it is worth mentioning that the factors released by PRP possibly modulating Cx expression and GJ functionality during myo-differentiation process remain to be identified as well as their potential modes of action. We have previously demonstrated that PRP contains vascular endothelial growth factor (VEGF)-A and that, through this factor linking its receptor-1 (VEGFR-1 or Flt-1), PRP antagonizes TGF-β1/Smad3, thus preventing fibroblast myo-differentiation [30,48]. Taking into consideration that VEGF may modulate the expression of Cx43 and/or GJ functionality in different cell types [99–101] we may speculate that GJs/Cx43 might represent a downstream target of VEGF-A/VEGFR-1 mediated signaling in our experimental cell model. Studies are ongoing in our lab to assess this hypothesis. Moreover, it is known that GJ assembly and disassembly are events highly regulated by a sequence of protein kinase activation and phosphorylation events. This kind of regulation, as extensively reported for Cx43, has a net effect of reducing GJ communication [102–104]. Therefore, we may also postulate that VEGF-A or other factors released by PRP may reduce GJ/Cx43 functionality affecting such phosphorylation events. In such a view it has been reported that insulin-like growth factor (IGF)-1 is able to decrease gap junctional communication by inducing activation of PKCγ, enhancing the interaction between PKCγ and Cx43 and the phosphorylation of Cx43 by PKCγ [105] in epithelial cells. Since IGF-1 has been reported to be contained in PRP [106] and has been supposed as a potential modulator of fibrogenic events and pathways [14,107,108], it is tempting to speculate that similar interactions may also occur in our cell system. Therefore, the capability of PRP to counteract fibroblast differentiation towards myofibroblasts and its ability to modulate GJIC could also involve the IGF-1 signaling pathway. A full characterization of the releasing profile of likely cross-talking factors present in PRP are required to understand the molecular mechanisms underpinning the action of this plasma product.

5. Conclusions

In conclusion, the results of the present in vitro study provide the first experimental evidence that upregulation of Cx43 and the parallel increase of voltage-dependent GJ functionality are important mechanisms by which TGF-β1 endorses fibroblast differentiation towards myofibroblast, and that PRP treatment hampers this effect.

The main limitations of this study rely on the in vitro experimentation on the NIH/3T3 cell line. Obviously, the in vitro experimentation eliminates many paracrine/juxtacrine mechanisms, possibly regulating in situ intercellular interactions and cell functionality as well as the mechanical forces exerted by the surrounding microenvironment, including ECM stiffness, affecting cell behavior [16,18,109]. NIH/3T3 cells represent a widely used, reliable model to study fibroblast biology. We previously demonstrated that these cells show similar behavior, in terms of differentiation marker expression and electrophysiological parameters, to primary fibroblasts, such as human dermal fibroblasts, skeletal, and cardiac fibroblasts [23,48,55,56]. Nevertheless, the growing evidence on functional heterogeneity and the origin-linked response of fibroblasts to stimuli must be taken into account [110–112]. Therefore, we acknowledge that a different experimental set using primary cultures of skeletal muscle-derived fibroblasts could have offered in vitro findings possibly more closely related to in vivo conditions of skeletal muscle disease and fibrosis.

Another limitation is represented by the lack of a full characterization of the growth factors released by PRP. This should be relevant to understand better PRP mechanisms of action in the modulation of fibroblast-myofibroblast transition and to achieve a therapeutic translation of this approach. Furthermore, standardization of PRP preparation techniques as well as application protocols would allow performing meaningful comparative analyses.

However, despite these aspects, this research contributes to add further insights into molecular and functional mechanisms regulating fibroblast-myofibroblast transition. It likewise supports the anti-fibrotic action of PRP by means of its ability to hamper myofibroblast generation, targeting GJs, thus providing cues to novel therapeutic targets.

Author Contributions: Conceptualization, R.S., F.C., E.I., A.T., and C.S.; formal analysis, R.S., F.C., E.I., A.T., and C.S.; investigation, R.S., F.C., E.I., A.T., R.G., S.P., and C.S.; resources, R.S., F.C., P.P., F.B., S.Z.-O., and C.S.; data curation, R.S., F.C., E.I., A.T., and C.S.; writing—original draft preparation, R.S., and C.S.; writing—review and editing, R.S., F.C., E.I., A.T., S.Z.-O., and C.S.; visualization, R.S., F.C., E.I., A.T., and C.S.; funding acquisition, R.S., F.C., S.Z.-O., and C.S. All authors have read and agreed to the published version of the manuscript."

References

1.   Yin, H.; Price, F.; Rudnicki, M.A. Satellite cells and the muscle stem cell niche. *Physiol. Rev.* **2013**, *93*, 23–67. [CrossRef]

2.   Doyle, M.J.; Zhou, S.; Tanaka, K.K.; Pisconti, A.; Farina, N.H.; Sorrentino, B.P.; Olwin, B.B. Abcg2 labels multiple cell types in skeletal muscle and participates in muscle regeneration. *J. Cell. Biol.* **2011**, *195*, 147–163. [CrossRef] [PubMed]

3.   Judson, R.N.; Zhang, R.H.; Rossi, F.M. Tissue-resident mesenchymal stem/progenitor cells in skeletal muscle: Collaborators or saboteurs? *FEBS J.* **2013**, *280*, 4100–4108. [CrossRef]

4.   Meng, J.; Chun, S.; Asfahani, R.; Lochmüller, H.; Muntoni, F.; Morgan, J. Human skeletal muscle-derived CD133(+) cells form functional satellite cells after intramuscular transplantation in immunodeficient host mice. *Mol. Ther.* **2014**, *22*, 1008–1017. [CrossRef] [PubMed]

5.   Scicchitano, B.M.; Sica, G.; Musarò, A. Stem Cells and Tissue Niche: Two Faces of the Same Coin of Muscle Regeneration. *Eur. J. Transl. Myol.* **2016**, *26*, 6125. [CrossRef] [PubMed]

6. Tonlorenzi, R.; Rossi, G.; Messina, G. Isolation and Characterization of Vessel-Associated Stem/Progenitor Cells from Skeletal Muscle. *Methods Mol. Biol.* **2017**, *1556*, 149–177. [CrossRef] [PubMed]

7. Dumont, N.A.; Wang, Y.X.; Rudnicki, M.A. Intrinsic and extrinsic mechanisms regulating satellite cell function. *Development* **2015**, *142*, 1572–1581. [CrossRef]

8. Forcina, L.; Miano, C.; Pelosi, L.; Musarò, A. An Overview about the Biology of Skeletal Muscle Satellite Cells. *Curr. Genomics* **2019**, *20*, 24–37. [CrossRef]

9. Sacco, A.; Puri, P.L. Regulation of Muscle Satellite Cell Function in Tissue Homeostasis and Aging. *Cell Stem Cell.* **2015**, *16*, 585–587. [CrossRef]

10. Mann, C.J.; Perdiguero, E.; Kharraz, Y.; Aguilar, S.; Serrano, A.L.; Muñoz-Cánoves, P. Aberrant repair and fibrosis development in skeletal muscle. *Skelet. Muscle* **2011**, *1*, 21. [CrossRef]

11. Farup, J.; Madaro, L.; Puri, P.L.; Mikkelsen, U.R. Interactions between muscle stem cells, mesenchymal-derived cells and immune cells in muscle homeostasis, regeneration and disease. *Cell Death Dis.* **2015**, *6*, e1830. [CrossRef] [PubMed]

12. Ceafalan, L.C.; Fertig, T.E.; Popescu, A.C.; Popescu, B.O.; Hinescu, M.E.; Gherghiceanu, M. Skeletal muscle regeneration involves macrophage-myoblast bonding. *Cell Adhes. Migr.* **2018**, *12*, 228–235. [CrossRef] [PubMed]

13. Malecova, B.; Gatto, S.; Etxaniz, U.; Passafaro, M.; Cortez, A.; Nicoletti, C.; Giordani, L.; Torcinaro, A.; De Bardi, M.; Bicciato, S.; et al. Dynamics of cellular states of fibro-adipogenic progenitors during myogenesis and muscular dystrophy. *Nat. Commun.* **2018**, *9*, 3670. [CrossRef] [PubMed]

14. Forcina, L.; Miano, C.; Scicchitano, B.M.; Musarò, A. Signals from the Niche: Insights into the Role of IGF-1 and IL-6 in Modulating Skeletal Muscle Fibrosis. *Cells* **2019**, *8*, 232. [CrossRef] [PubMed]

15. Manetti, M.; Tani, A.; Rosa, I.; Chellini, F.; Squecco, R.; Idrizaj, E.; Zecchi-Orlandini, S.; Ibba-Manneschi, L.; Sassoli, C. Morphological evidence for telocytes as stromal cells supporting satellite cell activation in eccentric contraction-induced skeletal muscle injury. *Sci. Rep.* **2019**, *9*, 14515. [CrossRef] [PubMed]

16. Hinz, B.; McCulloch, C.A.; Coelho, N.M. Mechanical regulation of myofibroblast phenoconversion and collagen contraction. *Exp. Cell Res.* **2019**, *379*, 119–128. [CrossRef]

17. Weiskirchen, R.; Weiskirchen, S.; Tacke, F. Organ and tissue fibrosis: Molecular signals, cellular mechanisms and translational implications. *Mol. Aspects Med.* **2019**, *65*, 2–15. [CrossRef]

18. Tomasek, J.J.; Gabbiani, G.; Hinz, B.; Chaponnier, C.; Brown, R.A. Myofibroblasts and mechano-regulation of connective tissue remodelling. *Nat. Rev. Mol. Cell. Biol.* **2002**, *3*, 349–363. [CrossRef]

19. Koivumäki, J.T.; Clark, R.B.; Belke, D.; Kondo, C.; Fedak, P.W.; Maleckar, M.M.; Giles, W.R. Na(+) current expression in human atrial myofibroblasts: Identity and functional roles. *Front. Physiol.* **2014**, *5*, 275. [CrossRef]

20. Zhan, H.; Zhang, J.; Jiao, A.; Wang, Q. Stretch-activated current in human atrial myocytes and Na+ current and mechano-gated channels' current in myofibroblasts alter myocyte mechanical behavior: A computational study. *Biomed. Eng. Online* **2019**, *18*, 104. [CrossRef]

21. Chilton, L.; Ohya, S.; Freed, D.; George, E.; Drobic, V.; Shibukawa, Y.; Maccannell, K.A.; Imaizumi, Y.; Clark, R.B.; Dixon, I.M.; et al. K+ currents regulate the resting membrane potential, proliferation, and contractile responses in ventricular fibroblasts and myofibroblasts. *Am. J. Physiol. Heart. Circ. Physiol.* **2005**, *288*, 2931–2939. [CrossRef] [PubMed]

22. Kaur, K.; Zarzoso, M.; Ponce-Balbuena, D.; Guerrero-Serna, G.; Hou, L.; Musa, H.; Jalife, J. TGF-β1, released by myofibroblasts, differentially regulates transcription and function of sodium and potassium channels in adult rat ventricular myocytes. *PLoS ONE* **2013**, *8*, e55391. [CrossRef] [PubMed]

23. Squecco, R.; Sassoli, C.; Garella, R.; Chellini, F.; Idrizaj, E.; Nistri, S.; Formigli, L.; Bani, D.; Francini, F. Inhibitory effects of relaxin on cardiac fibroblast-to-myofibroblast transition: An electrophysiological study. *Exp. Physiol.* **2015**, *100*, 652–666. [CrossRef] [PubMed]

24. Sassoli, C.; Chellini, F.; Squecco, R.; Tani, A.; Idrizaj, E.; Nosi, D.; Giannelli, M.; Zecchi-Orlandini, S. Low intensity 635 nm diode laser irradiation inhibits fibroblast-myofibroblast transition reducing TRPC1 channel expression/activity: New perspectives for tissue fibrosis treatment. *Lasers Surg. Med.* **2016**, *48*, 318–332. [CrossRef]

25. Xue, M.; Jackson, C.J. Extracellular Matrix Reorganization During Wound Healing and Its Impact on Abnormal Scarring. *Adv. Wound Care (New Rochelle).* **2015**, *4*, 119–136. [CrossRef] [PubMed]

26. Jun, J.I.; Lau, L.F. Resolution of organ fibrosis. *J. Clin. Investig.* **2018**, *128*, 97–107. [CrossRef] [PubMed]

27. Horowitz, J.C.; Thannickal, V.J. Mechanisms for the Resolution of Organ Fibrosis. *Physiology (Bethesda)* **2019**, *34*, 43–55. [CrossRef]

28. Bochaton-Piallat, M.L.; Gabbiani, G.; Hinz, B. The myofibroblast in wound healing and fibrosis: Answered and unanswered questions. *F1000Research* **2016**, *5*, F1000 Faculty Rev-752. [CrossRef]

29. Rosenbloom, J.; Macarak, E.; Piera-Velazquez, S.; Jimenez, S.A. Human Fibrotic Diseases: Current Challenges in Fibrosis Research. *Methods Mol. Biol.* **2017**, *1627*, 1–23. [CrossRef] [PubMed]

30. Chellini, F.; Tani, A.; Zecchi-Orlandini, S.; Sassoli, C. Influence of Platelet-Rich and Platelet-Poor Plasma on Endogenous Mechanisms of Skeletal Muscle Repair/Regeneration. *Int. J. Mol. Sci.* **2019**, *20*, 683. [CrossRef]

31. Vu, T.D.; Pal, S.N.; Ti, L.K.; Martinez, E.C.; Rufaihah, A.J.; Ling, L.H.; Lee, C.N.; Richards, A.M.; Kofidis, T. An autologous platelet-rich plasma hydrogel compound restores left ventricular structure, function and ameliorates adverse remodeling in a minimally invasive large animal myocardial restoration model: A translational approach: Vu and Pal "Myocardial Repair: PRP, Hydrogel and Supplements". *Biomaterials* **2015**, *45*, 27–35. [CrossRef] [PubMed]

32. Jang, H.Y.; Myoung, S.M.; Choe, J.M.; Kim, T.; Cheon, Y.P.; Kim, Y.M.; Park, H. Effects of autologous platelet-rich plasma on regeneration of damaged endometrium in female rats. *Yonsei Med. J.* **2017**, *58*, 1195–1203. [CrossRef] [PubMed]

33. Moghadam, A.; Khozani, T.T.; Mafi, A.; Namavar, M.R.; Dehghani, F. Effects of platelet-rich plasma on kidney regeneration in gentamicin-induced nephrotoxicity. *J. Korean Med. Sci.* **2017**, *32*, 13–21. [CrossRef] [PubMed]

34. Andia, I.; Martin, J.I.; Maffulli, N. Advances with platelet rich plasma therapies for tendon regeneration. *Expert. Opin. Biol. Ther.* **2018**, *18*, 389–398. [CrossRef] [PubMed]

35. Sanchez-Avila, R.M.; Merayo-Lloves, J.; Riestra, A.C.; Berisa, S.; Lisa, C.; Sánchez, J.A.; Muruzabal, F.; Orive, G.; Anitua, E. Plasma rich in growth factors membrane as coadjuvant treatment in the surgery of ocular surface disorders. *Medicine (Baltimore)* **2018**, *97*, e0242. [CrossRef] [PubMed]

36. Sayadi, L.R.; Obagi, Z.; Banyard, D.A.; Ziegler, M.E.; Prussak, J.; Tomlinson, L.; Evans, G.R.D.; Widgerow, A.D. Platelet-rich plasma, adipose tissue, and scar modulation. *Aesthet. Surg. J.* **2018**, *38*, 1351–1362. [CrossRef]

37. Shoeib, H.M.; Keshk, W.A.; Foda, A.M.; Abo El Noeman, S.E. A study on the regenerative effect of platelet-rich plasma on experimentally induced hepatic damage in albino rats. *Can. J. Physiol. Pharmacol.* **2018**, *96*, 630–636. [CrossRef]

38. Tavukcu, H.H.; Aytaç, Ö.; Atuğ, F.; Alev, B.; Çevik, Ö.; Bülbül, N.; Yarat, A.; Çetinel, S.; Sener, G.; Kulaksızoğlu, H. Protective effect of platelet-rich plasma on urethral injury model of male rats. *Neurourol. Urodyn.* **2018**, *37*, 1286–1293. [CrossRef]

39. Terada, S.; Ota, S.; Kobayashi, M.; Kobayashi, T.; Mifune, Y.; Takayama, K.; Witt, M.; Vadalà, G.; Oyster, N.; Otsuka, T.; et al. Use of an anti-fibrotic agent improves the effect of platelet-rich plasma on muscle healing after injury. *J. Bone Jt. Surg. Am.* **2013**, *95*, 980–988. [CrossRef]

40. Cunha, R.C.; Francisco, J.C.; Cardoso, M.A.; Matos, L.F.; Lino, D.; Simeoni, R.B.; Pereira, G.; Irioda, A.C.; Simeoni, P.R.; Guarita-Souza, L.C.; et al. Effect of platelet-rich plasma therapy associated with exercise training in musculoskeletal healing in rats. *Transpl. Proc.* **2014**, *46*, 1879–1881. [CrossRef]

41. Anitua, E.; Pelacho, B.; Prado, R.; Aguirre, J.J.; Sánchez, M.; Padilla, S.; Aranguren, X.L.; Abizanda, G.; Collantes, M.; Hernandez, M.; et al. Infiltration of plasma rich in growth factors enhances in vivo angiogenesis and improves reperfusion and tissue remodeling after severe hind limb ischemia. *J. Control. Release* **2015**, *202*, 31–39. [CrossRef] [PubMed]

42. Cianforlini, M.; Mattioli-Belmonte, M.; Manzotti, S.; Chiurazzi, E.; Piani, M.; Orlando, F.; Provinciali, M.; Gigante, A. Effect of platelet rich plasma concentration on skeletal muscle regeneration: An experimental study. *J. Biol. Regul. Homeost. Agents* **2015**, *29*, 47–55. [PubMed]

43. Denapoli, P.M.; Stilhano, R.S.; Ingham, S.J.; Han, S.W.; Abdalla, R.J. Platelet-Rich Plasma in a Murine Model: Leukocytes, Growth Factors, Flt-1, and Muscle Healing. *Am. J. Sports Med.* **2016**, *44*, 1962–1971. [CrossRef] [PubMed]

44. Li, H.; Hicks, J.J.; Wang, L.; Oyster, N.; Philippon, M.J.; Hurwitz, S.; Hogan, M.V.; Huard, J. Customized platelet-rich plasma with transforming growth factor β1 neutralization antibody to reduce fibrosis in skeletal muscle. *Biomaterials* **2016**, *87*, 147–156. [CrossRef] [PubMed]

45. Zanon, G.; Combi, F.; Combi, A.; Perticarini, L.; Sammarchi, L.; Benazzo, F. Platelet-rich plasma in the treatment of acute hamstring injuries in professional football players. *Joints* **2016**, *4*, 17–23. [CrossRef]

46. Contreras-Muñoz, P.; Torrella, J.R.; Serres, X.; Rizo-Roca, D.; De la Varga, M.; Viscor, G.; Martínez-Ibáñez, V.; Peiró, J.L.; Järvinen, T.A.H.; Rodas, G.; et al. Postinjury Exercise and Platelet-Rich Plasma Therapies Improve Skeletal Muscle Healing in Rats But Are Not Synergistic When Combined. *Am. J. Sports Med.* **2017**, *45*, 2131–2141. [CrossRef]

47. Anitua, E.; Troya, M.; Orive, G. Plasma rich in growth factors promote gingival tissue regeneration by stimulating fibroblast proliferation and migration and by blocking transforming growth factor-β1-induced myodifferentiation. *J. Periodontol.* **2012**, *83*, 1028–1037. [CrossRef]

48. Chellini, F.; Tani, A.; Vallone, L.; Nosi, D.; Pavan, P.; Bambi, F.; Zecchi Orlandini, S.; Sassoli, C. Platelet-Rich Plasma Prevents In Vitro Transforming Growth Factor-β1- Induced Fibroblast to Myofibroblast Transition: Involvement of Vascular Endothelial Growth Factor (VEGF)-A/VEGF Receptor- 1-Mediated Signaling. *Cells* **2018**, *7*, 142. [CrossRef]

49. Willebrords, J.; Crespo Yanguas, S.; Maes, M.; Decrock, E.; Wang, N.; Leybaert, L.; da Silva, T.C.; Veloso Alves Pereira, I.; Jaeschke, H.; Cogliati, B.; et al. Structure, Regulation and Function of Gap Junctions in Liver. *Cell. Commun. Adhes.* **2015**, *22*, 29–37. [CrossRef]

50. Valiunas, V.; Gemel, J.; Brink, P.R.; Beyer, E.C. Gap junction channels formed by coexpressed connexin40 and connexin43. *Am. J. Physiol. Heart. Circ. Physiol.* **2001**, *281*, H1675–H1689. [CrossRef]

51. Gaudesius, G.; Miragoli, M.; Thomas, S.P.; Rohr, S. Coupling of cardiac electrical activity over extended distances by fibroblasts of cardiac origin. *Circ. Res.* **2003**, *93*, 421–428. [CrossRef] [PubMed]

52. Chilton, L.; Giles, W.R.; Smith, G.L. Evidence of intercellular coupling between co-cultured adult rabbit ventricular myocytes and myofibroblasts. *J. Physiol.* **2007**, *583*, 225–236. [CrossRef] [PubMed]

53. Zlochiver, S.; Muñoz, V.; Vikstrom, K.L.; Taffet, S.M.; Berenfeld, O.; Jalife, J. Electrotonic myofibroblast-to-myocyte coupling increases propensity to reentrant arrhythmias in two-dimensional cardiac monolayers. *Biophys. J.* **2008**, *95*, 4469–4480. [CrossRef]

54. Kakkar, R.; Lee, R.T. Intramyocardial fibroblast myocyte communication. *Circ. Res.* **2010**, *106*, 47–57. [CrossRef] [PubMed]

55. Sassoli, C.; Chellini, F.; Pini, A.; Tani, A.; Nistri, S.; Nosi, D.; Zecchi-Orlandini, S.; Bani, D.; Formigli, L. Relaxin prevents cardiac fibroblast-myofibroblast transition via notch-1-mediated inhibition of TGF-β/Smad3 signaling. *PLoS ONE* **2013**, *8*, e63896. [CrossRef] [PubMed]

56. Sassoli, C.; Nosi, D.; Tani, A.; Chellini, F.; Mazzanti, B.; Quercioli, F.; Zecchi-Orlandini, S.; Formigli, L. Defining the role of mesenchymal stromal cells on the regulation of matrix metalloproteinases in skeletal muscle cells. *Exp. Cell Res.* **2014**, *323*, 297–313. [CrossRef]

57. Chellini, F.; Tani, A.; Vallone, L.; Nosi, D.; Pavan, P.; Bambi, F.; Zecchi-Orlandini, S.; Sassoli, C. Platelet-Rich Plasma and Bone Marrow-Derived Mesenchymal Stromal Cells Prevent TGF-β1-Induced Myofibroblast Generation but Are Not Synergistic when Combined: Morphological in vitro Analysis. *Cells Tissues Organs* **2018**, *206*, 283–295. [CrossRef]

58. Sassoli, C.; Vallone, L.; Tani, A.; Chellini, F.; Nosi, D.; Zecchi-Orlandini, S. Combined use of bone marrow-derived mesenchymal stromal cells (BM-MSCs) and platelet rich plasma (PRP) stimulates proliferation and differentiation of myoblasts in vitro: New therapeutic perspectives for skeletal muscle repair/regeneration. *Cell Tissue Res.* **2018**, *372*, 549–570. [CrossRef]

59. Squecco, R.; Sassoli, C.; Nuti, F.; Martinesi, M.; Chellini, F.; Nosi, D.; Zecchi-Orlandini, S.; Francini, F.; Formigli, L.; Meacci, E. Sphingosine 1-phosphate induces myoblast differentiation through Cx43 protein expression: A role for a gap junction-dependent and -independent function. *Mol. Biol. Cell.* **2006**, *17*, 4896–4910. [CrossRef]

60. Formigli, L.; Sassoli, C.; Squecco, R.; Bini, F.; Martinesi, M.; Chellini, F.; Luciani, G.; Sbrana, F.; Zecchi-Orlandini, S.; Francini, F.; et al. Regulation of transient receptor potential canonical channel 1 (TRPC1) by sphingosine 1-phosphate in C2C12 myoblasts and its relevance for a role of mechanotransduction in skeletal muscle differentiation. *J. Cell. Sci.* **2009**, *122*, 1322–1333. [CrossRef]

61. Pierucci, F.; Frati, A.; Squecco, R.; Lenci, E.; Vicenti, C.; Slavik, J.; Francini, F.; Machala, M. Meacci, E. Non-dioxin-like organic toxicant PCB153 modulates sphingolipid metabolism in liver progenitor cells: Its role in Cx43-formed gap junction impairment. *Arch. Toxicol.* **2017**, *91*, 749–760. [CrossRef] [PubMed]

62. Sassoli, C.; Formigli, L.; Bini, F.; Tani, A.; Squecco, R.; Battistini, C.; Zecchi-Orlandini, S.; Francini, F.; Meacci, E. Effects of S1P on skeletal muscle repair/regeneration during eccentric contraction. *J. Cell. Mol. Med.* **2011**, *15*, 2498–2511. [CrossRef] [PubMed]

63. Pappone, P.A.; Lee, S.C. Purinergic receptor stimulation increases membrane trafficking in brown adipocytes. *J. Gen. Physiol.* **1996**, *108*, 393–404. [CrossRef] [PubMed]

64. Formigli, L.; Meacci, E.; Sassoli, C.; Chellini, F.; Giannini, R.; Quercioli, F.; Tiribilli, B.; Squecco, R.; Bruni, P.; Francini, F.; et al. Sphingosine 1-phosphate induces cytoskeletal reorganization in C2C12 myoblasts: Physiological relevance for stress fibres in the modulation of ion current through stretch-activated channels. *J. Cell. Sci.* **2005**, *118*, 1161–1171. [CrossRef] [PubMed]

65. Meacci, E.; Bini, F.; Sassoli, C.; Martinesi, M.; Squecco, R.; Chellini, F.; Zecchi-Orlandini, S.; Francini, F.; Formigli, L. Functional interaction between TRPC1 channel and connexin-43 protein: A novel pathway underlying S1P action on skeletal myogenesis. *Cell. Mol. Life Sci.* **2010**, *67*, 4269–4285. [CrossRef] [PubMed]

66. Andia, I.; Abate, M. Platelet-rich plasma in the treatment of skeletal muscle injuries. *Expert. Opin. Biol.* **2015**, *15*, 987–999. [CrossRef]

67. Cole, B.J.; Seroyer, S.T.; Filardo, G.; Bajaj, S.; Fortier, L.A. Platelet-rich plasma: Where are we now and where are we going? *Sports Health* **2010**, *2*, 203–210. [CrossRef]

68. Delos, D.; Leineweber, M.J.; Chaudhury, S.; Alzoobaee, S.; Gao, Y.; Rodeo, S.A. The effect of platelet-rich plasma on muscle contusion healing in a rat model. *Am. J. Sports Med.* **2014**, *42*, 2067–2074. [CrossRef]

69. Dimauro, I.; Grasso, L.; Fittipaldi, S.; Fantini, C.; Mercatelli, N.; Racca, S.; Geuna, S.; Di Gianfrancesco, A.; Caporossi, D.; Pigozzi, F.; et al. Platelet-rich plasma and skeletal muscle healing: A molecular analysis of the early phases of the regeneration process in an experimental animal model. *PLoS ONE* **2014**, *9*, e102993. [CrossRef]

70. Reurink, G.; Goudswaard, G.J.; Moen, M.H.; Weir, A.; Verhaar, J.A.; Bierma-Zeinstra, S.M.; Maas, M.; Tol, J.L. Dutch HIT-study Investigators. Rationale, secondary outcome scores and 1-year follow-up of a randomised trial of platelet-rich plasma injections in acute hamstring muscle injury: The Dutch Hamstring Injection Therapy study. *Br. J. Sports Med.* **2015**, *49*, 1206–1212. [CrossRef]

71. Kelc, R.; Vogrin, M. Concerns about fibrosis development after scaffolded PRP therapy of muscle injuries: Commentary on an article by Sanchez et al.: Muscle repair: Platelet-rich plasma derivates as a bridge from spontaneity to intervention. *Injury* **2015**, *46*, 428. [CrossRef]

72. Guillodo, Y.; Madouas, G.; Simon, T.; Le Dauphin, H.; Saraux, A. Platelet-rich plasma (PRP) treatment of sports-related severe acute hamstring injuries. *Muscles Ligaments Tendons J.* **2016**, *5*, 284–288. [CrossRef]

73. Grassi, A.; Napoli, F.; Romandini, I.; Samuelsson, K.; Zaffagnini, S.; Candrian, C.; Filardo, G. Is Platelet-Rich Plasma (PRP) Effective in the Treatment of Acute Muscle Injuries? A Systematic Review and Meta-Analysis. *Sports Med.* **2018**, *48*, 971–989. [CrossRef] [PubMed]

74. Rossi, L.A.; Molina Rómoli, A.R.; Bertona Altieri, B.A.; Burgos Flor, J.A.; Scordo, W.E.; Elizondo, C.M. Does platelet-rich plasma decrease time to return to sports in acute muscle tear? A randomized controlled trial. *Knee Surg. Sports Traumatol. Arthrosc.* **2017**, *25*, 3319–3325. [CrossRef] [PubMed]

75. Tonogai, I.; Hayashi, F.; Iwame, T.; Takasago, T.; Matsuura, T.; Sairyo, K. Platelet-rich plasma does not reduce skeletal muscle fibrosis after distraction osteogenesis. *J Exp Orthop.* **2018**, *5*, 26. [CrossRef] [PubMed]

76. Anitua, E.; de la Fuente, M.; Muruzabal, F.; Riestra, A.; Merayo-Lloves, J.; Orive, G. Plasma rich in growth factors (PRGF) eye drops stimulates scarless regeneration compared to autologous serum in the ocular surface stromal fibroblasts. *Exp. Eye Res.* **2015**, *135*, 118–126. [CrossRef] [PubMed]

77. Van der Bijl, I.; Vlig, M.; Middelkoop, E.; de Korte, D. Allogeneic platelet-rich plasma (**PRP**) is superior to platelets or plasma alone in stimulating fibroblast proliferation and migration, angiogenesis, and chemotaxis as relevant processes for wound healing. *Transfusion* **2019**, *59*, 3492–3500. [CrossRef]

78. Verhoekx, J.S.N.; Verjee, L.S.; Izadi, D.; Chan, J.K.K.; Nicolaidou, V.; Davidson, D.; Midwood, K.S.; Nanchahal, J. Isometric contraction of Dupuytren's myofibroblasts is inhibited by blocking intercellular junctions. *J. Investig. Dermatol.* **2013**, *133*, 2664–2671. [CrossRef]

79. Tarzemany, R.; Jiang, G.; Jiang, J.X.; Larjava, H.; Häkkinen, L. Connexin 43 Hemichannels Regulate the Expression of Wound Healing-Associated Genes in Human Gingival Fibroblasts. *Sci. Rep.* **2017**, *7*, 14157. [CrossRef]

80. Au, S.R.; Au, K.; Saggers, G.C.; Karne, N.; Ehrlich, H.P. Rat mast cells communicate with fibroblasts via gap junction intercellular communications. *J. Cell. Biochem.* **2007**, *100*, 1170–1177. [CrossRef]

81. Pistorio, A.L.; Ehrlich, H.P. Modulatory effects of connexin-43 expression on gap junction intercellular communications with mast cells and fibroblasts. *J. Cell. Biochem.* **2011**, *112*, 1441–1449. [CrossRef] [PubMed]

82. Foley, T.T.; Ehrlich, H.P. Through gap junction communications, co-cultured mast cells and fibroblasts generate fibroblast activities allied with hypertrophic scarring. *Plast. Reconstr. Surg.* **2013**, *131*, 1036–1044. [CrossRef] [PubMed]

83. Santos-Miranda, A.; Noureldin, M.; Bai, D. Effects of temperature on transjunctional voltage-dependent gating kinetics in Cx45 and Cx40 gap junction channels. *J. Mol. Cell. Cardiol.* **2019**, *127*, 185–193. [CrossRef]

84. Lastwika, K.J.; Dunn, C.A.; Solan, J.L.; Lampe, P.D. Phosphorylation of connexin 43 at MAPK, PKC or CK1 sites each distinctly alter the kinetics of epidermal wound repair. *J. Cell. Sci.* **2019**, *132*, jcs234633. [CrossRef]

85. Asazuma-Nakamura, Y.; Dai, P.; Harada, Y.; Jiang, Y.; Hamaoka, K.; Takamatsu, T. Cx43 contributes to TGF-beta signaling to regulate differentiation of cardiac fibroblasts into myofibroblasts. *Exp. Cell. Res.* **2009**, *315*, 1190–1199. [CrossRef] [PubMed]

86. Paw, M.; Borek, I.; Wnuk, D.; Ryszawy, D.; Piwowarczyk, K.; Kmiotek, K.; Wójcik-Pszczoła, K.A.; Pierzchalska, M.; Madeja, Z.; Sanak, M.; et al. Connexin43 Controls the Myofibroblastic Differentiation of Bronchial Fibroblasts from Patients with Asthma. *Am. J. Respir. Cell. Mol. Biol.* **2017**, *57*, 100–110. [CrossRef]

87. Coutinho, P.; Qiu, C.; Frank, S.; Tamber, K.; Becker, D. Dynamic changes in connexin expression correlate with key events in the wound healing process. *Cell. Biol. Int.* **2003**, *27*, 525–541. [CrossRef]

88. Kretz, M.; Euwens, C.; Hombach, S.; Eckardt, D.; Teubner, B.; Traub, O.; Willecke, K.; Ott, T. Altered connexin expression and wound healing in the epidermis of connexin-deficient mice. *J. Cell. Sci.* **2003**, *116*, 3443–3452. [CrossRef]

89. Qiu, C.; Coutinho, P.; Frank, S.; Franke, S.; Law, L.Y.; Martin, P.; Green, C.R.; Becker, D.L. Targeting connexin43 expression accelerates the rate of wound repair. *Curr. Biol.* **2003**, *13*, 1697–1703. [CrossRef]

90. Nakano, Y.; Oyamada, M.; Dai, P.; Nakagami, T.; Kinoshita, S.; Takamatsu, T. Connexin43 knockdown accelerates wound healing but inhibits mesenchymal transition after corneal endothelial injury in vivo. *Investig. Ophthalmol. Vis. Sci.* **2008**, *49*, 93–104. [CrossRef]

91. Montgomery, J.; Ghatnekar, G.S.; Grek, C.L.; Moyer, K.E.; Gourdie, R.G. Connexin 43-Based Therapeutics for Dermal Wound Healing. *Int. J. Mol. Sci.* **2018**, *19*, 1778. [CrossRef]

92. Cogliati, B.; Mennecier, G.; Willebrords, J.; Da Silva, T.C.; Maes, M.; Pereira, I.V.A.; Crespo-Yanguas, S.; Hernandez-Blazquez, F.J.; Dagli, M.L.Z.; Vinken, M. Connexins, Pannexins, and Their Channels in Fibroproliferative Diseases. *J. Membr. Biol.* **2016**, *249*, 199–213. [CrossRef] [PubMed]

93. Laird, D.W.; Lampe, P.D. Therapeutic strategies targeting connexins. *Nat. Rev. Drug. Discov.* **2018**, *17*, 905–921. [CrossRef] [PubMed]

94. Kameritsch, P.; Pogoda, K.; Pohl, U. Channel-independent influence of connexin 43 on cell migration. *Biochim. Biophys. Acta.* **2012**, *1818*, 1993–2001. [CrossRef] [PubMed]

95. Riteau, N.; Gasse, P.; Fauconnier, L.; Gombault, A.; Couegnat, M.; Fick, L.; Kanellopoulos, J.; Quesniaux, V.F.; Marchand-Adam, S.; Crestani, B.; et al. Extracellular ATP Is a Danger Signal Activating P2X7 Receptor in Lung Inflammation and Fibrosis. *Am. J. Respir. Crit. Care Med.* **2010**, *182*, 774–783. [CrossRef] [PubMed]

96. Lu, D.; Soleymani, S.; Madakshire, R.; Insel, P.A. ATP released from cardiac fibroblasts via connexin hemichannels activates profibrotic P2Y2 receptor. *FASEB* **2012**, *26*, 2580–2591. [CrossRef]

97. Ferrari, D.; Gambari, R.; Idzko, M.; Müller, T.; Albanesi, C.; Pastore, S.; La Manna, G.; Robson, S.C.; Cronstein, B. Purinergic signaling in scarring. *FASEB J.* **2016**, *30*, 3–12. [CrossRef]

98. Hills, C.; Price, G.W.; Wall, M.J.; Kaufmann, T.J.; Chi-Wai Tang, S.; Yiu, W.H.; Squires, P.E. Transforming Growth Factor Beta 1 Drives a Switch in Connexin Mediated Cell-to-Cell Communication in Tubular Cells of the Diabetic Kidney. *Cell. Physiol. Biochem.* **2018**, *45*, 2369–2388. [CrossRef]

99. Iyer, R.K.; Odedra, D.; Chiu, L.L.; Vunjak-Novakovic, G.; Radisic, M. Vascular endothelial growth factor secretion by nonmyocytes modulates Connexin-43 levels in cardiac organoids. *Tissue Eng. Part. A.* **2012**, *18*, 1771–1783. [CrossRef]

100. Wuestefeld, R.; Chen, J.; Meller, K.; Brand-Saberi, B.; Theiss, C. Impact of vegf on astrocytes: Analysis of gap junctional intercellular communication, proliferation, and motility. *Glia* **2012**, *60*, 936–947. [CrossRef]

101. Li, L.; Liu, H.; Xu, C.; Deng, M.; Song, M.; Yu, X.; Xu, S.; Zhao, X. VEGF promotes endothelial progenitor cell differentiation and vascular repair through connexin 43. *Stem. Cell. Res. Ther.* **2017**, *8*, 237. [CrossRef] [PubMed]

102. Boeldt, D.S.; Grummer, M.A.; Yi, F.; Magness, R.R.; Bird, I.M. Phosphorylation of Ser-279/282 and Tyr-265 positions on Cx43 as possible mediators of VEGF-165 inhibition of pregnancy-adapted Ca2+ burst function in ovine uterine artery endothelial cells. *Mol. Cell. Endocrinol.* **2015**, *412*, 73–84. [CrossRef] [PubMed]

103. Nimlamool, W.; Andrews, R.M.; Falk, M.M. Connexin43 phosphorylation by PKC and MAPK signals VEGF-mediated gap junction internalization. *Mol. Biol. Cell.* **2015**, *26*, 2755–2768. [CrossRef]

104. Solan, J.L.; Lampe, P.D. Spatio-temporal regulation of connexin43 phosphorylation and gap junction dynamics. *Biochim. Biophys. Acta Biomembr.* **2018**, *1860*, 83–90. [CrossRef] [PubMed]

105. Lin, D.; Boyle, D.L.; Takemoto, D.J. IGF-I-induced phosphorylation of connexin 43 by PKCgamma: Regulation of gap junctions in rabbit lens epithelial cells. *Investig. Ophthalmol. Vis. Sci.* **2003**, *44*, 1160–1168. [CrossRef] [PubMed]

106. Qiao, J.; An, N.; Ouyang, X. Quantification of growth factors in different platelet concentrates. *Platelets* **2017**, *28*, 774–778. [CrossRef]

107. Dong, Y.; Lakhia, R.; Thomas, S.S.; Dong, Y.; Wang, X.H.; Silva, K.A.; Zhang, L. Interactions between p-Akt and Smad3 in injured muscles initiate myogenesis or fibrogenesis. *Am. J. Physiol. Endocrinol. Metab.* **2013**, *305*, E367–E375. [CrossRef]

108. Andrade, D.; Oliveira, G.; Menezes, L.; Nascimento, A.L.; Carvalho, S.; Stumbo, A.C.; Thole, A.; Garcia-Souza, É.; Moura, A.; Carvalho, L.; et al. Insulin-like growth factor-1 short-period therapy improves cardiomyopathy stimulating cardiac progenitor cells survival in obese mice. *Nutr. Metab. Cardiovasc. Dis.* **2020**, *30*, 151–161. [CrossRef]

109. Sassoli, C.; Pierucci, F.; Zecchi-Orlandini, S.; Meacci, E. Sphingosine 1-Phosphate (S1P)/ S1P Receptor Signaling and Mechanotransduction: Implications for Intrinsic Tissue Repair/Regeneration. *Int. J. Mol. Sci.* **2019**, *20*, 5545. [CrossRef]

110. Lynch, M.D.; Watt, F.M. Fibroblast heterogeneity: Implications for human disease. *J. Clin. Investig.* **2018**, *128*, 26–35. [CrossRef]

111. Foote, A.G.; Wang, Z.; Kendziorski, C.; Thibeault, S.L. Tissue specific human fibroblast differential expression based on RNA sequencing analysis. *BMC Genomics* **2019**, *20*, 308. [CrossRef] [PubMed]

112. LeBleu, V.S.; Neilson, E.G. Origin and functional heterogeneity of fibroblasts. *FASEB J.* **2020**, *34*, 3519–3536. [CrossRef] [PubMed]

mTORC1 Mediates Lysine-Induced Satellite Cell Activation to Promote Skeletal Muscle Growth

Cheng-long Jin [1], Jin-ling Ye [2], Jinzeng Yang [3], Chun-qi Gao [1], Hui-chao Yan [1], Hai-chang Li [4] and Xiu-qi Wang [1,*]

[1] College of Animal Science, South China Agricultural University/Guangdong Provincial Key Laboratory of Animal Nutrition Control/National Engineering Research Center for Breeding Swine Industry, Guangzhou 510642, China; jinchenglong1992@163.com (C.-l.J.); cqgao@scau.edu.cn (C.-q.G.); yanhc@scau.edu.cn (H.-c.Y.)

[2] Institute of Animal Science, Guangdong Academy of Agricultural Sciences, Guangzhou 510642, China; YEJL2014@163.com

[3] Department of Human Nutrition, Food and Animal Sciences, University of Hawaii, Honolulu, HI 96822, USA; jinzeng@hawaii.edu

[4] Department of Surgery, Davis Heart and Lung Research Institute, The Ohio State University, Columbus, OH 43210, USA; Haichang.Li@osumc.edu

* Correspondence: xqwang@scau.edu.cn;

Abstract: As the first limiting amino acid, lysine (Lys) has been thought to promote muscle fiber hypertrophy by increasing protein synthesis. However, the functions of Lys seem far more complex than that. Despite the fact that satellite cells (SCs) play an important role in skeletal muscle growth, the communication between Lys and SCs remains unclear. In this study, we investigated whether SCs participate directly in Lys-induced skeletal muscle growth and whether the mammalian target of rapamycin complex 1 (mTORC1) pathway was activated both in vivo and in vitro to mediate SC functions in response to Lys supplementation. Subsequently, the skeletal muscle growth of piglets was controlled by dietary Lys supplementation. Isobaric tag for relative and absolute quantitation (iTRAQ) analysis showed activated SCs were required for longissimus dorsi muscle growth, and this effect was accompanied by mTORC1 pathway upregulation. Furthermore, SC proliferation was governed by medium Lys concentrations, and the mTORC1 pathway was significantly enhanced in vitro. After verifying that rapamycin inhibits the mTORC1 pathway and suppresses SC proliferation, we conclude that Lys is not only a molecular building block for protein synthesis but also a signal that activates SCs to manipulate muscle growth via the mTORC1 pathway.

Keywords: lysine; mTORC1; satellite cells; proliferation; skeletal muscle growth

1. Introduction

Lysine (Lys) is the first limiting essential amino acid for mammals consuming a predominantly cereal-based diet [1,2]. The important role of Lys in promoting skeletal muscle growth has already been demonstrated in animal husbandry, and this effect was attributed to increased protein synthesis [3,4]. Moreover, the functions of Lys in preventing human illnesses, such as osteoporosis and maldevelopment, have been intensively studied to protect human health [5,6]. In contrast, a low Lys diet has been used to treat glutaric aciduria type I and pyridoxine-dependent epilepsy [7,8], despite the fact that Lys deficiency causes severe body growth restriction and a reduction in body weight [9]. Furthermore, to study the mechanism of Lys in governing skeletal muscle growth, it has been reported that the mammalian target of rapamycin complex 1 (mTORC1) pathway is activated by Lys in the skeletal muscle of rats [10]. Additionally, Lys suppresses protein degradation in C2C12 myotubes via greater mTORC1 pathway phosphorylation [11]. However, protein synthesis is controlled by DNA in the nucleus, such that a higher number of cell nuclei in myofibers means greater protein synthesis efficiency [12].

As muscle stem cells are involved in skeletal muscle growth, satellite cells (SCs) are distributed in the basal lamina and sarcolemma of skeletal muscle fibers [13,14]. It has already been established that through proliferation [14], migration [15] and fusion into myotubes to form new nuclei, SCs contribute considerably to muscle fiber hypertrophy [16]. Moreover, in the study of SCs, the mTORC1 pathway is an invaluable index [17,18]. First, mTORC1 is critical for SC participation in skeletal muscle regeneration [19]. Another study showed that mTORC1 is also necessary for RNA-induced mitochondrial restoration in SC activation [17]. Furthermore, the addition of leucine (Leu) could promote proliferation in rat SCs via increasing mammalian target of rapamycin (mTOR) and ribosomal protein S6 kinase 1 (S6K1) phosphorylation [20]. Alway et al. found that a metabolite of Leu, β-hydroxy-β-methylbutyrate (HMB), promotes SC proliferation but does not activate the mTORC1 pathway [21]. Thus, investigating whether Lys could function as a signal regulatory factor that regulates SC proliferation through the mTORC1 pathway to promote skeletal muscle growth is an important endeavor.

In the current work, we aimed to expand our understanding of the role of Lys in governing skeletal muscle growth. Our research was designed to determine the specific skeletal muscle growth of piglets with dietary Lys supplementation in greater detail than a previous study [22]. Importantly, isobaric tag for relative and absolute quantitation (iTRAQ) analysis of the longissimus dorsi muscle displayed differentially expressed proteins related to SCs and the mTORC1 pathway, indicating the potential communication between Lys, the mTORC1 pathway and SCs in skeletal muscle growth. Then, we investigated the changes in proliferation and protein synthesis by accurately controlling Lys supplementation in medium to demonstrate that SC proliferation relies on mTORC1 pathway activation. Moreover, rapamycin was used to confirm the indispensable role of the mTORC1 pathway in the proliferation of SCs with Lys re-supplementation.

2. Materials and Methods

2.1. Ethics Statement

All animal procedures were performed in accordance with the Guidelines for the Care and Use of Laboratory Animals of South China Agricultural University (Guangzhou, China), and the experiments were approved by the Animal Ethics Committee (SCAU#0158Ethic Committee Approval Number) of South China Agricultural University (Guangzhou, China).

2.2. Animals and Sample Collection

The design for the feeding experiment is shown in Table S1. Briefly, a total of 30 Duroc × Landrace × Large White, male, weaned piglets with similar weights were divided randomly into 2 groups from days 0 to 14: the control group was fed a diet containing 1.31% Lys (n = 12), and the Lys deficiency group was fed a diet containing 0.83% Lys (n = 18). On day 15, six piglets closest to the average weight of each group were selected to determine skeletal muscle growth. Then, the remaining piglets in the Lys deficiency group were divided randomly into two groups from days 15 to 28: the Lys deficiency group was fed a diet containing 0.83% Lys (n = 6), and the Lys rescue group was fed a diet containing 1.31% Lys (n = 6). In addition, the remaining piglets in the control group were fed a diet containing 1.31% Lys between days 15 and 28 (n = 6). On day 29, all piglets were slaughtered, and the weight of their skeletal muscle was measured. Longissimus dorsi muscle samples were collected from all of the piglets at days 15 and 29, flash-frozen with liquid nitrogen and stored at − 80 °C.

2.3. Amino Acid Detection

To determine the content and concentration of amino acids in longissimus dorsi muscle, samples containing 20 mg protein were weighed and hydrolyzed with 6 mol/L hydrochloric acid (HCL) at 110 °C for 22 h. Then, the hydrolyzed liquid was transferred into a 50 mL volumetric flask with ultrapure water. Then, 1 mL of hydrolyzed liquid was dried by distillation and re-dissolved in 0.02 mol/L HCL. Finally, the amino acid composition was analyzed by an amino acid analyzer (Hitachi L-8900, Tokyo, Japan).

2.4. Protein Extraction

Tissue samples (n = 3) were excised and transferred into new tubes containing tissue lysis buffer (1% SDS, 8 mol/L urea) and 1 mmol/L phenylmethanesulfonyl fluoride (PMSF, Sigma-Aldrich, St. Louis, MO, USA). Then, the lysates were homogenized for 4 min using a TissueLyser (CK1000, Thmorgan, Beijing, China) and incubated on ice for 30 min. The lysates were centrifuged at 12,000× g and 4 °C for 15 min, and the supernatants were collected. The concentration of proteins was quantified using a micro-bicinchoninic acid assay (BCA) kit (Thermo-Fisher, Waltham, MA, USA) and separated on sodium dodecyl sulfate polyacrylamide gel electrophoresis (SDS-PAGE) gels.

2.5. iTRAQ Proteome Analysis

Proteins were treated with tris-(2-carboxyethyl)-phosphine (TECP, Sigma-Aldrich, St. Louis, MO, USA) and iodoacetamide and digested with trypsin. Then, the peptide mixture was labeled using the 8-plex iTRAQ reagent according to the manufacturer's instructions (Applied Biosystems, Foster City, CA, USA). Because there were eight samples, the peptides were divided into two parts for subsequent detection. For the first peptide group, the control group samples were labeled 115/116, the Lys deficiency group samples were labeled 117, the Lys rescue group samples were labeled 118/119, and the mixture (total of nine samples) was labeled 121. For the second peptide group, the control group samples were labeled 115, the Lys deficiency group samples were labeled 116/118, the Lys rescue group samples were labeled 119, and the mixture (total of nine samples) was labeled 121. Then, equal amounts of peptides from each peptide group were mixed together and vacuum dried.

Then, the peptides were separated by ultra-performance liquid chromatography (UPLC) with a Nano Aquity UPLC system (Waters, Milford, MA, USA) and analyzed in combination with a quadrupole-orbitrap mass spectrometer (Q-Exactive, Thermo-Fisher, Waltham, MA, USA) and an Easy-nLC 1200 (Thermo-Fisher, Waltham, MA, USA) for Nano LC-MS/MS analysis. Finally, the MS/MS data were searched using Protein Discoverer Software 2.1 against the Sus scrofa musculus database (UniProt, https://www.UniProt.org). The false discovery rate (FDR) applied to the control peptide level was defined as lower than 1%. For quantitative analysis, the 0.66 < fold change < 1.5 and p-value < 0.05 were the threshold values used to identify the differentially expressed proteins.

All identified proteins were annotated and classified by Gene Ontology (GO, http://www.geneontology.org), and the differentially expressed proteins were then analyzed by GOATOOLS 0.6.5 (https://pypi.org/project/goatools/) for the GO enrichment analysis. Data are available via ProteomeXchange with identifier PXD016396.

2.6. Immunohistochemical Analysis

First, the muscle samples were dehydrated with a 20% sucrose solution for 24 h and embedded in Tissue Tek to prepare the cryosections (5 μm, with at least six sections collected from each sample). Then, the tissue slides were incubated with Pax7 (MAB1675, R&D, Minneapolis, MN, USA) and Ki67 (NB500-170, Novus, Miami, FL, USA) at 4 °C overnight. After the slides were washed three times with phosphate-buffered saline (PBS), they were incubated with Alexa Fluor® 488 AffiniPure goat anti-mouse IgG (115-545-003, Jackson, West Grove, PA, USA) and Cy3-AffiniPure Goat anti-rabbit IgG (111-165-045, Jackson, West Grove, PA, USA) at room temperature for 90 min. Next, the slides were washed 3 times with PBS and incubated with 4′,6-diamidino-2-phenylindole (DAPI, Sigma-Aldrich, St. Louis, MO, USA) at room temperature for 5 min. Images were obtained using an immunofluorescence microscope (Ti2-U, Nikon, Tokyo, Japan TYPE, COMPANY, CITY, COUNTRY).

2.7. Western Blotting

Protein was extracted from the longissimus dorsi muscle or SCs with lysis buffer (RIPA, BioTeke, Beijing, China) and PMSF (Sigma-Aldrich, St. Louis, MO, USA). Next, the samples were centrifuged at 12,000× g and 4 °C for 15 min, and the protein concentration was determined using a micro BCA protein assay kit (Thermo-Fisher, Waltham, MA, USA). A total of 10 μg of protein was separated on 8–10% sodium dodecyl sulfate polyacrylamide gel electrophoresis (SDS-PAGE) gels and then transferred onto polyvinylidene fluoride membranes (PVDF, Millipore, Darmstadt, Germany). After blocking, the membranes were incubated with specific primary and second antibodies (Table S2). Immunoreactivity was detected using an electrochemiluminescence (ECL) Plus chemiluminescence detection kit (Millipore, Darmstadt, Germany) and a Fluor Chem M system (Protein Simple, Santa Clara, CA, USA). The band density was analyzed using ImageJ Analysis Software (https://imagej.nih.gov) after excluding the background density (n = 3). The results were confirmed by three independent experiments with three samples per treatment.

2.8. Isolation and Culture of SCs

The method used to isolate, purify and identify the SCs was performed as described previously with modification [23]. In this study, SCs were isolated from the longissimus dorsi muscle of 5-day-old Landrace piglets and cultured in Dulbecco's modified Eagle's Medium/Nutrient Mixture F-12 (DMEM/F-12, Thermo-fisher, Waltham, MA, USA) supplemented with 10% fetal bovine serum (FBS, Thermo-fisher, Waltham, MA, USA) at 37 °C and 5% CO_2. The medium was changed every 48 h.

2.9. Lys Depletion and Supplementation

After a 24 h period to allow adhesion, cells were starved for 6 h in FBS- and Lys-free DMEM/F12 medium. Then, the cells were cultured in 500 μmol/L Lys (control) and 0 μmol/L Lys (Lys deficiency) DMEM/F12 medium with 10% FBS for 24, 48 and 72 h to investigate cell proliferation. For proliferation rescue, due to the extreme decrease in proliferation after Lys deficiency for 48 h, we added sufficient Lys for another 72 h at this point. Lys concentrations in DMEM/F12, FBS and culture medium are displayed in Table S3.

2.10. Cell Proliferation Assay

For the 3-(4,5-dimethylthiazol-2-yl)-2, 5-diphenyltetrazolium bromide (MTT) assay, 20 μL 5 mg/mL MTT solution (Sigma-Aldrich, St. Louis, MO, USA) was added to each well and incubated for 4 h. Then, the plates were centrifuged at 1400× g for 15 min at 25 °C. A total of 150 μL dimethylsulfoxide (DMSO) working solution was added to each well after the supernatants were carefully discarded. The OD value of the product was evaluated using a microplate reader (Bio-Rad, Hercules, CA, USA) at a wavelength of 490 nm (n = 20). For the cell count assay [14,24], SCs were trypsinized and washed with PBS 3 times, and viable cells were counted using a hemocytometer under an automated cell counter (Count Star, Shanghai, China, n = 10).

2.11. Flow Cytometry

SCs were seeded at a density of 5×10^5 cells/well in 6-well culture plates (Corning, Corning, NY, USA) to detect the cell cycle distribution. The cultivation process was carried out as described above and according to a method described previously [25]. After harvesting at 24, 48 and 72 h, the cells were fixed in 70% ice-cold ethanol at −20 °C for cell cycle analysis. Before the samples were analyzed by flow cytometry using a Becton Dickinson Fluorescence Activating Cell Sorter Aria (BD Biosciences,

San Diego, CA, USA), the cells were centrifuged at 200× g and 4 °C for 5 min, re-suspended in 1 mL PBS, treated with 100 μL 200 mg/mL DNase-free RNase, incubated at 37 °C for 30 min, and treated with 100 μL 1 mg/mL propidium iodide (PI, Sigma-Aldrich, St. Louis, MO, USA) at room temperature (25 °C) for 10 min (n = 6).

2.12. Protein Synthesis

To measure protein synthesis, a nonradioactive technique called surface sensing of translation (SUnSET) was used [26,27]. In this study, 1 μg/mL puromycin (Millipore, Waltham, MA, USA) was added to all wells for an additional 30 min of culture, and puromycin was detected by western blotting with an anti-puromycin antibody (Millipore, Waltham, MA, USA, Table S2). The total protein concentration was determined by BCA (Thermo-fisher, Waltham, MA, USA).

2.13. Immunofluorescence Staining

SCs were cultured for 96 h for the proliferation rescue assay and differentiation rescue assay. First, SCs were fixed in 4% paraformaldehyde for 30 min and then permeabilized with 0.1% Triton-X-100 for 10 min. After blocking with 1% bull serum albumin (BSA) and 10% goat serum for 30 min, the SCs were stained with primary antibodies for 90 min and then probed with goat anti-rabbit IgG (Table S2). In addition, the nuclei were labeled with 4',6-diamidino-2-phenylindole (DAPI, Sigma-Aldrich, St. Louis, MO, USA) for 5 min at room temperature. Images were obtained using immunofluorescence microscopy.

2.14. Rapamycin Inhibition

After Lys deficiency for 48 h, Lys rescue medium was added alone or combined with 20 or 50 nmol/L (nM) rapamycin for another 48 h. After a total of 96 h, cell viability was measured by MTT assay, and cell proliferation was measured by cell count assay. In addition, cell samples were collected to detect protein synthesis and the mTORC1 pathway by western blotting.

2.15. Statistical Analysis

The data were analyzed using Statistical Analysis System software (SAS, Version 9.2; SAS Institute, Cary, NC, USA). For control group and Lys deficiency group comparisons, the results were analyzed by t-test. For control group, Lys deficiency group and Lys rescue group comparisons, the mean data were assessed for significance using Tukey's test. The data are expressed as the mean ± S.E.M. Differences between treatments were considered statistically significant when $p < 0.05$ and extremely significant when $p < 0.01$.

3. Results

3.1. Skeletal Muscle Growth in Piglets Relies on Dietary Lys Supplementation

To determine the effects of dietary Lys supplementation on the skeletal muscle growth of weaned piglets, we developed the experimental design shown in Supplemental Table 1. After the piglets (initial body weight: control = 8.42 ± 0.11 kg versus Lys deficiency = 8.42 ± 0.08 kg) were fed the Lys-restricted diet for 14 d, we found that the growth of the piglets (final body weight: control = 11.91 ± 0.18 kg versus Lys deficiency = 11.33 ± 0.18 kg) was significantly suppressed (Table S4). In detail, compared with those of the control group, the relative weights of the longissimus dorsi muscle, extensor carpi radialis muscle, semimembranosus muscle, total forequarters muscle and total hindquarters muscle were significantly decreased by dietary Lys deficiency for 14 d (Table S4).

After dietary Lys deficiency for 14 d, the piglets received a diet we supplemented to match the level in the control diet for another 14 d. Obviously, the final weight of the piglets in the Lys rescue group was significantly increased compared with that of the piglets in the Lys deficiency group (Table 1). Moreover, compared with those after Lys deficiency for 28 d, the relative weights of the longissimus dorsi muscle, lateral head of triceps of brachii muscle, extensor carpi radialis muscle, biceps femoris muscle, semimembranosus muscle, semitendinosus muscle, cranial tibial muscle, soleus muscle, lateral head of gastrocnemius muscle and total hindquarters muscle were all increased in the Lys rescue group, which was subjected to dietary Lys deficiency for 14 d and re-supplemented for another 14 d (Table 1). Collectively, these findings suggest that skeletal muscle growth in piglets relies on dietary Lys supplementation.

Table 1. Effect of dietary Lys re-supplementation on the skeletal muscle growth of weaned piglets on 28 d (n = 5, %) [1].

Item	Control	Lys Deficiency	Lys Rescue	p-Value
Initial Weight (kg)	12.02 ± 0.29	11.32 ± 0.44	11.34 ± 0.35	0.336
Final Weight (kg)	17.95 ± 0.49 [a]	15.99 ± 0.30 [b]	17.44 ± 0.46 [a]	0.018
Longissimus Dorsi Muscle	2.00 ± 0.06 [ab]	1.86 ± 0.07 [b]	2.19 ± 0.06 [a]	0.018
Psoas Major Muscle	0.34 ± 0.01 [a]	0.28 ± 0.01 [b]	0.30 ± 0.01 [b]	0.014
Forequarters muscles				
Infraspinatus Muscle	0.24 ± 0.02	0.22 ± 0.01	0.21 ± 0.01	0.221
Supraspinatus Muscle	0.41 ± 0.02	0.40 ± 0.01	0.42 ± 0.02	0.538
Subclavius Muscle	0.23 ± 0.02	0.25 ± 0.01	0.22 ± 0.01	0.227
Latissimus Dorsi Muscle	0.26 ± 0.03	0.26 ± 0.04	0.27 ± 0.03	0.925
Long Head of Triceps of Brachii Muscle	0.63 ± 0.02	0.63 ± 0.01	0.67 ± 0.02	0.201
Lateral Head of Triceps of Brachii Muscle	0.17 ± 0.01 [a]	0.14 ± 0.004 [b]	0.18 ± 0.01 [a]	0.003
Extensor Carpi Radialis Muscle	0.13 ± 0.003 [a]	0.12 ± 0.002 [b]	0.13 ± 0.003 [a]	0.011
Extensor Muscle of Second- and Third-Digits	0.02 ± 0.001	0.02 ± 0.002	0.02 ± 0.002	0.684
Lateral Digital Extensor Muscle	0.02 ± 0.001	0.02 ± 0.001	0.02 ± 0.002	0.441
Total Forequarters Muscles	2.15 ± 0.07	2.02 ± 0.03	2.15 ± 0.03	0.111
Hindquarters muscles				
Middle Gluteus Medius Muscle	0.54 ± 0.02	0.48 ± 0.02	0.55 ± 0.03	0.102
Superficial Gluteal Muscle	0.17 ± 0.01	0.14 ± 0.01	0.15 ± 0.02	0.457
Biceps Femoris Muscle	1.15 ± 0.01 [a]	1.04 ± 0.04 [b]	1.21 ± 0.02 [a]	0.008
Semimembranosus Muscle	1.36 ± 0.06 [ab]	1.23 ± 0.05 [b]	1.46 ± 0.03 [a]	0.013
Semitendinosus Muscle	0.39 ± 0.02 [ab]	0.36 ± 0.01 [b]	0.41 ± 0.01 [a]	0.043
Tensor fascia Lata Muscle	0.18 ± 0.02	0.17 ± 0.01	0.20 ± 0.01	0.313
Cranial Tibial Muscle	0.04 ± 0.003 [a]	0.03 ± 0.001 [b]	0.04 ± 0.002 [a]	0.045
Long Peroneal Muscle	0.04 ± 0.003 [a]	0.03 ± 0.001 [b]	0.03 ± 0.002 [b]	0.035
Peroneus Tertius Muscle	0.08 ± 0.003	0.08 ± 0.002	0.08 ± 0.002	0.191
Gemelli Muscle	0.27 ± 0.01 [a]	0.23 ± 0.01 [b]	0.25 ± 0.01 [ab]	0.018
Soleus Muscle	0.23 ± 0.005 [a]	0.19 ± 0.01 [b]	0.23 ± 0.01 [a]	0.020
Lateral Head of Gastrocnemius Muscle	0.37 ± 0.005 [a]	0.31 ± 0.01 [b]	0.36 ± 0.02 [a]	0.027
Adductor Muscle	0.18 ± 0.02	0.19 ± 0.01	0.21 ± 0.01	0.301
Total Hindquarters Muscles	4.98 ± 0.12 [a]	4.49 ± 0.12 [b]	5.17 ± 0.11 [a]	0.004

[1] Values without the same small letters within the same line indicate a significant difference ($p < 0.05$).

3.2. Lys-induced Skeletal Muscle Growth in Relation to SC Activation Level

In addition to the great change in longissimus dorsi muscle mass with dietary Lys supplementation (Tables S1 and S4), we also found that the Lys concentration in the longissimus dorsi muscle was significantly reduced by dietary Lys deficiency for 14 d (Table S5), whereas it could be rescued by dietary Lys re-supplementation for an additional 14 d (Table 2). Furthermore, the concentrations of threonine (Thr), serine (Ser), glutamate (Glu) and arginine (Arg) showed the same changes as Lys (Tables S2 and S5).

Considering these findings, we collected muscle samples for iTRAQ analysis to learn more about the role of Lys in governing skeletal muscle growth (Figure 1). After GO enrichment analysis, we found that proteins related to the transition between slow and fast fibers, filamin binding, mitogen-activated protein kinase binding, cytoskeletal protein binding, actin cytoskeleton, microtubule binding, cytoskeleton organization, tubulin binding and muscle myosin complexes were enriched in the Lys deficiency versus control downregulated proteins (Figure 1A), indicating that the muscle structure was changed.

Table 2. Effect of dietary Lys re-supplementation on the concentrations of amino acids in the longissimus dorsi muscle on day 28 (freeze-dried basis, %) [1].

Item	Control	Lys Deficiency	Lys Rescue	p-Value
Aspartate	0.11 ± 0.003 [ab]	0.10 ± 0.006 [b]	0.12 ± 0.003 [a]	0.038
Threonine	0.06 ± 0.003 [a]	0.05 ± 0.003 [b]	0.06 ± 0.002 [a]	0.015
Serine	0.05 ± 0.000 [a]	0.04 ± 0.003 [b]	0.05 ± 0.002 [a]	0.002
Glutamate	0.21 ± 0.003 [a]	0.18 ± 0.012 [b]	0.21 ± 0.006 [a]	0.024
Glycine	0.07 ± 0.003	0.06 ± 0.000	0.07 ± 0.006	0.423
Alanine	0.07 ± 0.003	0.07 ± 0.006	0.08 ± 0.003	0.671
Valine	0.06 ± 0.003 [ab]	0.06 ± 0.003 [b]	0.07 ± 0.002 [a]	0.017
Isoleucine	0.07 ± 0.003 [ab]	0.06 ± 0.003 [b]	0.07 ± 0.002 [a]	0.025
Leucine	0.12 ± 0.003 [ab]	0.11 ± 0.009 [b]	0.13 ± 0.004 [a]	0.059
Tyrosine	0.05 ± 0.000	0.05 ± 0.003	0.05 ± 0.003	0.354
Phenylalanine	0.07 ± 0.000 [ab]	0.06 ± 0.006 [b]	0.07 ± 0.003 [a]	0.103
Lysine	0.11 ± 0.003 [a]	0.09 ± 0.006 [b]	0.11 ± 0.003 [a]	0.006
Histidine	0.05 ± 0.003	0.04 ± 0.003	0.05 ± 0.003	0.547
Arginine	0.09 ± 0.000 [a]	0.08 ± 0.006 [b]	0.10 ± 0.002 [a]	0.007

[1] Values without the same small letters within the same line indicate a significant difference ($p < 0.05$).

In addition, in the Lys deficiency versus control upregulated proteins, the enrichment of lipase inhibitor activity, negative regulation of homotypic cell-cell adhesion, negative regulation of cell activation, response to nutrients and negative regulation of wound healing were observed (Figure 1B), and these results suggested that the functions of the muscle cells were disturbed.

Furthermore, proteins related to protein kinase C inhibitor activity, protein Ser/Thr kinase inhibitor activity and cellular response to amino acid starvation were enriched in the Lys rescue versus control downregulated proteins (Figure 1C). Thus, the mTORC1 pathway may play a crucial role in Lys-controlled skeletal muscle growth.

More importantly, the results for the Lys rescue versus control upregulated proteins showed that the proteins related to the negative regulation of fat cell differentiation, regulation of fibroblast proliferation, regulation of lens fiber cell differentiation, positive regulation of cell proliferation, sarcolemma, basal plasma membrane, basolateral plasma membrane and cell-cell adhesion were enriched (Figure 1D). These data suggest that SCs may be activated.

Moreover, the results for the Lys rescue versus Lys deficiency downregulated proteins showed that the positive regulation of fibril organization, regulation of fibril organization and positive regulation of gap junction assembly were enriched (Figure 1E). The results for the Lys rescue versus Lys deficiency upregulated proteins showed that the muscle system process, negative regulation of fat cell differentiation, muscle hypertrophy, positive regulation of myoblast differentiation, regulation of myoblast differentiation, regulation of fibroblast proliferation, regulation of cell differentiation, positive regulation of muscle cell differentiation, regulation of muscle cell differentiation and regulation of developmental process were enriched (Figure 1F). In summary, these results indicate that skeletal muscle growth regulation by dietary Lys supplementation is possibly connected with the mTORC1 pathway and SCs.

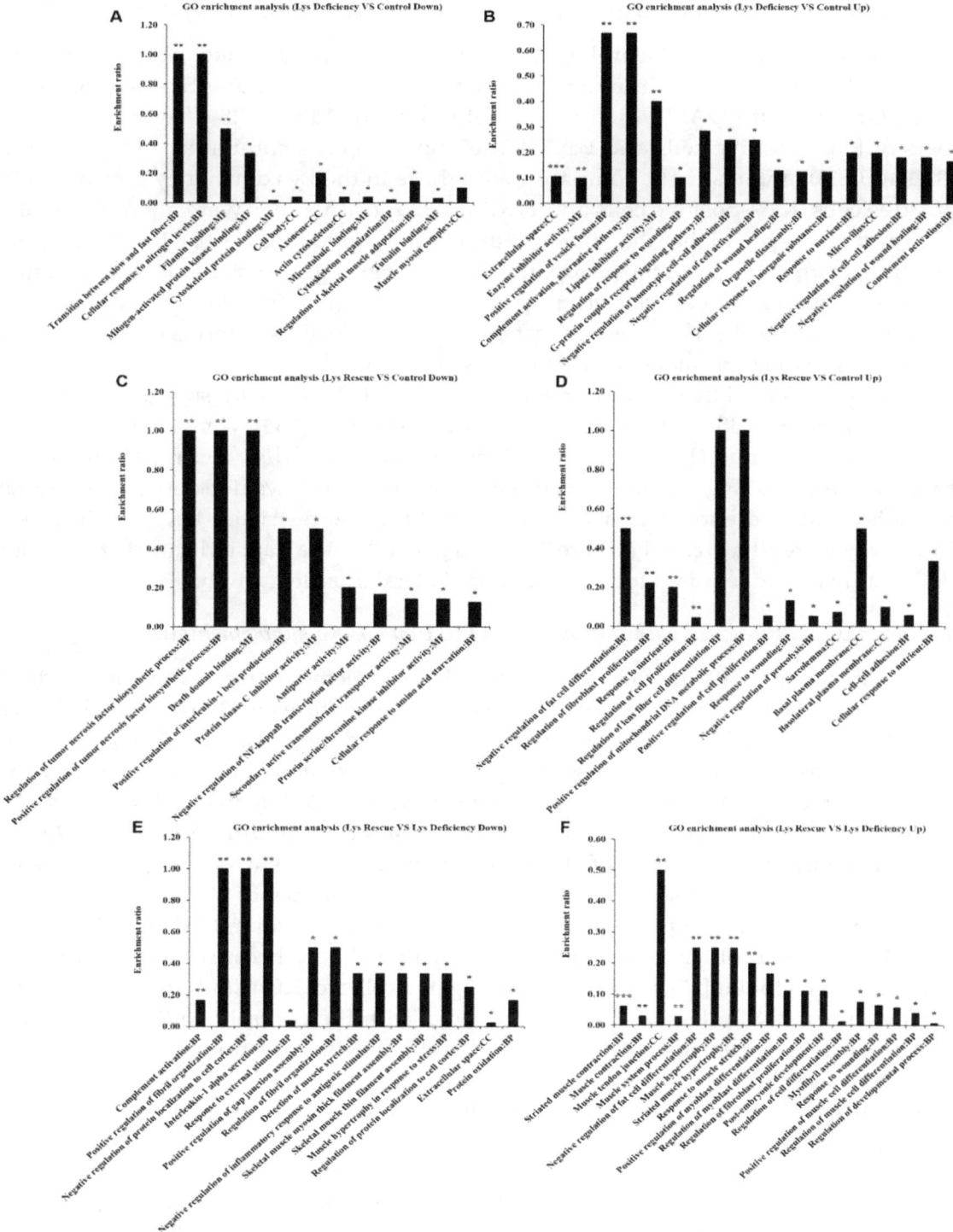

Figure 1. GO enrichment analysis of differentially expressed proteins in the longissimus dorsi muscle on day 28 according to iTRAQ analysis. (**A**) GO enrichment analysis results (Lys deficiency versus control) for downregulated proteins. (**B**) GO enrichment analysis results (Lys deficiency versus control) for upregulated proteins. (**C**) GO enrichment analysis results (Lys rescue versus control) for downregulated proteins. (**D**) GO enrichment analysis results (Lys rescue versus control) for upregulated proteins. (**E**) GO enrichment analysis results (Lys rescue versus Lys deficiency) for downregulated proteins. (**F**) GO enrichment analysis results (Lys rescue versus Lys deficiency) for upregulated proteins. The x-axis represents the different GO terms, and the y-axis represents the enrichment ratio (the ratio between the protein number enriched in the GO term and the protein number annotated to the GO term; the greater the ratio was, the greater the enrichment found was), * $p < 0.05$, ** $p < 0.01$, *** $p < 0.001$.

3.3. SCs and mTORC1 Activity Are Enhanced in Lys-induced Skeletal Muscle Growth

The specific marker Pax7 and the proliferation marker Ki67 were detected in SCs in the longissimus dorsi muscle on days 14 and 28 by immunohistochemical analysis (Figures S1A and S2A). Based on the total cells (stained with DAPI), dietary Lys deficiency for 14 d or 28 d significantly decreased the numbers of Pax7-positive cells and Pax7 + Ki67-positive cells compared with the control cells (Figures S1B and S2B). Interestingly, compared with those in the Lys deficiency group, the numbers of Pax7-positive cells, Ki67-positive cells and Pax7 + Ki67-positive cells were all increased in the Lys rescue group and were even higher than those in the control group (Figure 2B). In addition, compared with the control group and Lys rescue group, the Lys deficiency group had a decreased ratio of Pax7 + Ki67-positive cells to Pax7-positive cells, regardless of deficiency for 14 d or 28 d (Figures 1C and 2C). Taken together, these observations suggest that the status of SCs in terms of proliferation in the longissimus dorsi muscle is regulated by dietary Lys supplementation.

In addition, we observed that the key proteins in the mTORC1 pathway, such as p-mTOR (Ser2448), p-S6K1 (Thr389), p-S6 (Ser235), p-4EBP1 (Thr470) and eIF4E ($p = 0.083$), were all inhibited by dietary Lys deficiency for 14 d (Figure 1D,E), and this reduction was observed for samples from the group fed Lys-deficient diets for 28 d (Figure 2D,E). Fortunately, when dietary Lys deficiency was re-established to the control level at 14 d and sustained for another 14 d, the restricted key protein levels of the mTORC1 pathway were all increased (Figure 2D,E). In general, these data indicate that SCs, along with the mTORC1 pathway, are required for Lys-induced skeletal muscle growth.

3.4. Cell Proliferation Was Rescued with Increased mTORC1 by Lys Re-supplementation.

To gain further insight into the role of Lys in SCs, Lys supplementation treatment was designed as shown in Figure 3A. In addition, the Lys concentrations in cell culture are shown in Table S3. The MTT assay results showed that cell viability was significantly reduced under Lys deficiency for 48 h (Figures S2A and S3B), whereas cell viability was rescued by Lys re-supplementation for 48 h compared with Lys deficiency for 96 h (Figure 3B). The number of cells detected by an automated cell counter showed that SC proliferation was significantly decreased under Lys restriction conditions for 24 to 120 h (Figures S2B and S3C). In contrast, the number of SCs was increased after Lys was re-supplemented for 24 h after Lys deficiency (Figure 3C). However, cell viability and the number of SCs continued to increase at a slow rate in the deficiency group. This phenomenon might be explained by the existence of Lys in FBS (Figure S3). Because proliferation is determined by mitosis and because cell cycle distribution is a typically evaluated endpoint [25], we further investigated cell cycle distribution using flow cytometry after Lys deficiency for 48 h (Figure 2C–F). Compared with the control conditions, Lys deficiency resulted in an increased percentage of G1 cells at 48 h and 72 h, while the number of cells in the S phase was decreased (Figure 2E,F).

Moreover, because Lys plays an important role in protein synthesis, the SUnSET assay [26,27] was used to measure changes in protein synthesis in SCs. After Lys deficiency for 48 h, SCs evaluated by puromycin analysis showed an obvious decrease in protein synthesis (Figure S4A). However, protein synthesis was obviously increased after Lys was sufficiently supplemented for another 48 h (Figure 3D). Coomassie blue staining was used to verify equal protein loading (Figures 3E and 4B) [27]. Furthermore, a BCA assay was used to confirm the protein synthesis rate [28], and the results showed that total protein lysis in SCs cultured in Lys-deficient medium was extremely restricted at 48 h (Figure S4C) and was then enhanced after 48 h of Lys supplementation (Figure 3F).

Importantly, to investigate whether Lys-stimulated cell proliferation and protein synthesis were mediated by the mTORC1 pathway, the related proteins were analyzed by western blotting (Figures S4D,E and S3G,H). Compared with the levels in the control group, the levels of phosphorylated mTOR (Ser2448) and its downstream targets, phosphorylated S6K1 (Thr389), phosphorylated ribosomal protein S6 (S6, Ser235) and phosphorylated 4EBP1 (Thr70), and the levels of eukaryotic translation initiation factor 4E (eIF4E) were significantly decreased in the Lys deficiency group at 48 h and 96 h (Supplemental Figures 4E and 3H). However, compared with those under Lys deficiency for

96 h, the phosphorylated protein levels of mTOR and its downstream targets, such as 4EBP1 and S6K1, were restored by Lys supplementation for 48 h after Lys deficiency for 48 h (Figure 3H). Moreover, immunofluorescence staining further demonstrated that p-mTOR (Ser2448) expression was also increased after Lys supplementation (Figure S5). These data indicate that Lys-dependent SC proliferation and protein synthesis are related to mTORC1 pathways.

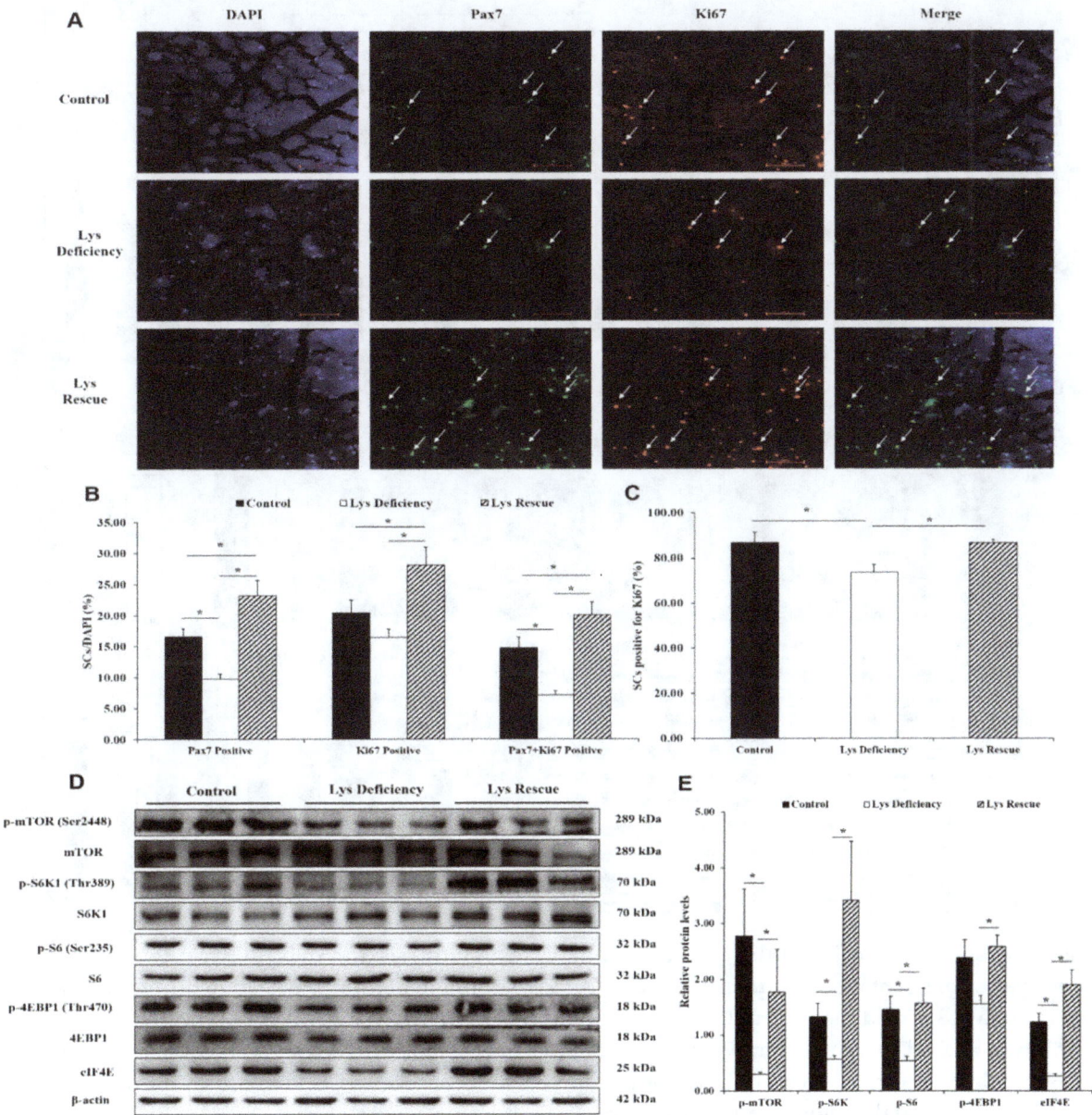

Figure 2. Activation of SCs and protein level of the mTORC1 pathway in the longissimus dorsi muscle on day 28. (**A**) Ki67 (red) and Pax7 (green) staining represents activated SCs during the proliferation period. Bar: 200×. (**B**) Percentage of cells positively stained for Ki67 (red), Pax7 (green) and Ki67 (red) + Pax7 (green) of the total cells (blue, DAPI). (**C**) Percentage of SCs positively stained for Ki67 (red) + Pax7 (green) to Pax7 (green). (**D**) Representative images of key proteins in the mTORC1 pathway detected by western blotting. (**E**) The values represent the ratio of the protein levels of p-mTOR (Ser2448), p-S6K1 (Thr389), p-S6 (Ser235) and p-4EBP1 (Thr470) to the total protein levels and the protein level of eIF4E to that of β-actin, n = 3. The results are shown as the means ± S.E.M. of three independent preparations. Statistical significance was assessed by ANOVA with Tukey's test, $* p < 0.05$.

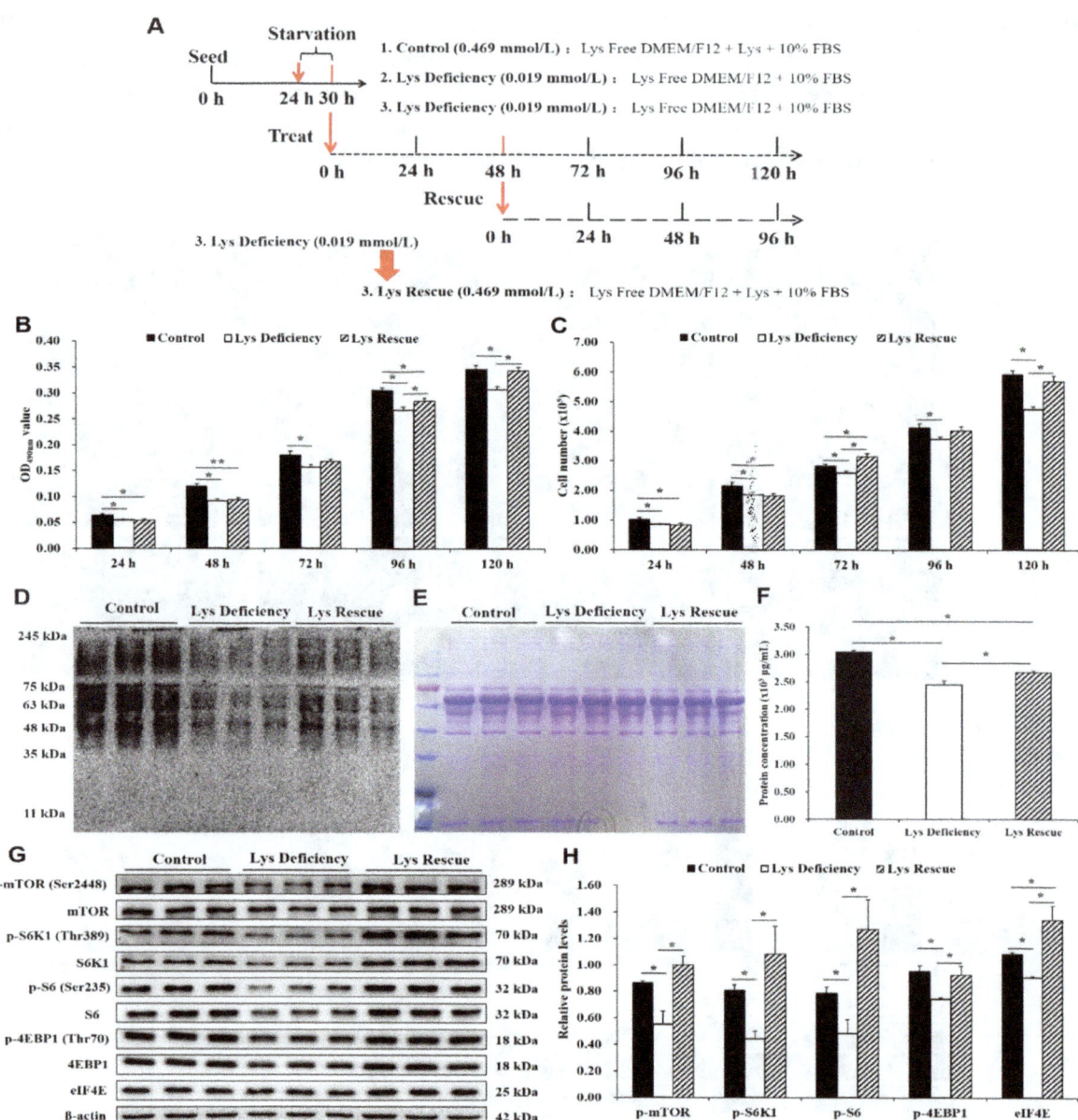

Figure 3. Changes in cell viability, proliferation, protein synthesis and mTORC1 pathway activation after Lys supplementation to sufficient levels. (**A**) Lys supplementation was changed from deficient to sufficient at 48 h, and the cells cultured for another 72 h. (**B**) MTT assays were used to measure cell viability, n = 20. (**C**) Cell proliferation was measured by cell counting assays, n = 10. (**D**) Representative image of the western blotting analyses for puromycin at 96 h, n = 3. (**E**) Coomassie blue staining was used to verify equal protein loading for puromycin measurements at 96 h, n = 3. (**F**) Total protein quantitation using bicinchoninic acid assays at 96 h, n = 3. (**G**) mTORC1 pathway-related proteins were measured by western blotting after Lys supplementation from deficiency for another 48 h (total 96 h). (**H**) The values represent the ratio of the phosphorylated protein levels to the total protein or β-actin level, n = 3. The bars are the means ± S.E.M. from the representative results of three independent experiments. Statistical significance was assessed by ANOVA and Tukey's test, * $p < 0.05$, ** $p < 0.01$.

3.5. Lys Rescue of SC Proliferation and mTORC1 Pathway Activation Were Inhibited by Rapamycin

To validate that mTORC1 pathway activity was crucial for Lys-regulated SC functions, SCs were treated with rapamycin under Lys rescue conditions for 48 h. As shown in Figure 4A, we found that the rescued cell viability by Lys re-supplementation was inhibited by the simultaneous addition of rapamycin and reduced to the Lys deficiency level. Moreover, Lys re-supplementation with rapamycin suppressed SC proliferation, and 50 nM rapamycin showed greater inhibition than 20 nM (Figure 4B). Furthermore, the SUnSET assay showed that 20 and 50 nM rapamycin restricted protein synthesis, which was rescued by Lys re-supplementation (Figure 4C). Protein amounts were also verified by Coomassie blue staining, and the results showed equal sample loading (Figure 4D). Apart from that, compared with the control group, all four other groups showed reductions in total protein concentrations (Figure 4E). Importantly, compared with Lys deficiency, Lys re-supplementation increased the total protein concentrations, whereas the increased protein concentrations were decreased by 20 ($p = 0.055$) and 50 nM ($p < 0.05$) rapamycin supplementation (Figure 4E). In addition, compared with control and Lys rescue conditions, Lys re-supplemented with rapamycin significantly decreased the protein levels of phosphorylated mTOR (Ser2448), phosphorylated S6K1 (Thr389), phosphorylated S6 (Ser235) and eIF4E (Figure 4F, G). Although there was no significant difference, the protein level of phosphorylated 4EBP1 (Thr70) was also decreased by 33.18% and 35.17% in the 20 and 50 nM rapamycin groups, respectively, compared to the Lys rescue group. Collectively, these results indicate that Lys-regulated SC functions are mediated by the mTORC1 pathway.

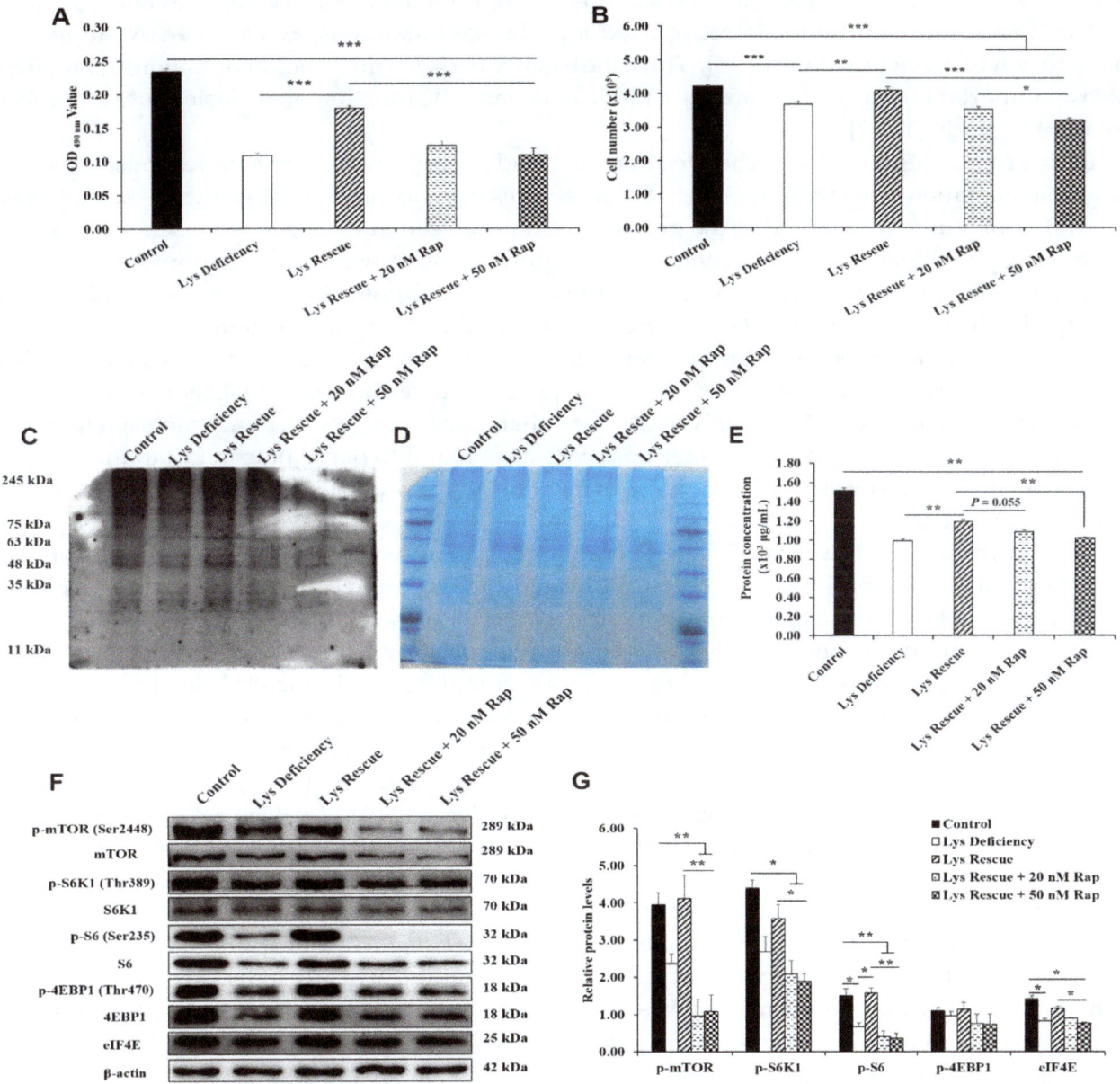

Figure 4. The increased cell viability, proliferation and protein synthesis induced by Lys rescue were inhibited by rapamycin, along with mTORC1 pathway downregulation. After Lys deficiency for

48 h, Lys was added to the medium alone or in combination with 20 or 50 nM rapamycin for another 48 h. (**A**) Cell viability was measured by MTT assays at 96 h, n = 20. (**B**) Cell counting assays were used to measure cell proliferation at 96 h, n = 10. (**C**) SUnSET measurements of protein synthesis were performed by incubating SCs in medium containing puromycin at 96 h. A representative image from the western blotting analyses for puromycin is shown, n = 3. (**D**) Coomassie blue staining was used to verify equal protein loading for puromycin measurements at 96 h, n = 3. (**E**) Total protein quantitation using bicinchoninic acid assays at 96 h is shown, n = 3. (**F**) Western blotting was used to detect the key proteins in the mTORC1 pathway at 96 h. (**G**) The values represent the ratio of the phosphorylated protein levels to the total protein or β-actin level, n = 3. The bars are the means ± S.E.M. from the representative results of three independent experiments. Statistical significance was assessed by ANOVA and Tukey's test, * $p < 0.05$, ** $p < 0.01$. *** $p < 0.001$.

4. Discussion

Lys is well known to be one of the most important essential amino acids for body growth [1,3,10,22,29]. However, the mechanisms through which Lys governs muscle mass are still debated. In addition, traditionally recognized muscle mass maintenance has been expanded from protein turnover to cell turnover [12,16]. Thus, the balance between myonuclear accretion and reduction is also an important factor in determining muscle mass, and the function of SC fusion into myotubes is important to study [16,30].

Early studies suggested that changes in whole-body weight were the main responses to dietary Lys supplementation or restriction [3,22,31]. Few studies have focused specifically on skeletal muscle growth. In our study, we found that the growth of almost all separated skeletal muscle was restricted during dietary Lys deficiency, while compensatory growth was shown after Lys supplementation was changed from deficient to sufficient [3,32]. In addition, some weights of specific skeletal muscles were unchanged, which could be caused by differences in myofiber type composition.

In previous studies, skeletal muscle mass accumulation was attributed to the relative efficiency between muscle protein synthesis and degradation [3,4,33]. Nevertheless, our GO enrichment analysis results obtained from the iTRAQ analysis showed that there were great changes in skeletal muscle structure and muscle cell function. Furthermore, SCs were found to participate in Lys-induced skeletal muscle growth. This is consistent with what was mentioned in a previous study, which did not provide compelling evidence [34].

To confirm the implications of the GO enrichment analysis for the longissimus dorsi muscle, we found that the SC proliferation ratios (indicated by Pax7 and Ki67 [35–37]) were accurately controlled by dietary Lys supplementation. Consistent with the compensatory growth of skeletal muscle, proliferation also showed the same tendency, especially Pax7 + Ki67-positive SCs. Taking these results together, we believe that SC turnover is required for Lys-induced skeletal muscle growth.

In the case of cell turnover, proliferation is the typical process by which cell numbers are increased by mitosis [14,24]. In this study, the suppressed Lys supply led to reduced cell numbers via changed cell cycle distribution such that there was an increased percentage of G1 phase cells and a decreased percentage of S phase cells. Similarly, a reduction in SC proliferation has also been detected in methionine (Met)- and cysteine (Cys)-restricted cell culture medium [38]. Furthermore, protein synthesis was suppressed directly by Lys deficiency and may thus ultimately cause muscle mass loss [31,32].

In addition to what we found under Lys deficiency conditions, the decrease in cell proliferation was suppressed by changing Lys supplementation from deficiency to sufficiency. These effects may be attributed to the function of Lys as an activator of cell mitotic activity [34]. Furthermore, protein synthesis was rescued by supplementing Lys to Lys-deficient cells. Despite the rescue growth effects of Lys supplementation found in our research, glycine seemed to suppress protein degradation weakly in cells in Lys-deficient medium [11]. These results could explain why Lys seems to play some special functions in life maintenance that have not been previously illustrated, that is, Lys is not used for only protein synthesis [29].

To obtain further insight from our findings, the mTORC1 pathway was measured to investigate the regulatory mechanisms of the Lys relationship with SCs and skeletal muscle growth. Notably, studies have shown that the mTORC1 pathway can be activated by energy, growth factors or nutrients, especially amino acids [38,39]. However, the function of Lys is not as defined as it is for Leu or Arg, as diets supplemented with Leu [40] or Arg [41] promote muscle growth and increase mTORC1 pathway activation. In fact, there has been little research on Lys interactions with mTORC1 in promoting muscle growth. In contrast, the key protein levels in the mTORC1 pathway were not altered after oral Lys administration in rats [33]. More importantly, previous studies showed that the mTORC1 pathway was activated by Lys to suppress protein degradation in vivo and in vitro [10,11]. In the present study, we found that the mTORC1 pathway was inhibited by reducing dietary Lys, and SC proliferation was likewise inhibited in Lys-deficient medium. Furthermore, the related proteins in the mTORC1 pathway were reactivated with complete Lys supplementation. In addition, the indispensable role of the mTORC1 pathway in Lys-governed SC function was verified by rapamycin [20]. We found that the inhibited proliferation and protein synthesis in the Lys deficiency group could be rescued by Lys re-supplementation, whereas these increases were suppressed by the simultaneous addition of rapamycin. Similar to our study, previous studies demonstrated that mTORC1 plays a crucial role in SC function [14,17–19]. Therefore, the mTORC1 pathway is necessary for Lys-induced SC activation in vivo and in vitro. However, the molecular mechanisms, such as extracellular Lys sensing in SCs and intracellular mTORC1 activation, need to be further studied.

5. Conclusions

In conclusion (Figure 5), our findings demonstrate that Lys supplementation exerts compensatory growth effects and that the functions of Lys in muscle mass accumulation are mediated by SCs and the mTORC1 pathway. Thus, Lys is not only a molecular building block for protein synthesis but also a signal that activates SCs to regulate muscle growth via the mTORC1 signaling pathway. These findings can provide us with a new target and therapeutic strategy for skeletal muscle regeneration and disease.

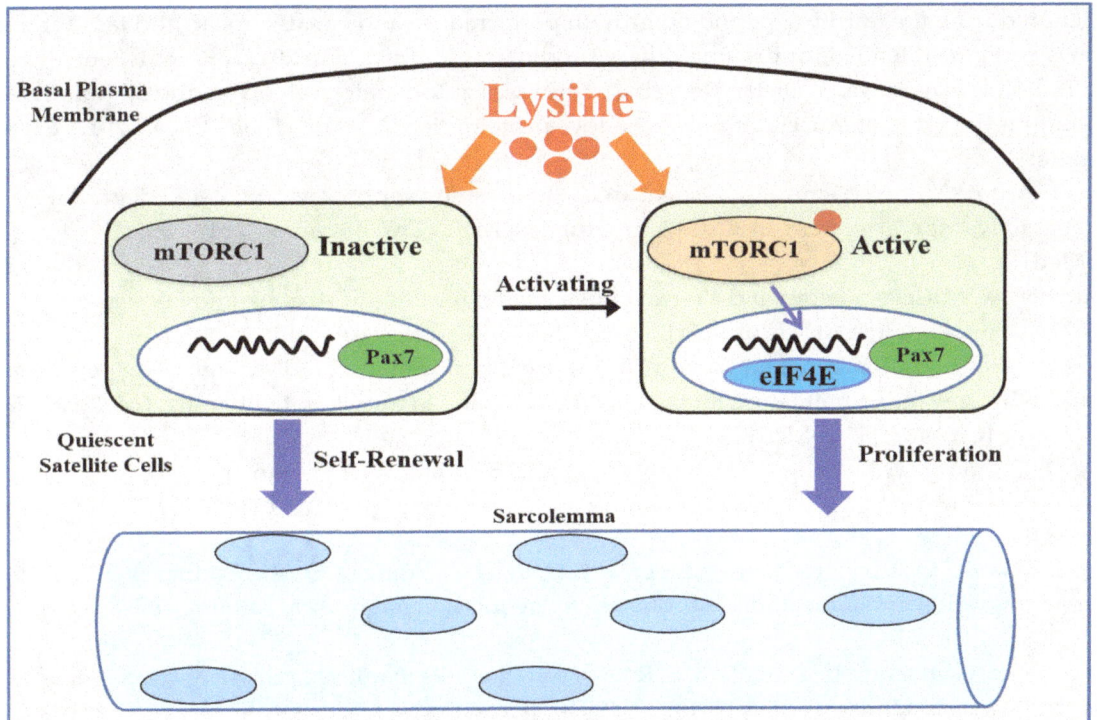

Figure 5. mTORC1 mediates Lys-induced SC activation to promote skeletal muscle growth. Lys supplementation activates the mTORC1 pathway to increase SC proliferation to enhance myogenic potential to promote skeletal muscle growth.

Author Contributions: Data curation, C.-l.J.; Formal analysis, C.-l.J. and J.-l.Y.; Funding acquisition, H.-c.Y. and X.-q.W.; Investigation, C.-l.J.; Methodology, C.-l.J., J.Y. and H.-c.L.; Project administration, C.-l.J. and C.-q.G.; Resources, X.-q.W.; Writing—original draft, C.-l.J.; Writing—review & editing, J.-l.Y., J.Y., C.-q.G., H.-c.L. and X.-q.W.

References

1. Li, P.F.; Zeng, Z.K.; Wang, D.; Xue, L.F.; Zhang, R.F.; Piao, X.S. Effects of the standardized ileal digestible lysine to metabolizable energy ratio on performance and carcass characteristics of growing-finishing pigs. *J. Anim. Sci. Biotechno.* **2012**, *3*, 9. [CrossRef]

2. Zeng, P.L.; Yan, H.C.; Wang, X.Q.; Zhang, C.M.; Zhu, C.; Shu, G.; Jiang, Q.Y. Effects of dietary lysine levels on apparent nutrient digestibility and serum amino acid absorption mode in growing pigs. *J. Anim. Sci.* **2013**, *26*, 1003–1011. [CrossRef]

3. Ishida, A.; Kyoya, T.; Nakashima, K.; Katsumata, M. Muscle protein metabolism during compensatory growth with changing dietary lysine levels from deficient to sufficient in growing rats. *J. Nutr. Sci. Vitaminol.* **2011**, *57*, 401–408. [CrossRef] [PubMed]

4. Mastellar, S.L.; Coleman, R.J.; Urschel, K.L. Controlled trial of whole body protein synthesis and plasma amino acid concentrations in yearling horses fed graded amounts of lysine. *Vet. J.* **2016**, *216*, 93–100. [CrossRef] [PubMed]

5. FAO/WHO/UNU Expert Consultation. Protein and amino acid requirements in human nutrition. World Health Organ. *Tech. Rep. Ser.* **2007**, *935*, 1–265.

6. Jennings, A.; MacGregor, A.; Spector, T.; Cassidy, A. Amino acid intakes are associated with bone mineral density and prevalence of low bone mass in women: Evidence from discordant monozygotic twins. *J. Bone Miner. Res.* **2016**, *31*, 326–335. [CrossRef]

7. Karnebeek, C.D.; Hartmann, H.; Jaggumantri, S.; Bok, L.A.; Cheng, B.; Connolly, M.; Coughlin, C.R.; Das, A.M.; Gospe, S.M.; Jakobs, C.; et al. Lysine restricted diet for pyridoxine-dependent epilepsy: First evidence and future trials. *Mol. Genet. Metab.* **2012**, *107*, 335–344. [CrossRef]

8. Boy, N.; Haege, G.; Heringer, J.; Assmann, B.; Mühlhausen, C.; Ensenauer, R.; Maier, E.M.; Lücke, T.; Hoffmann, G.F.; Müller, E.; et al. Low lysine diet in glutaric aciduria type I–effect on anthropometric and biochemical follow-up parameters. *J. Inherit. Metab. Dis.* **2013**, *36*, 525–533. [CrossRef]

9. Rodriguez, J.; Sanz, M.; Blanco, M.; Serrano, M.P.; Joy, M.; Latorre, M.A. The influence of dietary lysine restriction during the finishing period on growth performance and carcass, meat, and fat characteristics of barrows and gilts intended for dry-cured ham production. *J. Anim. Sci.* **2011**, *89*, 3651–3662. [CrossRef]

10. Sato, T.; Ito, Y.; Nagasawa, T. Dietary L-lysine suppresses autophagic proteolysis and stimulates Akt/mTOR signaling in the skeletal muscle of rats fed a low-protein diet. *J. Agric. Food. Chem.* **2015**, *63*, 8192–8198. [CrossRef]

11. Sato, T.; Ito, Y.; Nedachi, T.; Nagasawa, T. Lysine suppresses protein degradation through autophagic-lysosomal system in C2C12 myotubes. *Mol. Cell Biochem.* **2014**, *391*, 37–46. [CrossRef] [PubMed]

12. Gundersen, K. Muscle memory and a new cellular model for muscle atrophy and Hypertrophy. *J. Exp. Biol.* **2016**, *219*, 235–242. [CrossRef] [PubMed]

13. Ono, Y.; Calhabeu, F.; Morgan, J.E.; Katagiri, T.; Amthor, H.; Zammit, P.S. BMP signalling permits population expansion by preventing premature myogenic differentiation in muscle satellite cells. *Cell Death. Differ.* **2011**, *18*, 222–234. [CrossRef] [PubMed]

14. Wang, X.Q.; Yang, W.J.; Yang, Z.; Shu, G.; Wang, S.B.; Jiang, Q.Y.; Yuan, L.; Wu, T.S. The differential proliferative ability of satellite cells in Lantang and Landrace pigs. *PLoS ONE* **2012**, *7*, e32537. [CrossRef] [PubMed]

15. Wang, D.; Gao, C.Q.; Chen, R.Q.; Jin, C.L.; Li, H.C.; Yan, H.C.; Wang, X.Q. Focal adhesion kinase and paxillin promote migration and adhesion to fibronectin by swine skeletal muscle satellite cells. *Oncotarget* **2016**, *7*, 30845–30854. [CrossRef]

16. Pallafacchina, G.; Blaauw, B.; Schiaffino, S. Role of satellite cells in muscle growth and maintenance of muscle mass. *Nutr. Metab. Cardiovasc. Dis.* **2013**, *23*, 12–18. [CrossRef]

17. Jash, S.; Dhar, G.; Ghosh, U.; Adhya, S. Role of the mTORC1 complex in satellite cell activation by RNA-induced mitochondrial restoration: Dual control of cyclin D1 through microRNAs. *Mol. Cell Biol.* **2014**, *34*, 3594–3606. [CrossRef]

18. Gao, C.Q.; Zhi, R.; Yang, Z.; Li, H.C.; Yan, H.C.; Wang, X.Q. Low dose of IGF-I increases cell size of skeletal muscle satellite cells via Akt/S6K signaling pathway. *J. Cell Biochem.* **2015**, *116*, 2637–2648. [CrossRef]

19. Zhang, P.; Liang, X.; Shan, T.; Jiang, Q.; Deng, C.; Zheng, R.; Kuang, S. mTOR is necessary for proper satellite cell activity and skeletal muscle regeneration. *Biochem. Biophys. Res. Commun.* **2015**, *463*, 102–108. [CrossRef]

20. Dai, J.M.; Yu, M.X.; Shen, Z.Y.; Guo, C.Y.; Zhuang, S.Q.; Qiu, X.S. Leucine promotes proliferation and differentiation of primary preterm rat satellite cells in part through mTORC1 signaling pathway. *Nutrients* **2015**, *7*, 3387–3400. [CrossRef]

21. Alway, S.E.; Pereira, S.L.; Edens, N.K.; Hao, Y.; Bennett, B.T. β-Hydroxy-beta-methylbutyrate (HMB) enhances the proliferation of satellite cells in fast muscles of aged rats during recovery from disuse atrophy. *Exp. Gerontol.* **2013**, *48*, 973–984. [CrossRef] [PubMed]

22. Morales, A.; Garcia, H.; Arce, N.; Cota, M.; Zijlstra, R.T.; Araiza, B.A.; Cervantes, M. Effect of L-lysine on expression of selected genes, serum concentration of amino acids, muscle growth and performance of growing pigs. *J. Anim. Physiol. Anim. Nutr.* **2015**, *99*, 701–709. [CrossRef] [PubMed]

23. Jin, C.L.; Zhang, Z.M.; Ye, J.L.; Gao, C.Q.; Yan, H.C.; Li, H.C.; Yang, J.Z.; Wang, X.Q. Lysine-induced swine satellite cell migration is mediated by the FAK pathway. *Food Funct.* **2019**, *10*, 583–591. [CrossRef] [PubMed]

24. Ye, J.L.; Gao, C.Q.; Li, X.G.; Jin, C.L.; Wang, D.; Shu, G.; Wang, W.C.; Kong, X.F.; Yao, K.; Yan, H.C.; et al. EAAT3 promotes amino acid transport and proliferation of porcine intestinal epithelial cells. *Oncotarget* **2016**, *7*, 38681–38692. [CrossRef] [PubMed]

25. Li, X.G.; Sui, W.G.; Gao, C.Q.; Yan, H.C.; Yin, Y.L.; Li, H.C.; Wang, X.Q. L-Glutamate deficiency can trigger proliferation inhibition via down regulation of the mTOR/S6K1 pathway in pig intestinal epithelial cells. *J. Anim. Sci.* **2016**, *94*, 1541–1549. [CrossRef]

26. Schmidt, E.K.; Clavarino, G.; Ceppi, M.; Pierre, P. SUnSET, a nonradioactive method to monitor protein synthesis. *Nat. Methods.* **2009**, *6*, 275–277. [CrossRef]

27. Goodman, C.A.; Mabrey, D.M.; Frey, J.W.; Miu, M.H.; Schmidt, E.K.; Pierre, P.; Hornberger, T.A. Novel insights into the regulation of skeletal muscle protein synthesis as revealed by a new nonradioactive in vivo technique. *FASEB J.* **2011**, *25*, 1028–1039. [CrossRef]

28. McMillan, J.D.; Jennings, E.W.; Mohagheghi, A.; Zuccarello, M. Comparative performance of precommercial cellulases hydrolyzing pretreated corn stover. *Biotechnol. Biofuels.* **2011**, *4*, 29. [CrossRef]

29. Liao, S.F.; Wang, T.; Regmi, N. Lysine nutrition in swine and the related monogastric animals: Muscle protein biosynthesis and beyond. *Springerplus* **2015**, *4*, 147. [CrossRef]

30. Egner, I.M.; Bruusgaard, J.C.; Gundersen, K. Satellite cell depletion prevents fiber hypertrophy in skeletal muscle. *Development* **2016**, *143*, 2898–2906. [CrossRef]

31. Kim, J.; Lee, K.S.; Kwon, D.H.; Bong, J.J.; Jeong, J.Y.; Nam, Y.S.; Lee, M.S.; Liu, X.; Baik, M. Severe dietary lysine restriction affects growth and body composition and hepatic gene expression for nitrogen metabolism in growing rats. *J. Anim. Physiol. Anim. Nutr.* **2014**, *98*, 149–157. [CrossRef] [PubMed]

32. Yang, Y.X.; Guo, J.; Jin, Z.; Yoon, S.Y.; Choi, J.Y.; Wang, M.H.; Piao, X.S.; Kim, B.W.; Chae, B.J. Lysine restriction and realimentation affected growth, blood profiles and expression of genes related to protein and fat metabolism in weaned pigs. *J. Anim. Physiol. Anim. Nutr.* **2009**, *93*, 732–743. [CrossRef] [PubMed]

33. Sato, T.; Ito, Y.; Nagasawa, T. Regulation of skeletal muscle protein degradation and synthesis by oral administration of lysine in rats. *J. Nutr. Sci. Vitaminol.* **2013**, *59*, 412–419. [CrossRef] [PubMed]

34. Popha, S.; Mo, P.E.; Vieira, S.L. Satellite cell mitotic activity of broilers fed differing levels of lysine. *Int. J. Poult. Sci.* **2004**, *3*, 758–763.

35. Snijders, T.; Verdijk, L.B.; Smeets, J.S.J.; McKay, B.R.; Senden, J.M.G.; Hartgens, F.; Parise, G.; Greenhaff, P.; van Loon, L.J.C. The skeletal muscle satellite cell response to a single bout of resistance-type exercise is delayed with aging in men. *Age* **2014**, *36*, 9699. [CrossRef] [PubMed]

36. Mackey, A.L.; Andersen, L.L.; Frandsen, U.; Sjogaard, G. Strength training increases the size of the satellite cell pool in type I and II fibres of chronically painful trapezius muscle in females. *J. Physiol.* **2011**, *589*, 5503–5515. [CrossRef] [PubMed]

37. Snijders, T.; Verdijk, L.B.; Beelen, M.; McKay, B.R.; Parise, G.; Kadi, F.; van Loon, L.J.C. A single bout of exercise activates skeletal muscle satellite cells during subsequent overnight recovery. *Exp. Physiol.* **2012**, *97*, 762–773. [CrossRef]

38. Jewell, J.L.; Kim, Y.C.; Russell, R.C.; Yu, F.X.; Park, H.W.; Plouffe, S.W.; Tagliabracci, V.S.; Guan, K.L. Differential regulation of mTORC1 by leucine and glutamine. *Science* **2015**, *347*, 194–198. [CrossRef]

39. Wolfson, R.L.; Chantranupong, L.; Saxton, R.A.; Shen, K.; Scaria, S.M.; Cantor, J.R.; Sabatini, D.M. Sestrin2 is a leucine sensor for the mTORC1 pathway. *Science* **2016**, *351*, 43–48. [CrossRef]
40. Li, F.; Yin, Y.; Tan, B.; Kong, X.; Wu, G. Leucine nutrition in animals and humans: mTOR signaling and beyond. *Amino Acids* **2011**, *41*, 1185–1193. [CrossRef]
41. Yao, K.; Yin, Y.L.; Chu, W.Y.; Liu, Z.Q.; Deng, D.; Li, T.J.; Huang, R.L.; Zhang, J.S.; Tan, B.; Wang, W.C.; et al. Dietary arginine supplementation increases mTOR signaling activity in skeletal muscle of neonatal pigs. *J. Nutr.* **2008**, *138*, 867–872. [CrossRef] [PubMed]

6

"The Social Network" and Muscular Dystrophies: The Lesson Learnt about the Niche Environment as a Target for Therapeutic Strategies

Ornella Cappellari [†], Paola Mantuano [†] and Annamaria De Luca *

Section of Pharmacology, Department of Pharmacy-Drug Sciences, University of Bari "Aldo Moro", via Orabona 4—Campus, 70125 Bari, Italy; ornella.cappellari@uniba.it (O.C.); paola.mantuano@uniba.it (P.M.)
* Correspondence: annamaria.deluca@uniba.it;
† These authors contributed equally to this work.

Abstract: The muscle stem cells niche is essential in neuromuscular disorders. Muscle injury and myofiber death are the main triggers of muscle regeneration via satellite cell activation. However, in degenerative diseases such as muscular dystrophy, regeneration still keep elusive. In these pathologies, stem cell loss occurs over time, and missing signals limiting damaged tissue from activating the regenerative process can be envisaged. It is unclear what comes first: the lack of regeneration due to satellite cell defects, their pool exhaustion for degeneration/regeneration cycles, or the inhibitory mechanisms caused by muscle damage and fibrosis mediators. Herein, Duchenne muscular dystrophy has been taken as a paradigm, as several drugs have been tested at the preclinical and clinical levels, targeting secondary events in the complex pathogenesis derived from lack of dystrophin. We focused on the crucial roles that pro-inflammatory and pro-fibrotic cytokines play in triggering muscle necrosis after damage and stimulating satellite cell activation and self-renewal, along with growth and mechanical factors. These processes contribute to regeneration and niche maintenance. We review the main effects of drugs on regeneration biomarkers to assess whether targeting pathogenic events can help to protect niche homeostasis and enhance regeneration efficiency other than protecting newly formed fibers from further damage.

Keywords: muscle regeneration; muscle stem cells; stem cells niche; muscle homeostasis; neuromuscular disorders; Duchenne muscular dystrophy; pharmacological approach

1. The Muscle Tissue: Development and Insight

Skeletal muscle is a complex and heterogeneous tissue with a high regeneration potential and plasticity. Muscle regeneration recapitulates skeletal muscle ontogenesis for many aspects. Myogenesis can be divided into different phases, which comprehend embryonic (from E10.5 to E12.5 of mouse development) and fetal (from E14.5 to E17.5) phases [1]. First, muscle fibers are generated during embryonic myogenesis in the somites, transient mesodermal units, to which other fibers are subsequentially added for following differentiation into ventral sclerotome and a dorsal dermomyotome [2]. Myogenic progenitors appear at the end of the somitogenesis and respond to signals from the neural tube, such as Wnts (wingless-type MMTV integration site family) and Sonic hedgehog (Shh), which activate the basic helix–loop–helix transcription factors, such as myogenic factor 5 (Myf5) and myoblast determination protein 1 (MyoD) which commit cells to myogenesis [3]. The embryology of skeletal muscle is out of the scope of this review and excellent reviews on the topic are available [3].

Importantly, as previously stated, skeletal muscle is formed in successive and distinct, though overlapping waves, involving different types of myoblasts (embryonic, fetal myoblasts, and satellite cells). The progressive growth of muscles occurring during late embryonic (E10.5–12.5), fetal (E14.5–17.5), and postnatal life was recently attributed to a population of muscle progenitors that can be found already at embryonic stage [4–7]. These might derive from a paired box gene (*Pax*) 3/7 positive population of myogenic progenitors, residing in the central part of the dermomyotome. Around E11.5 of mouse development, embryonic myoblasts enter the myotome and fuse into myotubes. More or less at the same stage, during a phase referred to as primary myogenesis, myogenic progenitors (migrated from the dermomyotome to the limb), start to differentiate into multinucleated muscle fibers, commonly known as primary fibers. A second wave of myogenesis (from E14.5 and E17.5 in mouse) known as secondary myogenesis, is characterized by fetal myoblasts fusing with each other [8–10]. At the end of this phase, satellite cells can be morphologically identified as mononucleated cells located between the basal lamina and the sarcolemma. During perinatal and also postnatal development, satellite cells start dividing at a slow pace. Most of the progeny fuse with the adjacent fibers, with new nuclei contributing to growing muscle fibers (whose nuclei are not able to divide). Because of this process, it is possible to think that the majority of the nuclei of a mature muscle are probably derived from satellite cells. Then, when postnatal growth is finished, satellite cells enter a phase of quiescence, but they can be activated when the muscle tissue is damaged or in response to further growth demands. In these cases, satellite cells exit the quiescent state, and undergo a number of cells divisions, thereby producing fusion competent cells that are able either to fuse with damaged fibers or to form new ones. Moreover, part of the cells return instead to quiescence, thereby maintaining the progenitor pool. This ability has led to the suggestion that they represent a type of stem cells [11]. Many factors influence satellite cells' population during myogenesis, such as obesity, diabetes, and other metabolism-related problems. A very important one, for example, is represented by nutrient administration in the maternal stage, which seems to have a direct role in perinatal muscle growth, as extensively explained in Fiorotto and Davis [12].

2. Muscle Stem Cell Niche: Role in Tissue Homeostasis and Muscle Regeneration

Satellite cells occupy an exclusive niche within the muscle tissue, with both stem-like properties and demonstrated myogenic activities. As previously stated, satellite cells are able to remain quiescent or they can be activated in response either to growth/regenerative signal/injuries [13]. After this activation, they re-enter the cell cycle and undergo an asymmetric division to maintain self-renewal. Self-renewal is perpetuated via symmetric cell expansion (generating two identical daughter stem cells) or through an asymmetric cell division (generating both a stem cell and a committed progenitor daughter cell) [14].

Of the two formed daughter cells, one goes back replenishing the niche, then becoming quiescent again; meanwhile, the other participates in the muscle regeneration/growth/homeostasis process. This mechanism is finely regulated. In fact, satellite cell fate is tuned by mechanisms involving both cell-autonomous and external stimuli, in concert with the programmed expression and action of various transcription factors [15,16]. The complex processes governing satellite cell activation and myogenesis have attracted much interest over the years and have been beautifully revised [16,17]. Notably, the decision to undergo symmetric or asymmetric self-renewal is a critical step in satellite cell fate determination, and a deregulation of this process could potentially have detrimental consequences on the execution of a muscle regeneration program. Satellite cells are located beneath the basal lamina in a quiescent state, in which they express Pax7 and Myf5 [18]. When they are activated and differentiate into myoblasts, they express MyoD and myogenin (Myog). If a Pax7+ cell population is deleted, skeletal muscle regeneration is impaired, thereby reinforcing the importance of these cells in this process [19]. After muscle injury, there is a time-dependent and well-organized inflammatory response that happens together with satellite cell activation and through their differentiation process. The recruitment of immune cells to the site of injury is pivotal to obtaining complete skeletal muscle regeneration [20]. The acute inflammatory response following muscle injury usually begins with neutrophils infiltration [21]. This is usually followed by an infiltration of macrophages carrying an

M1 phenotype, which produces mostly inflammatory cytokines, such as tumor necrosis factor-alpha (TNF-α), interleukin 1 beta (IL-1β), and interferon-gamma (IFN-γ) [22].

The addition of these cytokines in primary myoblasts' culture remarkably increases cell proliferation, supporting the assumption that the early increase in M1 macrophage population and the first phase of inflammation actively participate in satellite cell activation [23]. Afterward, an important expansion of M2 macrophages does occur, which is associated with tissue repair and satellite cell differentiation [24]. In fact, M2 macrophages produce different cytokines, such as interleukins IL-4 and IL-10, which improve myoblast differentiation in vitro and increase Myog expression levels, the transcription factor that is essential for satellite cell terminal differentiation [25]. Therefore, M1 and M2 macrophages' kinetics are critical for the early steps of muscle regeneration.

Epigenetic regulation mechanisms can also play a role in satellite cell pool maintenance by modulating proliferation and differentiation. A complete epigenetic profiling of quiescent satellite cells, obtained by Liu and colleagues via chip-seq analysis, has shown that during quiescence, chromatin is maintained in a transcriptionally permissive state, thereby allowing various epigenetic modifications, leading to increased expression of genes involved in satellite cells' proliferation. In particular, DNA methylation of some genes promoters (e.g., *Notch*, Notch homolog 1, translocation-associated), has been found to cause changes in satellite cell renewal, maintenance, and homeostasis [26–28].

In addition, mitochondrial functions, particularly fission and fusion, have been recently reported to play a role in maintaining and dictating satellite cells' fates. In fact, mitochondria are strongly connected to metabolic programming during quiescence, activation, self-renewal, proliferation, and differentiation. Interestingly, mitochondrial adaptation might take place to modify satellite cells' fates and function in the presence of different environmental cues, and under different metabolic states [29,30]. Therefore, satellite cells' functional outcomes are strongly associated with mitochondrial energy output [31,32]. Mitochondrial functions are so broad that some of them, including regeneration, could be interesting targets for pharmacological therapy.

However, while muscle repair after damage is an efficient process in healthy muscle, its probability of success appears low in many muscle disorders. The maintenance of an efficient regeneration process is guaranteed by both satellite cells' niche environment and satellite cells' pool. By disrupting either one of the two or both, the impairment in muscle regeneration suddenly happens, as likely occurs in many muscular dystrophies. In Duchenne muscular dystrophy (DMD), the most frequent and most studied one, it is still unclear which phenomenon comes first, also in relation to the different roles that cytokines play on adult myofiber and satellite cells and their complex crosstalk. However, the plethora of data collected in DMD over the last decades, also with the extensive use and characterization of the *mdx* mouse, its main animal model [33]. allow a deeper insight into the possibility to improve regeneration efficiency as a consequence of therapeutic approaches, from classical drugs to cell therapy.

Pharmacological approaches, even if unable to restore the primary defect, can target disease pathophysiology and progression, by acting at different stages of the inflammatory cascade and therefore slowing down the necrotic process. Yet, the outcomes of such strategies on regeneration efficiency are still unclear. Similarly, other approaches aim at enhancing regeneration with a direct drug action on satellite cell activation and differentiation, although such an effect without a parallel mechanism to minimize the damage of mature myofiber appears to be weak. Herein, we critically revised some of the main approaches used preclinically and clinically in DMD in the attempt to assess their potential outcomes in maintaining or enhancing the regeneration potential, also in relation to the mechanism of action. The overview of these effects may help the community to go back to basic scientific research with a better understanding of the imbalance in the social network governing muscle repair and stem cell niche in relation to disease mechanisms to better address therapeutic intervention for tissue repair.

3. Duchenne Muscular Dystrophy: Is There a Role for Satellite Cells and Their Niche?

3.1. DMD General Picture

DMD is a lethal progressive pediatric muscle disorder. It is genetically inherited as an X-linked disease caused by mutations in the dystrophin gene. The *DMD* gene (which encodes the protein dystrophin) is affected by point mutations, duplications, and deletions of parts of the gene, causing alterations in the reading frame and consequent truncation of the dystrophin protein, which is then rapidly degraded. Dystrophin protein is mainly expressed in skeletal and cardiac muscle and to a lesser extent in smooth muscle and the brain. Dystrophin represents an essential component of the large oligomeric dystrophin-glycoprotein complex (DGC) [34,35]. The DGC acts as a connector between the actin cytoskeleton of the myofiber and the surrounding extracellular matrix (ECM) through the sarcolemma. In the absence of dystrophin, DGC assembly is impaired which weakens the muscle fibers, rendering them highly susceptible to injury. At this point, muscle contraction-induced stress results in constant cycles of degeneration and regeneration [36]. Eventual accumulation of inflammation and fibrosis lead to progressive muscle weakening and loss of muscle mass and function [37]. The efficiency of regeneration appears to be low [38]. This progressive muscle wasting condition leads to severe disability and follows with premature death in affected individuals due to respiratory and/or cardiac failure, typically by or before the age of 30.

3.2. DMD and Stem Cell Polarity

DMD has also been considered a stem cell disease, as a failing regeneration is a typical feature. In fact, there is still a debate about the main determinant of the regeneration failure; it is not clear whether the lack of dystrophin impairs satellite cells' ability to repair the muscle, or the disruption of the stem cells niche environment, or the two altogether. The role of the niche for stem cells in muscle repair is, in general, crucial. In the case of DMD, the niche environment is believed to be compromised by the cascade of events due to constant inflammation and muscle degeneration [39]. However, the absence of dystrophin can play a key role, by affecting asymmetric division. In general, cell cortex polarization and specification of the mitotic spindle orientation are critical steps for the asymmetric localization of cell fate determinants [40].

Importantly, dystrophin interacts with the cell polarity-regulating serine/threonine-protein kinase MARK2 at the muscle fiber membrane [41]. Moreover, it has been demonstrated that activated satellite cells also express dystrophin [42]. Interestingly, dystrophin protein expression has been found to be polarized in satellite cells, and apparently, it is expressed at a very high level when cells are about to undergo cell division. Therefore, dystrophin has a pivotal role in regulating polarity in asymmetric satellite cell division. In support of this view, Chang et al. described a significant reduction in asymmetric division, with a consequent progressive loss of myogenic progenitor, in myoblast-derived satellite cells isolated from *mdx* mouse [43]. This phenomenon seems due to the *mdx*-derived loss of polarity of *mdx* satellite cells, which then resulted in defective mitotic spindle orientation, causing an impairment in asymmetric cell division. This observation supports the hypothesis that the absence of dystrophin, even at the satellite cell level and during asymmetric division, is a significant contributing factor in the failing repair efficiency manifestation of DMD phenotype [43].

However, the niche surrounding environment can also play a key role in the effectiveness of regeneration. This will be addressed in the following paragraph. An important question that remains unaddressed is to determine what the fate is of dystrophic satellite cells that are unable to undergo proper cell division. In accordance with the observation that *mdx* satellite cells exhibit a reduced ability to commit to the myogenic program, another recent study found that satellite cells from *mdx* mice have reduced myogenic potential and initiate a fibrogenic program. It is conceivable that satellite cell dysfunction in DMD can also account for enhanced fibrosis.

3.3. Inflammation and Regeneration Efficiency in DMD

In DMD, muscle tissue goes through continuous cycles of degeneration/regeneration. In the latest stages of the pathology, muscle tissue is substituted by fibrotic and adipose tissue mostly due to the inability of satellite cells to repair muscle damage. Chronic inflammation is a typical hallmark of DMD and may contribute to impaired skeletal muscle regeneration. Although many cells are involved in chronic inflammation, one of the most important roles is played by macrophages, since these cells are associated not only to satellite cells' activation but also to the survival of fibro/adipogenic progenitors (FAPs), which outcompete the satellite cell population during inflammation [44]. By competing with satellite cells, FAPs can increment the fibrotic process; an imbalance between the two populations ultimately leads to the accumulation of FAPs in skeletal muscles with consequent aberrant production of pro-fibrotic factors (e.g., ECM components). Thus, a pharmacological reduction of FAP accumulation could potentially help in preserving satellite cells and their ability to repair injured muscles.

Adding to the role of macrophages in modulating satellite cell proliferation and differentiation, a recent study demonstrated that the cytokines, produced by both M1 and M2, infiltrated macrophages in the injured skeletal muscle, are able to modulate ECM production through FAPs [45]. In particular, it has been shown that in physiological condition, ECM components' production by FAPs was regulated by TNF-α or transforming growth factor-beta 1 (TGF-β1), which are both secreted by M1 and M2 macrophages. On top of that, the M1 and M2 macrophage kinetics after muscle damage supported the initial accumulation followed by FAP apoptosis, avoiding the aberrant deposition of ECM in skeletal muscle. In this regard, an increase in both cytokines can be responsible for excessive ECM accumulation, thereby leading to poor or non-effective skeletal muscle regeneration. Based on those previous studies, FAPs and macrophages have been characterized as some of cells associated with generation and maintenance of the microenvironment responsible for satellite cells' activation and differentiation, i.e., the satellite cell niche, pivotal during skeletal muscle regeneration process. Even though the acute inflammatory response is associated with proper skeletal muscle regeneration, chronic and non-resolute inflammation, which is observed in the skeletal muscle of idiopathic inflammatory myopathies, dystrophies, and aging, is strongly associated with the impaired functions of satellite cells, immune cells, and FAPs, leading then to fibrosis accumulation and poor skeletal muscle regeneration [45,46].

Regarding M1 macrophage over-activation, some in vitro studies show that higher levels of the cytokines produced by these cells (e.g., IL-1β, TNF-α, IFN-γ) are able to mitigate or abrogate myoblast proliferation [23,47]. Moreover, the continuous stimulation of myogenic progenitor cells by IFN-γ leads to the suppression of genes responsible for terminal differentiation. This suppression accounts for the activity of the histone methyltransferase EZH2, which is mediated by the class II major histocompatibility complex transactivator [48]. A chronic increase in IFN-γ and class II major histocompatibility complex transactivator levels repress the expression of genes related to the late stages of satellite cell differentiation by enhancing the promoter region of these genes [48]. Although the level and chronicity of IFN-γ required to start these epigenetics effects in vivo are unknown, these findings suggest that a persistent increase in M1 macrophages expressing IFN-γ for a long time can definitely impair skeletal muscle regeneration. Table 1 summarizes the main cytokines involved in the early and late damaging signals, and in the pro-fibrotic pathways.

Table 1. Cytokines involved in satellite cell regeneration. List of cytokines involved in the inflammatory pathway for muscle regeneration and maintenance. The listed cytokines take part either in proliferation or differentiation of the satellite cell population aiming to repair muscle tissue after injury. Their role in relation to the phase of regeneration is indicated.

Cytokines	Effects on Satellite Cells (Early Phase)	Effects on Myoblasts (Later Phases)	References
IL-1β	Pro-inflammatory; increases SCs proliferation and coordinates interactions between SCs and microenvironment	Reduces myogenic differentiation	[23,49]
IL-4	Improves myoblast differentiation in vitro and increases Myog expression	Plays a role in SCs fusion and growth	[50]
IL-6	Pro-inflammatory; induces SCs proliferation	Stimulates hypertrophy and promotes myoblast differentiation	[51]
IL-7	None reported	Possible involvement in inhibiting differentiation (limited data available)	[52]
IL-10	Anti-inflammatory, counteracts IL-6; no effects on proliferation	Stimulates differentiation	[53]
IL-13	Pro-inflammatory; increases SCs proliferation	Fusion-promoting activity	[48,54]
IFN-γ	Pro-inflammatory; increases SCs proliferation	Impairs differentiation via inhibition of Myog expression	[48]
TGF-β1	Pro-fibrotic; maintains and induces SCs quiescence	Inhibits differentiation	[55]
TNF-α	Pro-inflammatory; increases SCs proliferation, activates SCs to enter the cell cycle via p38 MAPK activation	Inhibits differentiation and fusion	[23]

Abbreviations: SCs, satellite cells; IL, interleukin; IFN-γ, interferon γ; Myog, myogenin; TGF-β1, transforming growth factor β1; TNF-α, tumor necrosis factor α.

4. Pharmacological Approaches Targeting Niche Homeostasis: What We Learned from DMD

For many years, scientists have been putting a lot of effort into finding an effective and definitive treatment for DMD patients. Although pharmacological and technological progress has been made, there is still no absolute cure for this severe disease. Several promising gene and molecular therapies are currently under investigation, aimed at targeting the primary defect. These include gene replacement, exon skipping, and suppression of stop codons [56–58]. More recently, the promising gene-editing tool CRISPR/Cas9 has been offering exciting perspectives for restoring dystrophin expression in patients with DMD [59–61].

In parallel, various therapeutic strategies have been explored with drugs able to target the complex secondary mechanisms responsible for DMD pathogenesis. The aim is to find drugs safer than the current standard of care represented by corticosteroids. Indeed, glucocorticoids are beneficial to prolonging ambulation in DMD boys and are initiated early before other symptomatic therapies. The main efficacy of steroids is believed to be related to the control of inflammation [62–65].

Along this line, a large number of drugs have been investigated in DMD, many of them aimed at reducing inflammation and fibrosis, and they are then able to shut down the pathological loop leading to progressive damage [58]. Among this surge of new experimental pharmacotherapies, in this review, we will revise available data to assess whether drugs can help to maintain a proper equilibrium in satellite cell self-renewal via direct action, or mainly by regulating the inflammatory response and controlling fibrosis. In fact, to date, it is still unclear whether there is a pharmacological treatment that can help in maintaining better muscle homeostasis and improving satellite cell efficiency.

4.1. Biomarkers of Regeneration in DMD: Advantages and Limitations

From the perspective of evaluating the potential ability of old and new pharmacological strategies to modulate skeletal muscle regeneration in DMD, it is crucial to rely on a robust panel of translational biomarkers to obtain a more complete view on and assessment of the regenerative process in preclinical research. Recently, besides several valuable indices commonly used to quantify regeneration, degeneration, and repair efficiency, the advances in technology offered many possibilities to implement the number of regenerative biomarkers to be assessed. All the identified biomarkers described in this paragraph are summarized in Table 2.

The histological evaluation of dystrophic muscles in DMD patients and animal models is the most traditional way to quantify and characterize damage and regeneration. The classical and standardized hematoxylin and eosin (H&E) staining protocol (TREAT-NMD Standard Operating Procedures for the *mdx* mouse model; DMD_M.1.2.007) enables evaluating histopathology. In this context, the proportion of centronucleated fibers (CNF) represents a common index of regeneration, in parallel to a morphological change in size of nascent muscle cells (DMD_M.1.2.001) [66]. However, this structural assessment of the regenerative process is characterized by intrinsic limitations and variables which can complicate data interpretation; e.g., concerning how the level of centronucleation is associated with a still efficient/non-efficient repair system, the identification of activated satellite cells and the amount of fibrosis depending on pathology stage. Part of these uncertainties can be solved with immunohistochemistry (IHC) and immunofluorescence (IF) techniques that allow us to appreciate the indices of satellite cell activation and regeneration, and the presence of specific markers of regeneration in fused myotubes. In this frame of knowledge, a robust regenerative biomarker in different muscles of *mdx* mice at different ages is the presence of developmental myosin heavy chains (embryonic and neonatal MyHCs), usually assessed by IF imaging [67].

High levels of MyHCs are also considered valuable indicators of disease severity which correlate well with functional impairment in DMD boys. However, this index is also subjected to misinterpretation, since MyHCs may be occasionally present in non-regenerating fibers and are differentially expressed throughout the regeneration process. IHC and IF can allow detecting the presence and cellular localization of any cytokine and transcription factor potentially involved in regeneration, and then help to quickly characterize the efficiency and extent of the process in natural disease history and as effects of therapeutics. qRT-PCR and gene array platforms, together with immunoblotting, ELISA, and proteomic arrays, are also widely used to detect regeneration biomarkers while researchers are intending to gain better insight into the mechanisms behind the regenerative process in DMD, and to assess whether drugs can modulate the expression of these indicators of regeneration in DMD. The transcription factor Pax7 is frequently assessed with various imaging and quantitative approaches, since its expression is directly related to the maintenance of the satellite cell pool, in parallel with the relative expression of other myogenic regulatory factors Myf5, MyoD, and Myog, in relation to the stage of the regenerative process [68,69].

A regeneration-associated biomarker of growing interest is represented by utrophin, an autosomal analogue of dystrophin (80% similarity between the two proteins), physiologically abundant in early developing muscles, and progressively replaced by dystrophin at the sarcolemma level towards birth. In DMD and *mdx* muscles, utrophin is upregulated because of the repairing process, but not to the extent to efficiently compensate for dystrophin absence [68]. As pointed out recently, utrophin sarcolemmal localization and the homogeneity of its signal across the whole muscle in correlation with ongoing regeneration, are critical to assess potential protection resulting from direct or indirect stimulation of its upregulation. Thus, the importance of combining imaging techniques to identify utrophin located at myofibers sarcolemma with the traditional assessment of regenerating fibers and their size is increasing [67,68,70,71].

Furthermore, since inflammation is crucial in modulating the muscle regeneration microenvironment, a more detailed view of the ongoing inflammatory process can be obtained by checking cytokine expression and their intracellular signaling, and by the parallel assessment and relative proportion of M1 and M2 macrophage phenotypes in relation to a drug treatment [68,72]. In parallel, considering the existing cross-talk between myogenesis and angiogenesis during muscle regeneration, orchestrated by restorative macrophages in vivo, the levels of growth factors and particularly of vascular endothelial growth factor (VEGF) along with its receptors, represent another set of biomarkers of interest to monitoring the progression of the microvasculature [73].

The multifunctional cell-surface protein neural cell adhesion molecule (NCAM) is expressed in activated satellite cells and during myogenic differentiation, representing a useful tool to evaluate active muscle regeneration following spontaneous and/or induced degeneration, and the proportion of adult myogenic cells already committed to differentiation [74,75].

Blood-circulating biomarkers are also becoming increasingly attractive for monitoring DMD disease progression and the efficacy of experimental therapeutic options. Among these, an emerging candidate for evaluating muscle regeneration in dystrophic animal models and DMD patients is serum osteopontin (OPN), an inflammatory cytokine and myogenic factor which has been recently found to be highly elevated in the early disease phase of CXMD$_J$ (canine X-linked muscular dystrophy) dogs in Japan. Importantly, high serum OPN levels correlate well with phenotypic severity in CXMD$_J$ dogs [76,77]. Similarly, in DMD patients, a single-nucleotide polymorphism (SNP, rs28357094T>G referred to as the G allele) in the promoter of OPN gene *SPP1* has been identified as a genetic modifier of disease severity by modifying OPN activity [78,79]. It has been recently reported that, in the *mdx* mouse, OPN exacerbates the dystrophic phenotype by skewing macrophage polarization and promoting TGF-β1 activation via matrix metalloproteinase-9 (MMP-9) [80]. This extracellular protease and its inhibitor TIMP-1 are also strongly suggested as DMD progression plasma biomarkers. In fact, high serum levels of both MMP-9 and TIMP-1 are associated with dystrophic pathology; however, only MMP-9 has been shown to increase age-dependently, thereby becoming a marker of late-stage disease in older, non-ambulant patients [81]. Importantly, although the precise mechanisms by which MMP-9 regulates dystrophic muscle regeneration are still unclear, the knock-out of MMP-9 in *mdx*$^{Mmp9-/-}$ mice has been found to augment satellite cell proliferation and transplanted myoblast engraftment in muscles, accompanied by a significant reduction of M1 macrophages with a concomitant increase in the number of pro-myogenic M2 macrophages [82].

Several microRNAs (miRNAs) are specifically expressed in healthy skeletal muscle fibers, playing a crucial role in muscle development; DMD patients and *mdx* mice share a common altered signature of muscle-specific miRNAs [83]. Consequently, miRNAs are attracting increasing interest in recent years. In particular, bloodstream levels of specific regeneration and degeneration miRNAs have been proposed as bona fide markers for DMD diagnosis and therapeutic outcome [84]. In particular, miR-1 and miR-133, normally expressed in mature muscle fibers, are 2-fold reduced in the DMD muscle signature, whereas the levels of regeneration miRNAs, including miR-206, are doubled in satellite cells and proliferating myoblasts of dystrophic muscles. In parallel, the high serum levels of all these miRNAs in DMD patients and animal models compared to controls derive from the intensive degeneration occurring in DMD muscles. Interestingly, high levels of circulating miRNAs correspond to poor ambulant activity in patients [84].

In addition, other less canonical biomarkers of regeneration can come from functional studies at the cellular level. For instance, the expression and function of specific ion channels in myofibers may be useful indicators of the repairing process, and of activation of myogenic process and myofiber differentiation. These include various voltage-gated ion channels, such as Nav1.4, Kir, Cav1.1 [85]. One of such biomarkers we had the chance to better characterize in the frame of degeneration/regeneration events in *mdx* muscles is the macroscopic conductance to ClC-1 muscle chloride channel (gCl). ClC-1 channel is a skeletal muscle-specific channel of key importance for its role in setting sarcolemmal excitability. Its expression and function are strictly developmentally, phenotypically, and nerve regulated. The gCl is directly sensitive to inflammation, as shown by its decrease in response to inflammatory cytokines, chronic exercise, and angiotensin II (ANGII) in wt and *mdx* animals. In parallel, gCl is increased during active regeneration phases and by regeneration-promoting factors, such as IGF-1, as also shown in response to drugs with anti-inflammatory properties, such as gold standard α-methylprednisolone (PDN) [86–88]. The main disadvantage of functional biophysical biomarkers resides in the complex and time-consuming methodology required, which limits validation.

Finally, the evaluation of the expression of main regulators of stem cells division and polarization (e.g., partitioning-defective Par1b and Pard3) to monitor the ability of satellite cells to enter the myogenic program, maintain cell polarity, and ensure a proper asymmetric division is of the utmost importance to assess the effects of pharmacological approaches on dystrophic muscle stem cell niche balance [42,88].

Since none of these biomarkers may unambiguously identify the regenerative state in dystrophic muscles, it is essential to complementarily use these indices and to implement research to identify new ones, with the final purpose of obtaining an exhaustive view of these highly-orchestrated mechanisms, their alteration in the pathology, and the effects of drugs. In light of these observations, the following paragraphs will review the most relevant results obtained by standard therapy (i.e., glucocorticoids) and novel pharmacological approaches in DMD, with a particular focus on preclinical findings highlighting the ability of these drugs to enhance regeneration efficiency in dystrophic muscles, via the analysis of predictive biomarkers. Considering the great amount of preclinical data available on the *mdx* mouse model and the plethora of new compounds proposed and repurposed as potentially effective treatments in DMD, specific attention has been devoted to describing the impacts of drugs targeting muscle stem cell niche homeostasis in the regenerative process, particularly of those directed against pro-inflammatory and pro-fibrotic mediators, and of drugs directly aimed at directly modulating satellite cell self-renewal.

Table 2. Biomarkers of regeneration in DMD. List of tissue and circulating biomarkers identified for the assessment of regeneration in dystrophic animal models and also in DMD patients. The main techniques to perform their assessment at the structural and molecular level and the meaning of each biomarker in the regenerative process in relation to disease stages are also indicated.

Regenerative Biomarkers in DMD					
Biomarker	Sample Type	Detection Method	Disease Phase	Role-Meaning	References
Centronucleation and variation in fiber size	Skeletal muscle	Histology (H&E)	Early stage	Index of degeneration/regeneration cycles	*TREAT-NMD SOPs DMD_M.1.2.007, DMD_M.1.2.001;* [66,68]
Embryonic and neonatal MyHCs	Skeletal muscle	IHC, IF imaging	Differential expression depending on muscle and age	Indicator of muscle damage; correlates with functional impairment	[67]
Macrophage phenotypes (M1, M2)	Skeletal muscle	IHC, IF imaging	Early stage	Immune response during degeneration/regeneration	[68,72]
Pax7, Myf5, MyoD, Myog	Skeletal muscle	IHC, IF imaging; qRT-PCR, gene arrays; WB, ELISA, protein arrays	Differential expression depending on myogenesis stage	Myogenic regulatory factors	[68,69]
Par1b, Pard3	Skeletal muscle	IHC, IF imaging; qRT-PCR, gene arrays; WB, ELISA, protein arrays	Early stage	Regulators of stem cells asymmetric division and polarization	[42,68]
Utrophin	Skeletal muscle	IHC, IF imaging (for sarcolemmal localization); qRT-PCR; WB	Early stage	Abundant in early developing muscles and during repair	[68]
NCAM	Skeletal muscle	IHC, IF imaging	Early stage	Marks adult myogenic cells committed to differentiation	[74,75]

Table 2. *Cont.*

		Regenerative Biomarkers in DMD			
Biomarker	Sample Type	Detection Method	Disease Phase	Role-Meaning	References
VEGF	Skeletal muscle	IHC, IF imaging	Early stage	Indicator of microvasculature progression	[73]
Osteopontin	Serum, Skeletal muscle	ELISA, IF imaging	Early stage	Secreted by myoblasts and macrophages after injury; correlates with disease severity	[76–78]
MMP-9, TIMP-1	Serum	ELISA	Late stage (age-dependent increase of MMP-9)	Remodeling of ECM; activation of latent TGF-β1; inhibition of MMP-9 increases SCs proliferation	[81,82,89]
MicroRNAs signature (miR-1, miR-133, and miR-206)	Serum, Skeletal muscle	qRT-PCR	Differential expression in plasma/muscle depending on regeneration level	Specifically expressed in muscle and released in the bloodstream as a consequence of fibers degeneration	[83,84]
Ion channel biophysics, i.e., macroscopic conductance to ClC-1 chloride channel (gCl)	Skeletal muscle	Intracellular recordings with glass microelectrodes	Early and late stages	Biophysical index directly sensitive to inflammation; increased by regeneration and anti-inflammatory drugs	[86,87]

Abbreviations: ELISA, enzyme-linked immunosorbent assay; H&E, hematoxylin and eosin; IF, immunofluorescence; IHC, immunohistochemistry; MMP-9, matrix metalloproteinase-9; Myf5, myogenic factor 5; MyHC, myosin heavy chain; MyoD, myoblast determination protein 1; NCAM, neural cell adhesion molecule; Par1b, partitioning-defective 1b; Pard3, partitioning-defective 3 homolog; Pax7, paired box protein 7; TIMP-1, tissue inhibitor of metalloproteinases 1; VEGF, vascular endothelial growth factor; WB, Western blot.

4.2. Glucocorticoids: Disease-Related Effects on Degeneration/Regeneration Efficiency for an Old Class

Glucocorticoids are currently the only established supportive therapy used in DMD boys at early pathology stages, although their severe side effects negatively impact on patients' quality of life. The beneficial effects of gold standard medications (i.e., prednisone, prednisolone, deflazacort) are well documented: they control inflammation, delay pathology progression, and increase loss of ambulation up to 2 years in young DMD patients [62,64,65]. Despite this, the precise molecular mechanisms behind their ability to alleviate DMD symptoms remain largely unknown. In this context, several preclinical and clinical studies suggest that glucocorticoids may exert their primary effects by controlling muscle inflammation and fibrosis, and regeneration. We and others collected extensive evidence about the effects of PDN administration to *mdx* mice and its impact on biomarkers of regeneration (see Table 3).

In multiple studies, we observed that treating *mdx* mice from 4–5 weeks of age with PDN (1 mg/kg; for 4 or 8 weeks), resulted in a potent anti-inflammatory action, as shown by the reduced levels of activated p65 nuclear factor-κB (NF-κB) by IHC, and in a marked reduction of reactive oxygen species (ROS), measured by dihydroethidium IF staining in dystrophic muscles. This was accompanied by a notable increase in extensor digitorum longus (EDL) myofibers gCl [86,87,90]. NF-κB modulation by PDN was also confirmed at transcript levels by qRT-PCR in other studies [91]. Importantly, PDN was also able to increase utrophin expression, measured by IF in *mdx* gastrocnemius (GC) muscle, as a direct index of improved regeneration; in parallel, α and β-dystroglycan were found increased by Western blot, as indices of improved membrane stability [71].

Table 3. Glucocorticoid therapy and degeneration-regeneration efficiency in DMD. Preclinical and clinical observations collected about the impact of glucocorticoid supportive treatments on biomarkers of regeneration in DMD. The observed direct and indirect effects on the regenerative process are briefly listed, and the techniques used for the detection.

Standards of Care for DMD and Regeneration		
Glucocorticoid Drugs	**Direct/Indirect Effects on Regenerative Biomarkers**	**References**
α-methyl-prednisolone (PDN)	4—8 weeks of treatment in *mdx* mice (from 4 weeks of age) • Reduced NF-κB expression and activation (qRT-PCR, IHC) • Increased utrophin expression (IF) • Increased EDL myofibers gCl (electrophysiology) • Increased α- and β-dystroglycan (WB) • Reduced macrophage infiltration (H&E)	[71,86,90]
prednisone	• Weekly treatment in 6-month-old *mdx* mice (for 4 weeks) increased expression of Annexins *A1, A6* (gene arrays) • 6-month treatment in **DMD patients** increased muscle satellite cells, reducing fibroblasts and dendritic cells (H&E)	[92,94]
deflazacort	• Weekly treatment in 6-month-old *mdx* mice (for 4 weeks) increased expression of Annexins *A1, A6* (gene arrays) • 3-month treatment in **DMD patients** increased the gene and protein expression of Pax7, Myf5, MyoD, C-MET and reduced neonatal MyHC, TNF-α and macrophage-related CD68 (qRT-PCR, IHC)	[92,93]

Abbreviations: c-MET, tyrosine-protein kinase Met; NF-κB, nuclear factor kappa-light-chain-enhancer of activated B cells.

Furthermore, in a recent study by McNally and colleagues, the weekly administration of prednisone or deflazacort to *mdx* mice was associated with more consistent expression of muscle repair markers Annexins *A1* and *A6* compared to daily treatment, in parallel to a reduction of inflammatory macrophage infiltration and fibrosis, suggesting that dystrophic muscle remodeling may be also regimen-specific; therefore an appropriate dose frequency could further enhance muscle recovery and proper regeneration, possibly reducing side effects [92].

In the clinical setting, muscle biopsies from DMD patients treated with deflazacort for 3 months, gene and protein expression analyses of selected regenerative, and regulatory biomarkers showed that the drug increased the most important mediators of myogenesis and myofiber regeneration (Pax7, Myf5, MyoD, C-MET) and reduced neonatal MyHC, indicating an improved maturation process. In parallel, deflazacort strongly decreased TNF-α and macrophage-related *CD68* [93]. Accordingly, a 6-month treatment with prednisone in DMD boys was associated with an increased number of satellite cells, paralleled by a decrease in fibroblasts and dendritic cells [94].

Interestingly, the SNP of *SPP1* identified as a determinant of DMD disease severity has been recently associated with an alteration in response to deflazacort treatment in patients, with an increase in serum OPN levels [79,95], further supporting the existence of a cross-talk between regenerative pathways and glucocorticoids pharmacological actions in dystrophic muscles.

All these findings suggest that the effect of glucocorticoid therapy in dystrophic muscles is at least partially mediated by an improved regeneration and that this effect is "paradoxical" compared to that observed in individuals with functional dystrophin, where glucocorticoids are known to trigger muscle atrophy.

4.3. Pharmacological Approaches Targeting Inflammatory Mediators and Pathways

Among the new therapeutic avenues explored to pharmacologically modulate secondary events in DMD pathogenesis, several attempts have been focused on drugs potentially more effective and safer than standard glucocorticoids, targeted against pro-inflammatory molecules (see Table 4). As already stated in previous paragraphs, some of these mediators are key players of regeneration efficiency due to their direct role in muscle wasting, and then, in the modulation of functional and structural indices. For most of them, a clear impact on regeneration efficiency is lacking, and in some cases, an expected, reduction of centronucleated myofibers has been observed, as a clear consequence of necrosis.

In this general frame, a key target is the transcription factor NF-κB, a key regulator of pro-inflammatory responses in skeletal muscle. Its active form, p65 NF-κB, is highly expressed in dystrophic muscles before symptoms onset. Vamorolone (VBP15)—a Δ9,11 glucocorticoid analogue now under evaluation in Phase II clinical trials on DMD boys (NCT02760264, NCT03038399, NCT02760277) acts as a dissociative steroid, a retaining membrane, and has anti-inflammatory properties of classical steroids but loses the transactivation sub-activity associated with their side effects. First identified by Kanneboyina Nagaraju and colleagues, VBP15 strongly reduced NF-κB and TNF-α expression and percentage of inflammatory foci in 8-week-old *mdx* mice muscles, with a parallel amelioration of functional readouts [91]. A specific search of regenerative biomarkers would be certainly useful to gain more insight into the clinical efficacy of this promising therapeutic agent. Other anti-inflammatory compounds of increasing interest for DMD are edasalonexent (formerly CAT-1004, now being tested in a Phase II trial), NCT02439216 [96], and CAT-1041, two inhibitors of the IκB kinase (IKK)/NF-κB complex. In 4-week-old *mdx* mice, a 20-week treatment with each drug reduced p65 NF-κB, interleukin-6 (IL-6) and OPN protein levels, without modifying utrophin expression.

Histopathology was ameliorated, with a reduction of the total area of damage and of inflammatory macrophage infiltrates, in parallel to in vivo and ex vivo functional indices [97]. In *mdx* mice, IKK conditional deletion clarified that NF-κB functions in activated macrophages to promote inflammation and muscle necrosis, reducing regeneration via inhibition of muscle progenitor cells [98]. In 5-week-old *mdx* mice muscles, a 4-week treatment with the IKK inhibitor NEMO-binding-domain (NBD) peptide, induced strong decreases in macrophage infiltration and p65 NF-κB, measured by electrophoretic mobility shift assay (EMSA). Interestingly, increments in embryonic MyHC positive myofibers and CNF proportion, measured by IF and H&E respectively, were here taken as positive indices of increased regenerative potential, since they were accompanied by a notable inhibition of damaging pathways [99,100].

Approved drugs targeting TNF-α have been evaluated for possibly repurposing DMD, with interesting findings concerning regeneration. A 4-week treatment with etanercept (Enbrel®), a chimaera compound bearing the TNF-α soluble receptor, improved EDL myofibers gCl in adult *mdx* mice, while the histological profile was only modestly ameliorated. Histopathology was also analyzed in GC muscles from *mdx* mice treated from two weeks of age, when the first spontaneous degeneration cycle occurred, showing a significant reduction in the proportion of degenerating fibers; however, no clear index of regeneration was observed [101].

Several studies have been performed to assess the role of non-steroidal anti-inflammatory drugs (NSAIDs), inhibitors of cyclooxygenase (COX) enzymes, in dystrophic muscles, considering the canonical role of prostanoids in sustaining early and chronic inflammation. However, the effects of these drugs in DMD are controversial, likely in relation to the differential and tissue-specific roles of COX-related prostanoids. In fact, the various prostaglandins (PGs) have differential and opposite effects on regeneration and myogenesis, which complicate the outcomes of drugs inhibiting either or both COX-1 and COX-2 isoforms. In *mdx* mice, NSAIDs and COXIBs (e.g., ibuprofen, flurbiprofen, parecoxib) contributed to reducing macrophage infiltration to a different extent, without affecting functional indices or the percentage of regenerating myofibers. Our group could not confirm these effects for meloxicam, a COX-2 selective inhibitor, in *mdx* mice, likely in relation to the inhibition of PGE_2, which exerts a key pro-myogenesis action [101,102]. PGD_2, unlike other prostaglandins, inhibits myogenesis and its metabolites are increased in DMD patients; therefore, increased muscle fiber regeneration can be achieved by specific PGD_2 inhibition. Recently, HQL-79, a potent selective inhibitor of hematopoietic PGD synthase (HPGDS), was found to suppress muscle necrosis in *mdx* mice, without interfering with cytoprotective PGE_2 and other pro-myogenic PGs [103]. A highly-selective HPGDS inhibitor, TAS-205, was found to reduce necrosis and improve locomotor activity in *mdx* mice [104]; although no more specific results are available on its regenerative potential, a recent Phase I trial provided early evidence of a modest if any, potential therapeutic activity in DMD population (NCT02246478).

An interesting drug target is IL-6, a myokine known to induce a harmful inflammatory milieu in human and murine dystrophic muscles, by promoting the transition from acute neutrophil infiltration to chronic mononuclear cell infiltration; however, IL-6 has also been reported to participate in muscle regeneration by promoting myoblast differentiation [105]. In 4-week-old *mdx* mice, the IL-6 pharmacological blockade via neutralizing antibody, ameliorated functional performance, modulated inflammation via NF-κB inhibition, and improved homeostatic maintenance of dystrophic muscles, as evidenced by the significant gene upregulation of *Pax7*, *MyoD1*, *Myog*, *IL-4*, and *Wnt7a*, a secreted factor which drives the "planar cell polarity pathway" to promote satellite stem cell expansion via symmetric division. In another study, IL-6 blockade increased inflammation with no functional improvement, suggesting that attention should be paid to its dual role in dystrophic muscles, concerning any possible drug intervention [106–108].

Additionally, compounds with anti-inflammatory properties related to multiple intracellular actions may exert clear effects on regeneration in DMD. Among these, flavocoxid, a mixed flavonoid with antioxidant and NF-κB inhibiting properties, was described to exert an early, remarkable morphological benefit evidenced by H&E staining in 5-week-old *mdx* mice muscles, by reducing necrosis and mononuclear cell infiltrate, with an increased regenerating area defined as an increase in the number of Myog-positive nuclei by IHC, while CNF were comparable to vehicle [109].

Another wide-acting drug is pentoxifylline (PTX), a non-selective phosphodiesterase inhibitor exerting anti-inflammatory, anti-cytokine, and anti-fibrotic actions linked to a specific ability to inhibit abnormal calcium entry in dystrophic myofibers [74]. We found that a 4-week treatment with PTX restored calcium homeostasis and reduced markers of oxidative stress in *mdx* mice. Histopathology and fibrosis were improved in a muscle-specific manner. Interestingly, although no significant variation in CNF percentage was observed, PTX significantly increased the NCAM-positive area in diaphragm (DIA) and GC. Then, a wide action of PTX can be envisaged: A reduction of muscle necrosis by controlling inflammation-related oxidative stress and calcium homeostasis, while stimulating regeneration via reducing pro-fibrotic signaling and activating satellite cells. In vitro experiments with PTX in C_2C_{12} cell cultures further supported the potential ability of PTX to directly activate satellite cells and promote their growth, likely resulting from cAMP increase in satellite cells [74]. Whitehead et al. provided evidence that the anti-oxidant compound *N*-acetylcysteine (NAC) ameliorates skeletal muscle pathophysiology in GC muscles from 8-week-old *mdx* mice, by reducing ROS production, NF-κB activation, and CNF, and importantly, increasing utrophin and β-dystroglycan levels at the sarcolemma [70].

4.4. Pharmacological Approaches Targeting Pro-Fibrotic Mediators

TGF-β1 is a multifunctional cytokine playing a role as a master regulator of both ECM remodeling and myogenesis. In healthy muscles, a timely activation of TGF-β1 and satellite cells is thought to be critical for muscle recovery and development. In DMD patients and *mdx* mice, high levels of TGF-β1 correlate with disease severity and induce excessive collagen deposition, contributing to fibrosis progression (see Table 4). In parallel, the TGF-β1-SMAD (small mother against decapentaplegic) 2/3 pathway can also inhibit the activation of myogenic regulatory factors, thereby inhibiting proliferation and differentiation of satellite cells [13,110]. Therefore, agents able to prevent fibrosis by reducing TGF-β1 pathway, either directly or via modulation of upstream activating signals or epigenetic mechanisms, may be potentially beneficial to improving regeneration in DMD.

A main anti-fibrotic action has been attempted with halofunginone (HT-100), an anti-coccidial drug that inhibits TGF-β1 downstream signaling. This drug was described to promote satellite cell activation and survival in vitro in cultured myofibers from 6-week-old *mdx* mice, as shown by increased MyoD expression, with parallel reduction of pro-apoptotic Bax and Bcl2 [111].

As previously discussed, MMP-9 is aberrantly regulated in both DMD patients and *mdx* mice and likely involved in the cross-talk between inflammation (NF-κB activation augments MMP-9 expression) and fibrosis (MMP-9 cleaves latent TGF-β1). Early 5-week treatment with the MMPs inhibitor batimastat (BB-94) was able to significantly reduce the mRNA expression of a variety of MMPs, including *MMP-9*, *NF-kB*, *TNF-α*, and *TGF-β1* in *mdx* mice; at the histological level, batimastat-treated GC muscles showed significantly reduced fibrosis; and accumulation of macrophages, CNF, and embryonic MyHC-stained myofibers, paralleled by an increase in utrophin protein expression, measured by Western blot [89,112]. TGF-β1-mediated fibrosis and prevention of proper muscle tissue regeneration is also sustained by the increased expression of connective tissue growth factor (CTGF/CCN2) in DMD patients and *mdx* mice, where CTGF is mainly detected in regenerating fibers and in the interstitium between damaged fibers [110]. FG-3019 is an anti-CTGF antibody, found to control muscle damage and improve function in *mdx* mice after a 2-month treatment. However, the ability of FG-3019 to reduce necrosis (less uptake of Evans Blue dye) and fibrosis, implied also a concomitant reduction of regenerating activity, as shown by decreased levels of embryonic MyHC and Myog [113]. FG-3019 is now being tested in Phase II clinical trials on DMD boys (NCT02606136); again, the search of biomarkers of regeneration in patients would be useful.

The pharmacological inhibition of TGF-β superfamily member myostatin is considered as another attractive therapeutic option for DMD patients, for both increasing muscle mass and helping regeneration via reduction of the non-permissive pro-fibrotic environment [114]. Very recently, Wagner et al. demonstrated that the delivery of a myostatin inhibitor (RK35) in tibialis anterior (TA) muscle of dystrophic *mdx*-5^{Cv} mice, mediated by a biological hydrogel scaffold, was able to modulate muscle's immune microenvironment, by promoting a pro-regenerative macrophage polarization, facilitating the M1 to M2 transition, and facilitating the consequent production of anti-inflammatory cytokine IL-10 [115].

In this general frame, also the epigenetic modulation of myostatin/follistatin axis via histone deacetylase inhibitors (HDACi) deserves attention. In particular, the HDACi givinostat was found to induce a functional improvement in vivo in *mdx* mice, and importantly, a reduction of neutrophil granulocytes evaluated by IF for myeloperoxidase in TA muscle used to quantitate the magnitude of inflammation associated with muscle degeneration [116]. In the clinical setting, a 12-month treatment with givinostat in a Phase II study on DMD boys, significantly decreased total fibrosis, necrosis, and adipose tissue replacement, in parallel to increasing myofibers size, although no direct regenerative biomarker was assessed. Now, a safety and efficacy Phase III multicentre study is ongoing in ambulant patients (NCT02851797; [117]). By the way, the ability of HDACi to enhance regeneration also via nitric oxide (NO) pathways [118] is a main working hypothesis that would deserve to be specifically verified at both preclinical and clinical levels.

Other important approaches to control dystrophic muscle fibrosis are those acting through a multifaceted mechanism or on prime signals in fibrotic pathways, such as angiotensin II-related ones [87]. In *mdx* mice, a 6-month treatment with the antihypertensive losartan, an angiotensin-II type 1 receptor blocker, was found to decrease angiotensin II-mediated TGF-β1 signaling, with marked in vivo functional improvement. At the histological level, it attenuated disease progression and improved regeneration, measured as an increase in neonatal MyHC [119]. Interestingly, we reported that early treatment in *mdx* mice with the ACE inhibitor enalapril exerted mainly an anti-oxidant and anti-inflammatory action (via NF-κB inhibition). CNF percentage was reduced in GC muscle of treated mice, while the increase in gCl of EDL muscle could be related to a reduction of the direct action of ANGII on ClC-1 channel, more than to an enhanced regeneration [86]. This underlines how the disease phase is relevant in determining a different drug response and to observe an effect on regeneration efficiency, which can be more likely to be appreciated after a long-lasting control of the niche environment.

This simple hypothesis is not fully supported by data with other drugs which may exert an anti-fibrotic action in dystrophic muscles. Metformin (MET), a well-known anti-diabetic drug, has been repurposed in combination with NO-donors in clinical trials on DMD patients (NCT01995032). Recent reports described the ability of MET to directly inhibit TGF-β1-SMAD 2/3 mediated fibrosis [120]. Accordingly, we disclosed that a 20-week treatment with MET in *mdx* mice exerted a potent, metabolism-independent anti-fibrotic action evidenced by a significant functional and structural improvement, accompanied by decreased TGF-β1 levels in GC muscle. However, no significant changes were observed on histological biomarkers of regeneration, i.e., CNF proportion. Then, it is feasible that the molecular mechanism underlying the anti-fibrotic action (still under clarification for MET) or other parallel mechanisms can define the outcome on regeneration efficiency [121]. Interestingly, Pavlidou et al. recently reported that, in C57BL/6 mice, MET delayed satellite cell activation and maintained quiescence (as shown by reduced Pax7 protein expression) [44].

In our laboratory, the effects on fibrosis and regeneration biomarkers in *mdx* mice were also investigated after a treatment of 4 or 12 weeks GLPG0492, a non-steroidal selective androgen receptor modulator (SARM), proposed as a potential anabolic therapy for DMD patients. GLPG0492 reduced fibrosis and TGF-β1 levels in DIA muscle; however, neither histological signs of regeneration nor an increase in the expression of regeneration-related genes (*Myog*, *follistatin*, or *IGF-1*) was found [122], in spite of the fact that androgen receptor modulation is supposed to enhance myogenesis [123]. In parallel, the anticancer drug tamoxifen, a selective oestrogen receptor modulator (SERM), was shown to act as a ROS scavenger and inhibitor of fibroblast proliferation. Dorchies et al. tested the effects of long-term treatment with tamoxifen in the *mdx-5*[Cv] strain, which was found to induce a slower dystrophic phenotype, by reducing DIA muscle fibrosis and increasing CNF proportion [124]. Tamoxifen has been granted the designation of orphan drug by European Medicines Agency in 2017, and is currently under evaluation in a Phase III multicentre trial in DMD patients (NCT03354039). The apparent controversial results can be due to the different pathways modulated by the drugs that need in turn to be interpreted in the frame of the pathology-related events. Interestingly, estrogen receptor EERα in skeletal muscle is known to be an auxiliary co-activator of PGC-1α in enhancing endogenous anti-oxidant response and mitochondrial oxidative metabolism [125–127]. A role of the latter in satellite cells' activation and stem cell niche has been proposed [127].

4.5. Pharmacological Approaches to Enhance Satellite Cell Myogenic Capacity

Besides cell-based therapies and gene replacement strategies aimed at satellite cell reprogramming in DMD, new pharmacological interventions have been recently explored to target muscle stem cell microenvironment and stimulating intrinsic repair (see Table 4). Asymmetric cell division plays a pivotal role in the maintenance of the satellite cell pool. The granulocyte colony-stimulating factor receptor (G-CSFR) is asymmetrically segregated during muscle stem cell division and the G-CSF/G-CSFR axis supports long-term muscle regeneration in mice. Filgrastim, a G-CSF analogue currently being tested for efficacy and safety in a Phase I study on DMD patients (NCT02814110), increased myocytes and improved regeneration in *mdx* mice [128].

A treatment with the secreted factor Wnt7a, which drives the symmetric expansion of satellite cells [129,130], resulted in increased specific muscle force and reduced contractile damage in *mdx* mice. In parallel, it induced hypertrophy and a shift toward slow-twitch in human primary myotubes [19].

β1-integrin is another essential niche molecule that maintains satellite cell homeostasis, sustaining the expansion and self-renewal of the stem cell pool during regeneration. The exogenous administration of β1-integrin enhanced regeneration in vitro and also muscle function in vivo in *mdx* mice [131].

Interesting preclinical results were also obtained via pharmacological inhibition of p38MAPK, which is aberrantly regulated in regenerating dystrophic muscles, although the exact mechanism and the link with regeneration and myogenesis remains to be better determined. Treatment with the p38MAPK-inhibitor SB731445 in the $Sgcd^{-/-}$ mouse model was able to ameliorate the dystrophic phenotype and to improve the self-renewal of satellite cells [132].

Finally, unacylated ghrelin (UnAG) is a circulating hormone that protects muscle from atrophy, promotes myoblast differentiation, and enhances ischemia-induced muscle regeneration. UnAG was found to reduce muscle degeneration, improve muscle function, and increase dystrophin-null SC self-renewal in *mdx* mice, maintaining the satellite cell pool [133]. These first preclinical observations support the use of drugs aiming to directly restore polarity and proper mitotic division of satellite cells, as part of DMD therapy in the future, although a larger body of evidence regarding the mechanisms underlying their effects in dystrophic muscles will be needed to improve data translatability.

Table 4. Pharmacological approaches targeting niche homeostasis in DMD. Synthetic overview of drugs, new or repurposed, targeting the muscle stem cell niche microenvironment in dystrophic muscles by acting on inflammation, fibrosis, or self-renewal, and of their effects on regenerative biomarkers in *mdx* mice muscles. For drugs translated into clinical settings, the stage of development in DMD patients is indicated, and for repurposed drugs, the approval for other pathological conditions. * ClinicalTrials.Gov identifiers.

Some Novel Pharmacological Strategies Potentially Targeting the Niche Microenvironment in DMD				
Drug	**Molecular Target**	**Direct/Indirect Effects on Regeneration (*mdx* Mouse Model)**	**Clinical Status**	**References**
Inhibition of inflammation				
vamorolone (VBP15)	NF-κB	• Reduced NF-κB and TNF-α expression (qRT-PCR, IF) • Reduction of inflammatory foci (H&E)	Phase II NCT02760264, NCT03038399, NCT02760277 *	[91]
CAT-1004 (edasalonexent) CAT-1041	IκB kinase/NF-κB complex	• Reduced activated p65 NF-κB, IL-6 and osteopontin protein expression (WB)	Phase II (edasalonexent) NCT02439216	[96,97]
NEMO-binding-domain peptide	IκB kinase	• Reduced activated p65 NF-κB (EMSA) • Reduced macrophage infiltrates (H&E)	-	[99,100]
etanercept (Enbrel®)	TNF-α	• Increased EDL myofibers gCl (electrophysiology) • No direct regeneration index observed	FDA-approved for rheumatoid arthritis and psoriasis, no trials for DMD	[101]

Table 4. *Cont.*

Some Novel Pharmacological Strategies Potentially Targeting the Niche Microenvironment in DMD				
Drug	**Molecular Target**	**Direct/Indirect Effects on Regeneration (*mdx* Mouse Model)**	**Clinical Status**	**References**
NSAIDs and COXIBs	COX1 and/or COX2	• Reduced macrophage infiltrates (H&E) • No confirmed effects on regeneration • Meloxicam: possible interference with cytoprotective prostaglandin PGE$_2$	Anti-inflammatory agents	[101,102]
HQL-79, TAS-205	hematopoietic prostaglandin D synthase	• Suppressed muscle necrosis (H&E) • No interference with myogenic PGs • No specific results available on their regenerative potential	Phase I (TAS-205) NCT02246478	[103,104]
IL-6 neutralizing antibody	IL-6	• Improved the homeostatic maintenance (upregulation of *Pax7*, *MyoD1*, *Myog*, *IL-4*, and *Wnt7a* gene expression) • Increased inflammation with no functional improvement also reported	-	[106,108]
IL-1Ra anakinra (Kineret®)	IL-1β pathway	• No significant modification of disease-related regenerative parameters	FDA-approved for arthritis	[134]
flavocoxid	COX1, COX2, 5-lipoxygenase	• Reduced necrosis and macrophage infiltrates; no variation in CNF percentage (H&E) • Increased number of Myog-positive nuclei (IHC)	-	[109]
pentoxifylline	phosphodiesterase enzymes	• Improved histopathology with no variation in CNF percentage (H&E) • Increased NCAM-positive area (IHC) • Increased cAMP in satellite cells in vitro	Antithrombotic agent	[74]
N-acetylcysteine	wide anti-oxidant action	• Reduced NF-κB activation and ROS • Reduced CNF percentage (H&E) • Increased utrophin and β-dystroglycan levels at sarcolemma	Mainstay therapy for acetaminophen toxicity	[70]

Table 4. *Cont.*

Some Novel Pharmacological Strategies Potentially Targeting the Niche Microenvironment in DMD				
Drug	Molecular Target	Direct/Indirect Effects on Regeneration (*mdx* Mouse Model)	Clinical Status	References
Inhibition of Fibrosis				
halofunginone (HT-100)	TGF-β1 signalling	• Promoted satellite cell activation (increased MyoD protein expression) and survival (reduced Bax, Bcl2 protein expression) in vitro (IF, WB)	Anti-coccidial agent	[111]
batimastat (BB-94)	MMP-9	• Reduced mRNA expression of *MMP-9*, *NF-kB*, *TNF-α* and *TGF-β1* (qRT-PCR) • Reduced MMP-9 enzymatic activity • Reduced fibrosis, macrophage infiltrates and CNF (H&E, Sirius Red) • Reduced embryonic MyHC and increased utrophin expression (WB)	Anticancer agent	[89,112]
FG-3019 antibody	CTGF	• Reduced muscle necrosis (Evans Blue) • Decreased regeneration (lower levels of embryonic MyHC and Myog)	Phase II NCT02606136	[113]
RK35	myostatin	• Biological scaffold–mediated delivery • Promoted M1 to M2 macrophage transition and increased IL-10 release (IHC, IF, qRT-PCR, in vivo/in vitro assays)	-	[115]
givinostat	histone deacetylase (HDAC)	• Reduction of neutrophil granulocytes (IF for myeloperoxidase) • In DMD boys: successfully completed Phase II study; no direct biomarker of regeneration assessed	Phase III NCT02851797	[116–118]
losartan	ANG II type 1 receptor blocker	• Decreased ANG II-mediated TGF-β1 signalling pathway • Increased neonatal MyHC (H&E, IF)	Antihypertensive agent	[119]
enalapril	angiotensin-converting enzyme	• Early treatment reduced CNF (H&E) • Increased EDL myofibers gCl	Antihypertensive agent	[86]

Table 4. *Cont.*

Some Novel Pharmacological Strategies Potentially Targeting the Niche Microenvironment in DMD				
Drug	**Molecular Target**	**Direct/Indirect Effects on Regeneration (*mdx* Mouse Model)**	**Clinical Status**	**References**
metformin	AMPK	• Decreased muscular TGF-β1 (ELISA) • No changes in structural regenerative biomarkers (e.g., CNF proportion) • Maintained quiescence and reduced Pax 7 in healthy mice (IF, WB)	Phase III NCT01995032	[44,121]
GLPG0492	androgen receptor	• Reduced muscular TGF-β1(ELISA) • No increase of *Myog, follistatin* or *IGF-1* (qRT-PCR)	-	[122]
tamoxifen	oestrogen receptor	• Reduced muscle fibrosis and increased CNF proportion (H&E)	EMA Orphan Drug Designation (2017) Phase III NCT03354039	[124]
Promotion of Self-renewal				
filgrastim (G-CSF analogue)	G-CSFR	• Increased satellite cells and Pax 7 (IF)	Phase I NCT02814110	[128]
Wnt7a	activation of "planar cell polarity pathway"	• Hypertrophy and slow-twitch fiber shift (in human myoblasts cultures)	-	[129]
β1-integrin	MAPK Erk, AKT	• Enhanced regeneration in vitro • Maintained the responsiveness of the niche to Fgf2	-	[131]
SB731445	p38MAPK	• Treatment in the *Sgcd*−/− dystrophic mouse model improved satellite cells self-renewal	-	[132]
unacylated ghrelin	GHS-R; pleiotropic, tissue-specific hormonal activity	• Reduced muscle degeneration • Preserved the satellite cell pool at later stage of pathology	-	[133]

Abbreviations: ANG II, angiotensin II; AMPK, AMP-dependent protein kinase; Bax, Bcl-2-associated X protein; Bcl2, B-cell lymphoma 2; CNF, centronucleated fibers; COX1, COX2, cyclooxygenase 1 and 2; COXIBs, cyclooxygenase 2 inhibitors; CTGF, connective tissue growth factor; EMSA, electrophoretic mobility shift assay; Fgf2, fibroblast growth factor 2; G-CSFR, granulocyte colony stimulating factor; GHS-R, growth hormone secretagogue receptor; IL-1Ra, interleukin 1 receptor antagonist; NSAIDs, nonsteroidal anti-inflammatory drugs; PG, prostaglandin; ROS, reactive oxygen species; Wnt7a, wingless-type MMTV integration site family, member 7A.

5. Discussion

Satellite cells are muscle-committed stem cells resident in skeletal muscle, importantly contributing to muscle growth and differentiation, and allowing an efficient repair process after damage. Multiple intrinsic and extrinsic factors are involved in the orchestration of this complex process, thereby fascinating scientists for potential applications in the field of regenerative medicine, and for developing drugs able to counter progressive muscle wasting disorders, by enhancing an efficient repairing process in inherited or acquired conditions. DMD is a prototype of the efforts in this field, due to the intense research aimed at identifying potential therapies. DMD in fact has no cure; the progressive muscle degeneration is directly related to the events following the primary defect, which are related in a complex cross-talk, to the inefficient regeneration process. Accordingly, satellite cells are believed to be pivotal in determining disease outcome, since the exhaustion of the satellite cell pool causes the absence of a turning point of this muscle disorder. Intrinsic defects of satellite cells, due to the absence of dystrophin, have been described, and the role of the niche in the exhaustion of the satellite cell pool is still debated. As a matter of fact, the niche environment seems to be paramount in the ability of satellite cells to repair the continuous cycles of degeneration/regeneration happening in DMD [15,17,20]. Satellite cells' niche is disrupted over time by the inflammation and fibrosis occurring as the disease progress. Therefore, while the effort to treat the primary defect is still the main target of the scientific community, drugs able to act on muscle environment deserve to be taken into consideration. This approach concerns both novel drugs and repurposed ones, the latter having the additional advantage of a more rapid translational potential from bench to clinic. Drugs with the best clinical potential would ideally target main pathogenic events, reducing damage in parallel, making repair efficient. Knowing all that, we took advantage of the large amount of preclinical data obtained in our and other laboratories with the main aim of summarizing the available evidence of a potential drug action on regenerative efficiency via a direct or indirect action on stem cell niche and satellite cells.

As reviewed here, there are many promising compounds able to improve muscle regeneration, and even glucocorticoids have a positive outcome in improving myofiber regeneration and enhancing the maturation process, mostly in relation to the regimen approach, which may in part account for their clinical efficacy. Importantly, the complex and not fully clear action of glucocorticoids in dystrophic muscle, and mostly in the satellite cell niche, deserves to be better investigated, as these drugs are able to counter degeneration while sustaining the regeneration process.

In particular, drugs acting on different ILs and other inflammatory cytokines are promising [90, 100,104] and should be investigated in more depth. These drugs can take advantage of studies performed in DMD patients, and possibly gain better insight by looking at biomarkers of regeneration. Importantly, great progress has been made to identify reliable non-invasive biomarkers of both pathology progression and regeneration and drug efficacy. These will greatly help the translational assessment of therapy efficacy in the stem cell niche [42,66–83]. In a general situation, even if it is not clear yet whether is the exhaustion of the satellite cell pool or niche disruption drives the pathological progression, we know that drugs acting either on the amelioration of the niche environment or satellite cells' asymmetric division could be good candidates to slow down DMD.

At the same time, what we have learned from a complex disease such as DMD is that the outcome of drug action on regeneration efficiency is not always straightforward in spite of robust hypotheses and a clear mechanism of action. Interestingly, among novel potential therapies, our analysis of literature data enlightened that drugs purely directed against inflammatory molecules (e.g., TNF-α, NF-κB) are mostly able to reduce muscle damage but not improve regeneration, whilst several therapeutic interventions inhibiting or modulating molecules with a pleiotropic action seem to positively impact regenerative biomarkers, in parallel with controlling damage. These molecules, i.e., myokine IL-6, pro-fibrotic TGF-β1, c-AMP dependent pathways and estrogen receptors, and all self-renewal mediators (e.g., G-CSF, Wnt7a, β1-integrin, p38MAPK, ghrelin derivatives), represent potential therapeutic targets of new/repurposed drugs for DMD to specifically support regeneration efficiency, via a direct action on satellite cells or by improving niche environment. In parallel, the effects on regeneration via the pharmacological modulation of other promising targets, e.g., HDACs and ANGII pathways, need to be further explored. In particular, this topic will grant further insight into the specific roles in the regeneration process of different HDAC isoenzymes, and roles in alternative pathways of the RAS system, such as those mediated by ANG 1-7 via MAS receptor [86,87,118].

Then, we still need to understand key aspects of this multi-actor process that in turn have to be approached at different levels. In fact, there are major key players in disease progression and homeostasis maintenance, and it is reductive to assess that the disease progression is caused by the exhaustion of the satellite cells' niche. Then, combined strategies may work in synergy and such synergy may also occur with innovative molecular or cell therapies able to restore dystrophin expression. In fact, drugs able to address regeneration efficiency, although they will not cure, create ideal circumstances to sustain therapies aimed at correcting primary DMD defects, by creating a healthier environment. This has not been done yet, and the possible outcomes are not predictable, although they would ideally be of high clinical relevance.

In addition, the possibility to enhance our understanding of drug targetable events in myogenesis may also help to improve the in vitro approach of tissue engineering for building up both experimental platforms for drug discovery and simulation of reparative medicine.

References

1. Tajbakhsh, S. Skeletal muscle stem cells in developmental versus regenerative myogenesis. *J. Intern. Med.* **2009**, *266*, 372–389. [CrossRef] [PubMed]
2. Sambasivan, R.; Tajbakhsh, S. Skeletal muscle stem cell birth and properties. *Semin. Cell Dev. Biol.* **2007**, *18*, 870–882. [CrossRef] [PubMed]
3. Biressi, S.; Molinaro, M.; Cossu, G. Cellular heterogeneity during vertebrate skeletal muscle development. *Dev. Biol.* **2007**, *308*, 281–293. [CrossRef]
4. Gros, J.; Manceau, M.; Thomé, V.; Marcelle, C. A common somitic origin for embryonic muscle progenitors and satellite cells. *Nature* **2005**, *435*, 954–958. [CrossRef] [PubMed]
5. Kassar-Duchossoy, L.; Giacone, E.; Gayraud-Morel, B.; Jory, A.; Gomès, D.; Tajbakhsh, S. Pax3/Pax7 mark a novel population of primitive myogenic cells during development. *Genes Dev.* **2005**, *19*, 1426–1431. [CrossRef] [PubMed]
6. Relaix, F.; Rocancourt, D.; Mansouri, A.; Buckingham, M. A Pax3/Pax7-dependent population of skeletal muscle progenitor cells. *Nature* **2005**, *435*, 948–953. [CrossRef]
7. Schienda, J.; Engleka, K.A.; Jun, S.; Hansen, M.S.; Epstein, J.A.; Tabin, C.J.; Kunkel, L.M.; Kardon, G. Somitic origin of limb muscle satellite and side population cells. *Proc. Natl. Acad. Sci. USA* **2006**, *103*, 945–950. [CrossRef] [PubMed]
8. Duxson, M.J.; Usson, Y.; Harris, A.J. The origin of secondary myotubes in mammalian skeletal muscles: Ultrastructural studies. *Dev. Camb. Engl.* **1989**, *107*, 743–750.
9. Dunglison, G.F.; Scotting, P.J.; Wigmore, P.M. Rat embryonic myoblasts are restricted to forming primary fibres while later myogenic populations are pluripotent. *Mech. Dev.* **1999**, *87*, 11–19. [CrossRef]
10. Evans, D.; Baillie, H.; Caswell, A.; Wigmore, P. During fetal muscle development, clones of cells contribute to both primary and secondary fibers. *Dev. Biol.* **1994**, *162*, 348–353. [CrossRef] [PubMed]
11. Collins, C.A.; Partridge, T.A. Self-renewal of the adult skeletal muscle satellite cell. *Cell Cycle* **2005**, *4*, 1338–1341. [CrossRef] [PubMed]
12. Fiorotto, M.L.; Davis, T.A. Critical Windows for the Programming Effects of Early-Life Nutrition on Skeletal Muscle Mass. *Nestle Nutr. Inst. Workshop Ser.* **2018**, *89*, 25–35. [CrossRef]
13. Forcina, L.; Miano, C.; Musarò, A. The physiopathologic interplay between stem cells and tissue niche in muscle regeneration and the role of IL-6 on muscle homeostasis and diseases. *Cytokine Growth Factor Rev.* **2018**, *41*, 1–9. [CrossRef] [PubMed]
14. Yin, H.; Price, F.; Rudnicki, M.A. Satellite cells and the muscle stem cell niche. *Physiol. Rev.* **2013**, *93*, 23–67. [CrossRef] [PubMed]
15. Chargé, S.B.P.; Rudnicki, M.A. Cellular and molecular regulation of muscle regeneration. *Physiol. Rev.* **2004**, *84*, 209–238. [CrossRef] [PubMed]
16. Mashinchian, O.; Pisconti, A.; Le Moal, E.; Bentzinger, C.F. The Muscle Stem Cell Niche in Health and Disease. *Curr. Top. Dev. Biol.* **2018**, *126*, 23–65. [CrossRef] [PubMed]

17. Hardy, D.; Besnard, A.; Latil, M.; Jouvion, G.; Briand, D.; Thépenier, C.; Pascal, Q.; Guguin, A.; Gayraud-Morel, B.; Cavaillon, J.-M.; et al. Comparative Study of Injury Models for Studying Muscle Regeneration in Mice. *PLoS ONE* **2016**, *11*, e0147198. [CrossRef]

18. Gayraud-Morel, B.; Chrétien, F.; Jory, A.; Sambasivan, R.; Negroni, E.; Flamant, P.; Soubigou, G.; Coppée, J.-Y.; Di Santo, J.; Cumano, A.; et al. Myf5 haploinsufficiency reveals distinct cell fate potentials for adult skeletal muscle stem cells. *J. Cell Sci.* **2012**, *125*, 1738–1749. [CrossRef]

19. Von Maltzahn, J.; Jones, A.E.; Parks, R.J.; Rudnicki, M.A. Pax7 is critical for the normal function of satellite cells in adult skeletal muscle. *Proc. Natl. Acad. Sci. USA* **2013**, *110*, 16474–16479. [CrossRef]

20. Tidball, J.G. Regulation of muscle growth and regeneration by the immune system. *Nat. Rev. Immunol.* **2017**, *17*, 165–178. [CrossRef]

21. Schneider, B.S.P.; Tiidus, P.M. Neutrophil infiltration in exercise-injured skeletal muscle: How do we resolve the controversy? *Sports Med.* **2007**, *37*, 837–856. [CrossRef]

22. Mosser, D.M.; Edwards, J.P. Exploring the full spectrum of macrophage activation. *Nat. Rev. Immunol.* **2008**, *8*, 958–969. [CrossRef]

23. Otis, J.S.; Niccoli, S.; Hawdon, N.; Sarvas, J.L.; Frye, M.A.; Chicco, A.J.; Lees, S.J. Pro-inflammatory mediation of myoblast proliferation. *PLoS ONE* **2014**, *9*, e92363. [CrossRef] [PubMed]

24. Chazaud, B.; Sonnet, C.; Lafuste, P.; Bassez, G.; Rimaniol, A.-C.; Poron, F.; Authier, F.-J.; Dreyfus, P.A.; Gherardi, R.K. Satellite cells attract monocytes and use macrophages as a support to escape apoptosis and enhance muscle growth. *J. Cell Biol.* **2003**, *163*, 1133–1143. [CrossRef] [PubMed]

25. Meadows, E.; Cho, J.-H.; Flynn, J.M.; Klein, W.H. Myogenin regulates a distinct genetic program in adult muscle stem cells. *Dev. Biol.* **2008**, *322*, 406–414. [CrossRef] [PubMed]

26. Liu, L.; Cheung, T.H.; Charville, G.W.; Hurgo, B.M.C.; Leavitt, T.; Shih, J.; Brunet, A.; Rando, T.A. Chromatin modifications as determinants of muscle stem cell quiescence and chronological aging. *Cell Rep.* **2013**, *4*, 189–204. [CrossRef]

27. Segalés, J.; Perdiguero, E.; Muñoz-Cánoves, P. Epigenetic control of adult skeletal muscle stem cell functions. *FEBS J.* **2015**, *282*, 1571–1588. [CrossRef]

28. Terragni, J.; Zhang, G.; Sun, Z.; Pradhan, S.; Song, L.; Crawford, G.E.; Lacey, M.; Ehrlich, M. Notch signaling genes: Myogenic DNA hypomethylation and 5-hydroxymethylcytosine. *Epigenetics* **2014**, *9*, 842–850. [CrossRef]

29. Katajisto, P.; Döhla, J.; Chaffer, C.L.; Pentinmikko, N.; Marjanovic, N.; Iqbal, S.; Zoncu, R.; Chen, W.; Weinberg, R.A.; Sabatini, D.M. Stem cells. Asymmetric apportioning of aged mitochondria between daughter cells is required for stemness. *Science* **2015**, *348*, 340–343. [CrossRef]

30. Bhattacharya, D.; Scimè, A. Mitochondrial Function in Muscle Stem Cell Fates. *Front. Cell Dev. Biol.* **2020**, *8*, 480. [CrossRef]

31. Lyons, C.N.; Leary, S.C.; Moyes, C.D. Bioenergetic remodeling during cellular differentiation: Changes in cytochrome c oxidase regulation do not affect the metabolic phenotype. *Biochem. Cell Biol.* **2004**, *82*, 391–399. [CrossRef]

32. Folmes, C.D.L.; Dzeja, P.P.; Nelson, T.J.; Terzic, A. Mitochondria in control of cell fate. *Circ. Res.* **2012**, *110*, 526–529. [CrossRef]

33. Grounds, M.D.; Radley, H.G.; Lynch, G.S.; Nagaraju, K.; De Luca, A. Towards developing standard operating procedures for pre-clinical testing in the mdx mouse model of Duchenne muscular dystrophy. *Neurobiol. Dis.* **2008**, *31*, 1–19. [CrossRef] [PubMed]

34. Campbell, K.P.; Kahl, S.D. Association of dystrophin and an integral membrane glycoprotein. *Nature* **1989**, *338*, 259–262. [CrossRef] [PubMed]

35. Ervasti, J.M.; Ohlendieck, K.; Kahl, S.D.; Gaver, M.G.; Campbell, K.P. Deficiency of a glycoprotein component of the dystrophin complex in dystrophic muscle. *Nature* **1990**, *345*, 315–319. [CrossRef]

36. Petrof, B.J.; Shrager, J.B.; Stedman, H.H.; Kelly, A.M.; Sweeney, H.L. Dystrophin protects the sarcolemma from stresses developed during muscle contraction. *Proc. Natl. Acad. Sci. USA* **1993**, *90*, 3710–3714. [CrossRef] [PubMed]

37. Kharraz, Y.; Guerra, J.; Pessina, P.; Serrano, A.L.; Muñoz-Cánoves, P. Understanding the Process of Fibrosis in Duchenne Muscular Dystrophy. *BioMed Res. Int.* **2014**, *2014*, 965631. [CrossRef]

38. Pascual Morena, C.; Martinez-Vizcaino, V.; Álvarez-Bueno, C.; Fernández Rodríguez, R.; Jiménez López, E.; Torres-Costoso, A.I.; Cavero-Redondo, I. Effectiveness of pharmacological treatments in Duchenne muscular dystrophy: A protocol for a systematic review and meta-analysis. *BMJ Open* **2019**, *9*, e029341. [CrossRef]

39. Boldrin, L.; Zammit, P.S.; Morgan, J.E. Satellite cells from dystrophic muscle retain regenerative capacity. *Stem Cell Res.* **2015**, *14*, 20–29. [CrossRef]

40. Dewey, E.B.; Taylor, D.T.; Johnston, C.A. Cell Fate Decision Making through Oriented Cell Division. *J. Dev. Biol.* **2015**, *3*, 129–157. [CrossRef]

41. Yamashita, K.; Suzuki, A.; Satoh, Y.; Ide, M.; Amano, Y.; Masuda-Hirata, M.; Hayashi, Y.K.; Hamada, K.; Ogata, K.; Ohno, S. The 8th and 9th tandem spectrin-like repeats of utrophin cooperatively form a functional unit to interact with polarity-regulating kinase PAR-1b. *Biochem. Biophys. Res. Commun.* **2010**, *391*, 812–817. [CrossRef] [PubMed]

42. Dumont, N.A.; Wang, Y.X.; von Maltzahn, J.; Pasut, A.; Bentzinger, C.F.; Brun, C.E.; Rudnicki, M.A. Dystrophin expression in muscle stem cells regulates their polarity and asymmetric division. *Nat. Med.* **2015**, *21*, 1455–1463. [CrossRef] [PubMed]

43. Chang, N.C.; Chevalier, F.P.; Rudnicki, M.A. Satellite Cells in Muscular Dystrophy—Lost in Polarity. *Trends Mol. Med.* **2016**, *22*, 479–496. [CrossRef] [PubMed]

44. Pavlidou, T.; Marinkovic, M.; Rosina, M.; Fuoco, C.; Vumbaca, S.; Gargioli, C.; Castagnoli, L.; Cesareni, G. Metformin Delays Satellite Cell Activation and Maintains Quiescence. *Stem Cells Int.* **2019**, *2019*, 5980465. [CrossRef]

45. Lemos, D.R.; Babaeijandaghi, F.; Low, M.; Chang, C.-K.; Lee, S.T.; Fiore, D.; Zhang, R.-H.; Natarajan, A.; Nedospasov, S.A.; Rossi, F.M.V. Nilotinib reduces muscle fibrosis in chronic muscle injury by promoting TNF-mediated apoptosis of fibro/adipogenic progenitors. *Nat. Med.* **2015**, *21*, 786–794. [CrossRef]

46. Perandini, L.A.; Chimin, P.; da Lutkemeyer, D.S.; Câmara, N.O.S. Chronic inflammation in skeletal muscle impairs satellite cells function during regeneration: Can physical exercise restore the satellite cell niche? *FEBS J.* **2018**, *285*, 1973–1984. [CrossRef]

47. Li, Y.-P. TNF-alpha is a mitogen in skeletal muscle. *Am. J. Physiol. Cell Physiol.* **2003**, *285*, C370–C376. [CrossRef]

48. Londhe, P.; Davie, J.K. Interferon-γ resets muscle cell fate by stimulating the sequential recruitment of JARID2 and PRC2 to promoters to repress myogenesis. *Sci. Signal.* **2013**, *6*, ra107. [CrossRef]

49. Chaweewannakorn, C.; Tsuchiya, M.; Koide, M.; Hatakeyama, H.; Tanaka, Y.; Yoshida, S.; Sugawara, S.; Hagiwara, Y.; Sasaki, K.; Kanzaki, M. Roles of IL-1α/β in regeneration of cardiotoxin-injured muscle and satellite cell function. *Am. J. Physiol. Regul. Integr. Comp. Physiol.* **2018**, *315*, R90–R103. [CrossRef]

50. Van de Vyver, M.; Myburgh, K.H. Cytokine and satellite cell responses to muscle damage: Interpretation and possible confounding factors in human studies. *J. Muscle Res. Cell Motil.* **2012**, *33*, 177–185. [CrossRef]

51. Kurosaka, M.; Machida, S. Interleukin-6-induced satellite cell proliferation is regulated by induction of the JAK2/STAT3 signalling pathway through cyclin D1 targeting. *Cell Prolif.* **2013**, *46*, 365–373. [CrossRef] [PubMed]

52. Haugen, F.; Norheim, F.; Lian, H.; Wensaas, A.J.; Dueland, S.; Berg, O.; Funderud, A.; Skålhegg, B.S.; Raastad, T.; Drevon, C.A. IL-7 is expressed and secreted by human skeletal muscle cells. *Am. J. Physiol. Cell Physiol.* **2010**, *298*, C807–C816. [CrossRef] [PubMed]

53. Deng, B.; Wehling-Henricks, M.; Villalta, S.A.; Wang, Y.; Tidball, J.G. IL-10 triggers changes in macrophage phenotype that promote muscle growth and regeneration. *J. Immunol.* **2012**, *189*, 3669–3680. [CrossRef] [PubMed]

54. Fu, X.; Xiao, J.; Wei, Y.; Li, S.; Liu, Y.; Yin, J.; Sun, K.; Sun, H.; Wang, H.; Zhang, Z.; et al. Combination of inflammation-related cytokines promotes long-term muscle stem cell expansion. *Cell Res.* **2015**, *25*, 655–673. [CrossRef] [PubMed]

55. Rathbone, C.R.; Yamanouchi, K.; Chen, X.K.; Nevoret-Bell, C.J.; Rhoads, R.P.; Allen, R.E. Effects of transforming growth factor-beta (TGF-β1) on satellite cell activation and survival during oxidative stress. *J. Muscle Res. Cell Motil.* **2011**, *32*, 99–109. [CrossRef]

56. Aartsma-Rus, A.; Ginjaar, I.B.; Bushby, K. The importance of genetic diagnosis for Duchenne muscular dystrophy. *J. Med. Genet.* **2016**, *53*, 145–151. [CrossRef]

57. Duan, D. Systemic AAV Micro-dystrophin Gene Therapy for Duchenne Muscular Dystrophy. *Mol. Ther. J. Am. Soc. Gene Ther.* **2018**, *26*, 2337–2356. [CrossRef]

58. Waldrop, M.A.; Flanigan, K.M. Update in Duchenne and Becker muscular dystrophy. *Curr. Opin. Neurol.* **2019**, *32*, 722–727. [CrossRef] [PubMed]

59. Salmaninejad, A.; Valilou, S.F.; Bayat, H.; Ebadi, N.; Daraei, A.; Yousefi, M.; Nesaei, A.; Mojarrad, M. Duchenne muscular dystrophy: An updated review of common available therapies. *Int. J. Neurosci.* **2018**, *128*, 854–864. [CrossRef]

60. Amoasii, L.; Hildyard, J.C.W.; Li, H.; Sanchez-Ortiz, E.; Mireault, A.; Caballero, D.; Harron, R.; Stathopoulou, T.-R.; Massey, C.; Shelton, J.M.; et al. Gene editing restores dystrophin expression in a canine model of Duchenne muscular dystrophy. *Science* **2018**, *362*, 86–91. [CrossRef]

61. Koo, T.; Lu-Nguyen, N.B.; Malerba, A.; Kim, E.; Kim, D.; Cappellari, O.; Cho, H.-Y.; Dickson, G.; Popplewell, L.; Kim, J.-S. Functional Rescue of Dystrophin Deficiency in Mice Caused by Frameshift Mutations Using Campylobacter jejuni Cas9. *Mol. Ther.* **2018**, *26*, 1529–1538. [CrossRef] [PubMed]

62. Birnkrant, D.J.; Bushby, K.; Bann, C.M.; Apkon, S.D.; Blackwell, A.; Brumbaugh, D.; Case, L.E.; Clemens, P.R.; Hadjiyannakis, S.; Pandya, S.; et al. Diagnosis and management of Duchenne muscular dystrophy, part 1: Diagnosis, and neuromuscular, rehabilitation, endocrine, and gastrointestinal and nutritional management. *Lancet Neurol.* **2018**, *17*, 251–267. [CrossRef]

63. McDonald, C.M.; Henricson, E.K.; Abresch, R.T.; Duong, T.; Joyce, N.C.; Hu, F.; Clemens, P.R.; Hoffman, E.P.; Cnaan, A.; Gordish-Dressman, H.; et al. Long-term effects of glucocorticoids on function, quality of life, and survival in patients with Duchenne muscular dystrophy: A prospective cohort study. *Lancet Lond. Engl.* **2018**, *391*, 451–461. [CrossRef]

64. Bushby, K.; Finkel, R.; Birnkrant, D.J.; Case, L.E.; Clemens, P.R.; Cripe, L.; Kaul, A.; Kinnett, K.; McDonald, C.; Pandya, S.; et al. Diagnosis and management of Duchenne muscular dystrophy, part 2: Implementation of multidisciplinary care. *Lancet Neurol.* **2010**, *9*, 177–189. [CrossRef]

65. Birnkrant, D.J.; Bushby, K.; Bann, C.M.; Apkon, S.D.; Blackwell, A.; Colvin, M.K.; Cripe, L.; Herron, A.R.; Kennedy, A.; Kinnett, K.; et al. Diagnosis and management of Duchenne muscular dystrophy, part 3: Primary care, emergency management, psychosocial care, and transitions of care across the lifespan. *Lancet Neurol.* **2018**, *17*, 445–455. [CrossRef]

66. Willmann, R.; Luca, A.D.; Nagaraju, K.; Rüegg, M.A. Best Practices and Standard Protocols as a Tool to Enhance Translation for Neuromuscular Disorders. *J. Neuromuscul. Dis.* **2015**, *2*, 113–117. [CrossRef]

67. Guiraud, S.; Edwards, B.; Squire, S.E.; Moir, L.; Berg, A.; Babbs, A.; Ramadan, N.; Wood, M.J.; Davies, K.E. Embryonic myosin is a regeneration marker to monitor utrophin-based therapies for DMD. *Hum. Mol. Genet.* **2019**, *28*, 307–319. [CrossRef]

68. Guiraud, S.; Davies, K.E. Regenerative biomarkers for Duchenne muscular dystrophy. *Neural Regen. Res.* **2019**, *14*, 1317–1320. [CrossRef]

69. Ribeiro, A.F.; Souza, L.S.; Almeida, C.F.; Ishiba, R.; Fernandes, S.A.; Guerrieri, D.A.; Santos, A.L.F.; Onofre-Oliveira, P.C.G.; Vainzof, M. Muscle satellite cells and impaired late stage regeneration in different murine models for muscular dystrophies. *Sci. Rep.* **2019**, *9*, 11842. [CrossRef]

70. Whitehead, N.P.; Pham, C.; Gervasio, O.L.; Allen, D.G. N-Acetylcysteine ameliorates skeletal muscle pathophysiology in mdx mice. *J. Physiol.* **2008**, *586*, 2003–2014. [CrossRef]

71. Tamma, R.; Annese, T.; Capogrosso, R.F.; Cozzoli, A.; Benagiano, V.; Sblendorio, V.; Ruggieri, S.; Crivellato, E.; Specchia, G.; Ribatti, D.; et al. Effects of prednisolone on the dystrophin-associated proteins in the blood-brain barrier and skeletal muscle of dystrophic mdx mice. *Lab. Investig.* **2013**, *93*, 592–610. [CrossRef] [PubMed]

72. Villalta, S.A.; Nguyen, H.X.; Deng, B.; Gotoh, T.; Tidball, J.G. Shifts in macrophage phenotypes and macrophage competition for arginine metabolism affect the severity of muscle pathology in muscular dystrophy. *Hum. Mol. Genet.* **2009**, *18*, 482–496. [CrossRef] [PubMed]

73. Latroche, C.; Weiss-Gayet, M.; Muller, L.; Gitiaux, C.; Leblanc, P.; Liot, S.; Ben-Larbi, S.; Abou-Khalil, R.; Verger, N.; Bardot, P.; et al. Coupling between Myogenesis and Angiogenesis during Skeletal Muscle Regeneration Is Stimulated by Restorative Macrophages. *Stem Cell Rep.* **2017**, *9*, 2018–2033. [CrossRef]

74. Burdi, R.; Rolland, J.-F.; Fraysse, B.; Litvinova, K.; Cozzoli, A.; Giannuzzi, V.; Liantonio, A.; Camerino, G.M.; Sblendorio, V.; Capogrosso, R.F.; et al. Multiple pathological events in exercised dystrophic mdx mice are targeted by pentoxifylline: Outcome of a large array of in vivo and ex vivo tests. *J. Appl. Physiol. (1985)* **2009**, *106*, 1311–1324. [CrossRef] [PubMed]

75. Capkovic, K.L.; Stevenson, S.; Johnson, M.C.; Thelen, J.J.; Cornelison, D.D.W. Neural cell adhesion molecule (NCAM) marks adult myogenic cells committed to differentiation. *Exp. Cell Res.* **2008**, *314*, 1553–1565. [CrossRef] [PubMed]

76. Kuraoka, M.; Kimura, E.; Nagata, T.; Okada, T.; Aoki, Y.; Tachimori, H.; Yonemoto, N.; Imamura, M.; Takeda, S. Serum Osteopontin as a Novel Biomarker for Muscle Regeneration in Duchenne Muscular Dystrophy. *Am. J. Pathol.* **2016**, *186*, 1302–1312. [CrossRef] [PubMed]

77. Hathout, Y.; Liang, C.; Ogundele, M.; Xu, G.; Tawalbeh, S.M.; Dang, U.J.; Hoffman, E.P.; Gordish-Dressman, H.; Conklin, L.S.; van den Anker, J.N.; et al. Disease-specific and glucocorticoid-responsive serum biomarkers for Duchenne Muscular Dystrophy. *Sci. Rep.* **2019**, *9*, 12167. [CrossRef]

78. Pegoraro, E.; Hoffman, E.P.; Piva, L.; Gavassini, B.F.; Cagnin, S.; Ermani, M.; Bello, L.; Soraru, G.; Pacchioni, B.; Bonifati, M.D.; et al. SPP1 genotype is a determinant of disease severity in Duchenne muscular dystrophy. *Neurology* **2011**, *76*, 219–226. [CrossRef]

79. Kyriakides, T.; Pegoraro, E.; Hoffman, E.P.; Piva, L.; Cagnin, S.; Lanfranchi, G.; Griggs, R.C.; Nelson, S.F. SPP1 genotype is a determinant of disease severity in Duchenne muscular dystrophy: Predicting the severity of Duchenne muscular dystrophy: Implications for treatment. *Neurology* **2011**, *77*, 1858. [CrossRef]

80. Kramerova, I.; Kumagai-Cresse, C.; Ermolova, N.; Mokhonova, E.; Marinov, M.; Capote, J.; Becerra, D.; Quattrocelli, M.; Crosbie, R.H.; Welch, E.; et al. Spp1 (osteopontin) promotes TGFβ processing in fibroblasts of dystrophin deficient muscles through matrix metalloproteinases. *Hum. Mol. Genet.* **2019**. [CrossRef]

81. Nadarajah, V.D.; van Putten, M.; Chaouch, A.; Garrood, P.; Straub, V.; Lochmüller, H.; Ginjaar, H.B.; Aartsma-Rus, A.M.; van Ommen, G.J.B.; den Dunnen, J.T.; et al. Serum matrix metalloproteinase-9 (MMP-9) as a biomarker for monitoring disease progression in Duchenne muscular dystrophy (DMD). *Neuromuscul. Disord. NMD* **2011**, *21*, 569–578. [CrossRef]

82. Hindi, S.M.; Shin, J.; Ogura, Y.; Li, H.; Kumar, A. Matrix metalloproteinase-9 inhibition improves proliferation and engraftment of myogenic cells in dystrophic muscle of mdx mice. *PLoS ONE* **2013**, *8*, e72121. [CrossRef] [PubMed]

83. Greco, S.; De Simone, M.; Colussi, C.; Zaccagnini, G.; Fasanaro, P.; Pescatori, M.; Cardani, R.; Perbellini, R.; Isaia, E.; Sale, P.; et al. Common micro-RNA signature in skeletal muscle damage and regeneration induced by Duchenne muscular dystrophy and acute ischemia. *FASEB J.* **2009**, *23*, 3335–3346. [CrossRef] [PubMed]

84. Cacchiarelli, D.; Legnini, I.; Martone, J.; Cazzella, V.; D'Amico, A.; Bertini, E.; Bozzoni, I. miRNAs as serum biomarkers for Duchenne muscular dystrophy. *EMBO Mol. Med.* **2011**, *3*, 258–265. [CrossRef] [PubMed]

85. Hoffman, E.P. Voltage-gated ion channelopathies: Inherited disorders caused by abnormal sodium, chloride, and calcium regulation in skeletal muscle. *Annu. Rev. Med.* **1995**, *46*, 431–441. [CrossRef]

86. Cozzoli, A.; Nico, B.; Sblendorio, V.T.; Capogrosso, R.F.; Dinardo, M.M.; Longo, V.; Gagliardi, S.; Montagnani, M.; De Luca, A. Enalapril treatment discloses an early role of angiotensin II in inflammation- and oxidative stress-related muscle damage in dystrophic mdx mice. *Pharmacol. Res.* **2011**, *64*, 482–492. [CrossRef]

87. Cozzoli, A.; Liantonio, A.; Conte, E.; Cannone, M.; Massari, A.M.; Giustino, A.; Scaramuzzi, A.; Pierno, S.; Mantuano, P.; Capogrosso, R.F.; et al. Angiotensin II modulates mouse skeletal muscle resting conductance to chloride and potassium ions and calcium homeostasis via the AT1 receptor and NADPH oxidase. *Am. J. Physiol. Cell Physiol.* **2014**, *307*, C634–C647. [CrossRef]

88. Pierno, S.; Camerino, G.M.; Cannone, M.; Liantonio, A.; De Bellis, M.; Digennaro, C.; Gramegna, G.; De Luca, A.; Germinario, E.; Danieli-Betto, D.; et al. Paracrine effects of IGF-1 overexpression on the functional decline due to skeletal muscle disuse: Molecular and functional evaluation in hindlimb unloaded MLC/mIgf-1 transgenic mice. *PLoS ONE* **2014**, *8*, e65167. [CrossRef]

89. Ogura, Y.; Tajrishi, M.M.; Sato, S.; Hindi, S.M.; Kumar, A. Therapeutic potential of matrix metalloproteinases in Duchenne muscular dystrophy. *Front. Cell Dev. Biol.* **2014**, *2*, 11. [CrossRef]

90. Capogrosso, R.F.; Cozzoli, A.; Mantuano, P.; Camerino, G.M.; Massari, A.M.; Sblendorio, V.T.; De Bellis, M.; Tamma, R.; Giustino, A.; Nico, B.; et al. Assessment of resveratrol, apocynin and taurine on mechanical-metabolic uncoupling and oxidative stress in a mouse model of duchenne muscular dystrophy: A comparison with the gold standard, α-methyl prednisolone. *Pharmacol. Res.* **2016**, *106*, 101–113. [CrossRef]

91. Heier, C.R.; Damsker, J.M.; Yu, Q.; Dillingham, B.C.; Huynh, T.; Van der Meulen, J.H.; Sali, A.; Miller, B.K.; Phadke, A.; Scheffer, L.; et al. VBP15, a novel anti-inflammatory and membrane-stabilizer, improves muscular dystrophy without side effects. *EMBO Mol. Med.* **2013**, *5*, 1569–1585. [CrossRef] [PubMed]

92. Quattrocelli, M.; Barefield, D.Y.; Warner, J.L.; Vo, A.H.; Hadhazy, M.; Earley, J.U.; Demonbreun, A.R.; McNally, E.M. Intermittent glucocorticoid steroid dosing enhances muscle repair without eliciting muscle atrophy. *J. Clin. Investig.* **2017**, *127*, 2418–2432. [CrossRef] [PubMed]

93. Jensen, L.; Petersson, S.J.; Illum, N.O.; Laugaard-Jacobsen, H.C.; Thelle, T.; Jørgensen, L.H.; Schrøder, H.D. Muscular response to the first three months of deflazacort treatment in boys with Duchenne muscular dystrophy. *J. Musculoskelet. Neuronal Interact.* **2017**, *17*, 8–18. [PubMed]

94. Hussein, M.R.A.; Abu-Dief, E.E.; Kamel, N.F.; Mostafa, M.G. Steroid therapy is associated with decreased numbers of dendritic cells and fibroblasts, and increased numbers of satellite cells, in the dystrophic skeletal muscle. *J. Clin. Pathol.* **2010**, *63*, 805–813. [CrossRef] [PubMed]

95. Vianello, S.; Pantic, B.; Fusto, A.; Bello, L.; Galletta, E.; Borgia, D.; Gavassini, B.F.; Semplicini, C.; Sorarù, G.; Vitiello, L.; et al. SPP1 genotype and glucocorticoid treatment modify osteopontin expression in Duchenne muscular dystrophy cells. *Hum. Mol. Genet.* **2017**, *26*, 3342–3351. [CrossRef] [PubMed]

96. Donovan, J.M.; Zimmer, M.; Offman, E.; Grant, T.; Jirousek, M. A Novel NF-κB Inhibitor, Edasalonexent (CAT-1004), in Development as a Disease-Modifying Treatment for Patients With Duchenne Muscular Dystrophy: Phase 1 Safety, Pharmacokinetics, and Pharmacodynamics in Adult Subjects. *J. Clin. Pharmacol.* **2017**, *57*, 627–639. [CrossRef] [PubMed]

97. Hammers, D.W.; Sleeper, M.M.; Forbes, S.C.; Coker, C.C.; Jirousek, M.R.; Zimmer, M.; Walter, G.A.; Sweeney, H.L. Disease-modifying effects of orally bioavailable NF-κB inhibitors in dystrophin-deficient muscle. *JCI Insight* **2016**, *1*, e90341. [CrossRef]

98. Acharyya, S.; Villalta, S.A.; Bakkar, N.; Bupha-Intr, T.; Janssen, P.M.L.; Carathers, M.; Li, Z.-W.; Beg, A.A.; Ghosh, S.; Sahenk, Z.; et al. Interplay of IKK/NF-kappaB signaling in macrophages and myofibers promotes muscle degeneration in Duchenne muscular dystrophy. *J. Clin. Investig.* **2007**, *117*, 889–901. [CrossRef]

99. Reay, D.P.; Yang, M.; Watchko, J.F.; Daood, M.; O'Day, T.L.; Rehman, K.K.; Guttridge, D.C.; Robbins, P.D.; Clemens, P.R. Systemic delivery of NEMO binding domain/IKKγ inhibitory peptide to young mdx mice improves dystrophic skeletal muscle histopathology. *Neurobiol. Dis.* **2011**, *43*, 598–608. [CrossRef] [PubMed]

100. Peterson, J.M.; Kline, W.; Canan, B.D.; Ricca, D.J.; Kaspar, B.; Delfín, D.A.; DiRienzo, K.; Clemens, P.R.; Robbins, P.D.; Baldwin, A.S.; et al. Peptide-Based Inhibition of NF-κB Rescues Diaphragm Muscle Contractile Dysfunction in a Murine Model of Duchenne Muscular Dystrophy. *Mol. Med.* **2011**, *17*, 508–515. [CrossRef] [PubMed]

101. Pierno, S.; Nico, B.; Burdi, R.; Liantonio, A.; Didonna, M.P.; Cippone, V.; Fraysse, B.; Rolland, J.-F.; Mangieri, D.; Andreetta, F.; et al. Role of tumour necrosis factor alpha, but not of cyclo-oxygenase-2-derived eicosanoids, on functional and morphological indices of dystrophic progression in mdx mice: A pharmacological approach. *Neuropathol. Appl. Neurobiol.* **2007**, *33*, 344–359. [CrossRef] [PubMed]

102. Serra, F.; Quarta, M.; Canato, M.; Toniolo, L.; De Arcangelis, V.; Trotta, A.; Spath, L.; Monaco, L.; Reggiani, C.; Naro, F. Inflammation in muscular dystrophy and the beneficial effects of non-steroidal anti-inflammatory drugs. *Muscle Nerve* **2012**, *46*, 773–784. [CrossRef]

103. Mohri, I.; Aritake, K.; Taniguchi, H.; Sato, Y.; Kamauchi, S.; Nagata, N.; Maruyama, T.; Taniike, M.; Urade, Y. Inhibition of Prostaglandin D Synthase Suppresses Muscular Necrosis. *Am. J. Pathol.* **2009**, *174*, 1735–1744. [CrossRef]

104. Hoxha, M. Duchenne muscular dystrophy: Focus on arachidonic acid metabolites. *Biomed. Pharmacother. Biomedecine Pharmacother.* **2019**, *110*, 796–802. [CrossRef] [PubMed]

105. Muñoz-Cánoves, P.; Scheele, C.; Pedersen, B.K.; Serrano, A.L. Interleukin-6 myokine signaling in skeletal muscle: A double-edged sword? *Febs J.* **2013**, *280*, 4131–4148. [CrossRef] [PubMed]

106. Pelosi, L.; Berardinelli, M.G.; De Pasquale, L.; Nicoletti, C.; D'Amico, A.; Carvello, F.; Moneta, G.M.; Catizone, A.; Bertini, E.; De Benedetti, F.; et al. Functional and Morphological Improvement of Dystrophic Muscle by Interleukin 6 Receptor Blockade. *EBioMedicine* **2015**, *2*, 285–293. [CrossRef] [PubMed]

107. Guadagnin, E.; Mázala, D.; Chen, Y.-W. STAT3 in Skeletal Muscle Function and Disorders. *Int. J. Mol. Sci.* **2018**, *19*, 2265. [CrossRef] [PubMed]

108. Kostek, M.C.; Nagaraju, K.; Pistilli, E.; Sali, A.; Lai, S.-H.; Gordon, B.; Chen, Y.-W. IL-6 signaling blockade increases inflammation but does not affect muscle function in the mdx mouse. *BMC Musculoskelet. Disord.* **2012**, *13*, 106. [CrossRef] [PubMed]

109. Messina, S.; Bitto, A.; Aguennouz, M.; Mazzeo, A.; Migliorato, A.; Polito, F.; Irrera, N.; Altavilla, D.; Vita, G.L.; Russo, M.; et al. Flavocoxid counteracts muscle necrosis and improves functional properties in mdx mice: A comparison study with methylprednisolone. *Exp. Neurol.* **2009**, *220*, 349–358. [CrossRef]

110. Ismaeel, A.; Kim, J.-S.; Kirk, J.S.; Smith, R.S.; Bohannon, W.T.; Koutakis, P. Role of Transforming Growth Factor-β in Skeletal Muscle Fibrosis: A Review. *Int. J. Mol. Sci.* **2019**, *20*, 2446. [CrossRef]

111. Barzilai-Tutsch, H.; Bodanovsky, A.; Maimon, H.; Pines, M.; Halevy, O. Halofuginone promotes satellite cell activation and survival in muscular dystrophies. *Biochim. Biophys. Acta* **2016**, *1862*, 1–11. [CrossRef]

112. Kumar, A.; Bhatnagar, S.; Kumar, A. Matrix metalloproteinase inhibitor batimastat alleviates pathology and improves skeletal muscle function in dystrophin-deficient mdx mice. *Am. J. Pathol.* **2010**, *177*, 248–260. [CrossRef] [PubMed]

113. Morales, M.G.; Gutierrez, J.; Cabello-Verrugio, C.; Cabrera, D.; Lipson, K.E.; Goldschmeding, R.; Brandan, E. Reducing CTGF/CCN2 slows down mdx muscle dystrophy and improves cell therapy. *Hum. Mol. Genet.* **2013**, *22*, 4938–4951. [CrossRef]

114. Harish, P.; Malerba, A.; Lu-Nguyen, N.; Forrest, L.; Cappellari, O.; Roth, F.; Trollet, C.; Popplewell, L.; Dickson, G. Inhibition of myostatin improves muscle atrophy in oculopharyngeal muscular dystrophy (OPMD). *J. Cachexia Sarcopenia Muscle* **2019**, *10*, 1016–1026. [CrossRef] [PubMed]

115. Estrellas, K.M.; Chung, L.; Cheu, L.A.; Sadtler, K.; Majumdar, S.; Mula, J.; Wolf, M.T.; Elisseeff, J.H.; Wagner, K.R. Biological scaffold–mediated delivery of myostatin inhibitor promotes a regenerative immune response in an animal model of Duchenne muscular dystrophy. *J. Biol. Chem.* **2018**, *293*, 15594–15605. [CrossRef] [PubMed]

116. Consalvi, S.; Mozzetta, C.; Bettica, P.; Germani, M.; Fiorentini, F.; Del Bene, F.; Rocchetti, M.; Leoni, F.; Monzani, V.; Mascagni, P.; et al. Preclinical studies in the mdx mouse model of duchenne muscular dystrophy with the histone deacetylase inhibitor givinostat. *Mol. Med. Camb. Mass* **2013**, *19*, 79–87. [CrossRef] [PubMed]

117. Bettica, P.; Petrini, S.; D'Oria, V.; D'Amico, A.; Catteruccia, M.; Pane, M.; Sivo, S.; Magri, F.; Brajkovic, S.; Messina, S.; et al. Histological effects of givinostat in boys with Duchenne muscular dystrophy. *Neuromuscul. Disord. NMD* **2016**, *26*, 643–649. [CrossRef]

118. Colussi, C.; Mozzetta, C.; Gurtner, A.; Illi, B.; Rosati, J.; Straino, S.; Ragone, G.; Pescatori, M.; Zaccagnini, G.; Antonini, A.; et al. HDAC2 blockade by nitric oxide and histone deacetylase inhibitors reveals a common target in Duchenne muscular dystrophy treatment. *Proc. Natl. Acad. Sci. USA* **2008**, *105*, 19183–19187. [CrossRef]

119. Cohn, R.D.; van Erp, C.; Habashi, J.P.; Soleimani, A.A.; Klein, E.C.; Lisi, M.T.; Gamradt, M.; ap Rhys, C.M.; Holm, T.M.; Loeys, B.L.; et al. Angiotensin II type 1 receptor blockade attenuates TGF-beta-induced failure of muscle regeneration in multiple myopathic states. *Nat. Med.* **2007**, *13*, 204–210. [CrossRef]

120. Juban, G.; Saclier, M.; Yacoub-Youssef, H.; Kernou, A.; Arnold, L.; Boisson, C.; Ben Larbi, S.; Magnan, M.; Cuvellier, S.; Théret, M.; et al. AMPK Activation Regulates LTBP4-Dependent TGF-β1 Secretion by Pro-inflammatory Macrophages and Controls Fibrosis in Duchenne Muscular Dystrophy. *Cell Rep.* **2018**, *25*, 2163.e6–2176.e6. [CrossRef]

121. Mantuano, P.; Sanarica, F.; Conte, E.; Morgese, M.G.; Capogrosso, R.F.; Cozzoli, A.; Fonzino, A.; Quaranta, A.; Rolland, J.-F.; De Bellis, M.; et al. Effect of a long-term treatment with metformin in dystrophic mdx mice: A reconsideration of its potential clinical interest in Duchenne muscular dystrophy. *Biochem. Pharmacol.* **2018**, *154*, 89–103. [CrossRef] [PubMed]

122. Cozzoli, A.; Capogrosso, R.F.; Sblendorio, V.T.; Dinardo, M.M.; Jagerschmidt, C.; Namour, F.; Camerino, G.M.; De Luca, A. GLPG0492, a novel selective androgen receptor modulator, improves muscle performance in the exercised-mdx mouse model of muscular dystrophy. *Pharmacol. Res.* **2013**, *72*, 9–24. [CrossRef] [PubMed]

123. Singh, R.; Artaza, J.N.; Taylor, W.E.; Braga, M.; Yuan, X.; Gonzalez-Cadavid, N.F.; Bhasin, S. Testosterone Inhibits Adipogenic Differentiation in 3T3-L1 Cells: Nuclear Translocation of Androgen Receptor Complex with β-Catenin and T-Cell Factor 4 May Bypass Canonical Wnt Signaling to Down-Regulate Adipogenic Transcription Factors. *Endocrinology* **2006**, *147*, 141–154. [CrossRef] [PubMed]

124. Dorchies, O.M.; Reutenauer-Patte, J.; Dahmane, E.; Ismail, H.M.; Petermann, O.; Patthey- Vuadens, O.; Comyn, S.A.; Gayi, E.; Piacenza, T.; Handa, R.J.; et al. The anticancer drug tamoxifen counteracts the pathology in a mouse model of duchenne muscular dystrophy. *Am. J. Pathol.* **2013**, *182*, 485–504. [CrossRef] [PubMed]

125. Jung, S.; Kim, K. Exercise-induced PGC-1α transcriptional factors in skeletal muscle. *Integr. Med. Res.* **2014**, *3*, 155–160. [CrossRef]

126. Dinulovic, I.; Furrer, R.; Beer, M.; Ferry, A.; Cardel, B.; Handschin, C. Muscle PGC-1α modulates satellite cell number and proliferation by remodeling the stem cell niche. *Skelet. Muscle* **2016**, *6*, 39. [CrossRef]

127. Furrer, R.; Handschin, C. Optimized Engagement of Macrophages and Satellite Cells in the Repair and Regeneration of Exercised Muscle. In *Hormones, Metabolism and the Benefits of Exercise*; Spiegelman, B., Ed.; Springer: Cham, Switzerland, 2017; ISBN 978-3-319-72789-9.

128. Hayashiji, N.; Yuasa, S.; Miyagoe-Suzuki, Y.; Hara, M.; Ito, N.; Hashimoto, H.; Kusumoto, D.; Seki, T.; Tohyama, S.; Kodaira, M.; et al. G-CSF supports long-term muscle regeneration in mouse models of muscular dystrophy. *Nat. Commun.* **2015**, *6*, 6745. [CrossRef]

129. Le Grand, F.; Jones, A.E.; Seale, V.; Scimè, A.; Rudnicki, M.A. Wnt7a Activates the Planar Cell Polarity Pathway to Drive the Symmetric Expansion of Satellite Stem Cells. *Cell Stem Cell* **2009**, *4*, 535–547. [CrossRef]

130. Brack, A.S.; Rando, T.A. Tissue-specific stem cells: Lessons from the skeletal muscle satellite cell. *Cell Stem Cell* **2012**, *10*, 504–514. [CrossRef]

131. Rozo, M.; Li, L.; Fan, C.-M. Targeting β1-integrin signaling enhances regeneration in aged and dystrophic muscle in mice. *Nat. Med.* **2016**, *22*, 889–896. [CrossRef]

132. Wissing, E.R.; Boyer, J.G.; Kwong, J.Q.; Sargent, M.A.; Karch, J.; McNally, E.M.; Otsu, K.; Molkentin, J.D. P38α MAPK underlies muscular dystrophy and myofiber death through a Bax-dependent mechanism. *Hum. Mol. Genet.* **2014**, *23*, 5452–5463. [CrossRef] [PubMed]

133. Reano, S.; Angelino, E.; Ferrara, M.; Malacarne, V.; Sustova, H.; Sabry, O.; Agosti, E.; Clerici, S.; Ruozi, G.; Zentilin, L.; et al. Unacylated Ghrelin Enhances Satellite Cell Function and Relieves the Dystrophic Phenotype in Duchenne Muscular Dystrophy mdx Model. *Stem Cells Dayt. Ohio* **2017**, *35*, 1733–1746. [CrossRef] [PubMed]

134. Klimek, M.E.; Sali, A.; Rayavarapu, S.; Van der Meulen, J.H.; Nagaraju, K. Effect of the IL-1 Receptor Antagonist Kineret® on Disease Phenotype in mdx Mice. *PLoS ONE* **2016**, *11*, e0155944. [CrossRef]

7

Parkin Overexpression Attenuates Sepsis-Induced Muscle Wasting

Jean-Philippe Leduc-Gaudet [1,2,3,4,5], Dominique Mayaki [1], Olivier Reynaud [2,3,4,5],
Felipe E. Broering [1,2], Tomer J. Chaffer [1], Sabah N. A. Hussain [1,2,*,†]
and Gilles Gouspillou [2,3,4,5,6,*,†]

1   Meakins-Christie Laboratories and Translational Research in Respiratory Diseases Program,
     Research Institute of the McGill University Health Centre, Department of Critical Care,
     McGill University Health Centre, Montréal, QC H4A 3J1, Canada;
     jean-philippe.leduc-gaudet@mail.mcgill.ca (J.-P.L.-G.); dominique.mayaki@muhc.mcgill.ca (D.M.);
     felipe.broering@mail.mcgill.ca (F.E.B.); jordichaffer@gmail.com (T.J.C.)
2   Division of Experimental Medicine, McGill University, Montréal, QC H4A 3J1, Canada;
     oreynaud26@gmail.com
3   Département des sciences de l'activité physique, Faculté des Sciences, UQAM, Montréal,
     QC H2X 1Y4, Canada
4   Groupe de recherche en Activité Physique Adaptée, Montréal, QC H2X 1Y4, Canada
5   Département des sciences biologiques, Faculté des Sciences, UQAM, Montréal, QC H2X 1Y4, Canada
6   Centre de Recherche de l'Institut Universitaire de Gériatrie de Montréal, Montréal, QC H3W 1W5, Canada
*   Correspondence: sabah.hussain@muhc.mcgill.ca (S.N.A.H.); gouspillou.gilles@uqam.ca (G.G.);
†   These authors contributed equally to this work as senior authors.

Abstract: Sepsis elicits skeletal muscle weakness and fiber atrophy. The accumulation of injured mitochondria and depressed mitochondrial functions are considered as important triggers of sepsis-induced muscle atrophy. It is unclear whether mitochondrial dysfunctions in septic muscles are due to the inadequate activation of quality control processes. We hypothesized that overexpressing Parkin, a protein responsible for the recycling of dysfunctional mitochondria by the autophagy pathway (mitophagy), would confer protection against sepsis-induced muscle atrophy by improving mitochondrial quality and content. Parkin was overexpressed for four weeks in the limb muscles of four-week old mice using intramuscular injections of adeno-associated viruses (AAVs). The cecal ligation and perforation (CLP) procedure was used to induce sepsis. Sham operated animals were used as controls. All animals were studied for 48 h post CLP. Sepsis resulted in major body weight loss and myofiber atrophy. Parkin overexpression prevented myofiber atrophy in CLP mice. Quantitative two-dimensional transmission electron microscopy revealed that sepsis is associated with the accumulation of enlarged and complex mitochondria, an effect which was attenuated by Parkin overexpression. Parkin overexpression also prevented a sepsis-induced decrease in the content of mitochondrial subunits of NADH dehydrogenase and cytochrome C oxidase. We conclude that Parkin overexpression prevents sepsis-induced skeletal muscle atrophy, likely by improving mitochondrial quality and contents.

Keywords: muscle atrophy; septicemia; mitochondria; mitochondrial fusion; mitochondrial fission

1. Introduction

Sepsis is a complex syndrome characterized by an overwhelming infection that results in a severe systemic inflammatory response. Sepsis causes diverse vascular, metabolic and endocrine abnormalities that lead to multiple organ failure, and often result in death [1]. Amongst the very deleterious effects of sepsis is severe weakness, which involves both respiratory and limb skeletal muscles [2–5]. In the short term, sepsis-induced respiratory muscle weakness leads to difficulty removing patients from mechanical ventilation, increases the risk of the recurrence of respiratory failure, prolonged hospitalization and increased mortality [6]. In sepsis survivors discharged from the intensive care unit, the long-term ramifications of sepsis-induced limb muscle weakness included functional impairment, limited physical activity and poor quality of life [7].

There is currently a lack of effective therapies to either prevent or treat sepsis-induced skeletal muscle weakness, due in large part to the fact that its molecular and cellular bases are poorly understood. However, one clue lies at the ultrastructural level, where significant accumulations of damaged and dysfunctional mitochondria are characteristic of sepsis-induced muscle dysfunction [8,9]. Indeed, Bready et al. showed that, in human skeletal muscle, sepsis results in decreased complex I activity (a key enzyme of the mitochondrial electron transfer system) and declined the ATP/ADP ratio in skeletal muscles [10]. These defects in muscle bioenergetics were also observed in a rat model of sepsis [11]. By studying biopsies obtained from septic patients, Fredriksson K et al. described a 30% decrease in complex IV activity in limb skeletal muscles [12]. Several studies on experimental animals also reported that sepsis results in decreased mitochondrial respiration [13–16] and an increase in the mitochondrial production of reactive oxygen species (ROS) in skeletal muscle [17,18]. Sepsis has also been shown to increase the levels of morphologically abnormal mitochondria, such as those with disorganized cristae, translucent vacuoles and even myelin-like structures [13,19–21]. Recently, Owen et al. showed that persistent muscle weakness in mice that have survived sepsis is associated with abnormal mitochondrial ultrastructure, decreased respiration, decreased activity of complexes of the mitochondrial electron transfer system and persistent oxidative damage to muscle proteins [21].

In healthy muscles, damaged or dysfunctional mitochondria are selectively recycled in a process, known as mitophagy (selective autophagy of mitochondria), which is primarily regulated through the PINK1-Parkin pathway. Parkin, an E3 ubiquitin ligase encoded by the *Park2* gene, is a 465 amino acid protein that translocates to depolarized mitochondria to initiate mitophagy. Parkin-dependent mitophagy is regulated by PTEN-induced kinase 1 (PINK1), which acts upstream from Parkin. In healthy mitochondria, PINK1 is imported into the inner mitochondrial membrane and cleaved by PARL [22]. Cleaved PINK1 is then released into the cytosol where it is degraded by the proteasome system. In depolarized mitochondria, the importation of PINK1 into the inner mitochondrial membrane is blocked. PINK1 is no longer degraded and becomes phosphorylated and stabilized on the outer mitochondrial membrane [23–26]. Phosphorylated PINK1 triggers the recruitment of Parkin to the mitochondria. Parkin then ubiquitinates outer mitochondrial membrane proteins, including the fusion proteins MFN1, MFN2, MIRO and TOMM20 [27]. The degradation of MFN1 and MFN2 triggers mitochondrial fission and fragmentation, both of which are important to the recycling of mitochondria by the mitophagy pathway [28]. The functional importance of the PINK1-Parkin mitophagy pathway in regulating skeletal muscle mitochondrial function and quality in sepsis remains unknown. Recently, we reported that the genetic deletion of Parkin leads to the poor recovery of cardiac function in septic mice and increased sepsis-induced mitochondrial dysfunction in the heart [29]. We also demonstrated that autophagy is significantly induced in the skeletal muscles of septic mice and that the induction of autophagy is associated with increased muscle Parkin levels, suggesting that mitophagy was induced [20,30]. However, several morphologically and functionally abnormal mitochondria were observed in the electron micrographs of septic muscles, indicating that the mitophagy that was induced was likely insufficient to the task of completely recycling defective mitochondria [20,30]. Based on this reasoning, we hypothesized that enhancing mitophagy through Parkin overexpression would attenuate the impact of sepsis on skeletal muscles and their mitochondria. To test this hypothesis, Parkin was overexpressed for four weeks in the skeletal muscles of young mice using intramuscular injections of adeno-associated viruses (AAVs). The cecal ligation and perforation (CLP) procedure, a widely used model of sepsis [31], was used to induce sepsis. Sham-operated animals served as controls. We found that Parkin overexpression prevents sepsis-induced mitochondrial morphological injury and reverses the decline in mitochondrial protein content. We also found that Parkin overexpression protects against sepsis-induced myofiber atrophy. These findings indicate that defective mitophagy in sepsis can be therapeutically manipulated as a means of counteracting sepsis-induced muscle dysfunction.

2. Materials and Methods

2.1. Animal Procedures

All experiments were approved (#2014-7549) by the Research Ethics Board of the Research Institute of the McGill University Health Centre (MUHC-RI) and are in accordance with the principles outlined by the Canadian Council of Animal Care. Three-week-old male wild-type C57BL/6J mice (Charles River Laboratories, Saint-Constant, QC, Canada) were used for our experiments. All mice were group-housed under a standard 12:12 h light/dark cycle with food and water available ad libitum.

2.2. AAV Injections in Skeletal Muscle

All of the adeno-associated viruses (AAVs) used in our experiments were purchased from Vector Biolabs (Malvern, PA, USA) and were of Serotype 1, a serotype highly effective in transducing skeletal muscle cells [32]. Four-week-old mice were first anesthetized with an isoflurane (2.5 to 3.5%), and AAV1s containing a muscle specific promoter (muscle creatine kinase), a sequence coding for the reporter protein GFP and a sequence coding for Parkin (details on the AAV1 construction are available in Supplementary Figure S1) were then intramuscularly injected (25 μL per site; 1.5×10^{11} gc) into the gastrocnemius (GAS) muscles in the right leg. In this AAV1 construction, the sequences coding for Parkin and GFP were separated by a sequence coding for the auto-cleavable 2A peptide, allowing for the separation of the Parkin and GFP proteins once translated. Control AAV1s containing only the GFP sequence under the control of the MCK promoter were injected into the contralateral leg. Because the AAV1 recombination site in the wild-type AAV1s was deleted in these recombined AAV1s, both GFP and Parkin expression comprised episomal expression without integration into the host DNA.

2.3. Cecal Ligation and Perforation

After four weeks of AAV1 injection, the mice were subjected to cecal ligation and perforation or sham surgery. The cecal ligation and puncture (CLP) model, which closely mimics the clinical features of human sepsis [31], was performed to induce polymicrobial sepsis as described previously [30,33] with minor modifications. Briefly, the mice were first anesthetized with isoflurane (~3%; Piramal Critical Care). A midline abdominal incision (~2 cm) was then performed. The cecum was carefully ligated at ~1 cm from its distal portion. The ligated cecum was perforated by a through-and-through puncture performed with $25^{1/2}$ gauge needle in a sterile environment. Next, the ligated cecum was gently compressed to extrude a small amount of the cecal contents through the punctured holes. The cecum was then replaced in the abdominal cavity. The peritoneum was then closed in two separate layers using 3–0 absorbable polyfilament interrupted sutures. The skin was finally closed with a surgical staple (9 mm AutoClip® System, Fine Scientific tools, North Vancouver, BC, Canada). All of the animals received subcutaneous injections of buprenorphine (0.05 to 0.2 mg/kg in 1 mL of 0.9% saline) immediately after surgery. To minimize pain, buprenorphine was administered every 12 h (0.05 mg/kg in ~100 μL of 0.9% saline). The sham-operated mice were subjected to identical procedures with the exception of the cecum ligation and puncture. All of the animals were closely monitored for signs of excessive pain or distress, such as lack of movement, agonal breathing or excessive body loss (20%), by investigators and by the vivarium staff from the IR-MUHC. Any mouse reaching endpoint criteria was immediately euthanized.

2.4. Tissue Collection

Mice were anesthetized with isoflurane and subsequently euthanized by cervical dislocation 48 h after sham or CLP procedures. The gastrocnemius (GAS) muscles were carefully removed from both legs and cut in half; one half was mounted for histology and small strips were prepared for transmission electron microscope (TEM) analyses, as previously described [34]. The rest of the GAS was quickly frozen in liquid nitrogen and stored −80 °C until use for immunoblotting and qPCR experiments.

2.5. Fiber Size Determination

Muscles samples were mounted on plastic blocks in tragacanth gum and frozen in liquid isopentane cooled in liquid nitrogen. The samples were then stored until use at −80 °C. The samples were cut into 10 μm cross-sections using a cryostat (Leica Biosystem Inc., Concord, ON, Canada) at −20 °C and then mounted on lysine coated slides (Superfrost) to assess muscle fiber size, as described in [32,34]. To this end, the muscle cross-sections were first allowed to reach room temperature and were rehydrated with phosphate buffered saline (PBS, pH 7.2) and then blocked with goat serum (10% in PBS). The sections were then incubated with primary rabbit IgG polyclonal anti-laminin antibody (MilliporeSigma, Oakville, ON, Canada, L9393, 1:750) for 1 h at room temperature. The sections were then washed three times in PBS before being incubated for 1 h at room temperature with an Alexa Fluor 594 goat anti-rabbit IgG antibody (Invitrogen, Burlington, ON, Canada A-11037, 1:500). The sections were then washed three times in PBS and the slides were cover-slipped using Prolong Gold (Invitrogen, P36930) as mounting medium. The slides were imaged with a Zeiss Axio Imager 2 fluorescence microscope (Zeiss, Dorval, QC, Canada). The median minimum Feret's diameter of the muscle fibers, a reliable marker of myofiber size [35], was determined for each muscle sample using at least 200 fibers per muscle sample (average number ± SD of fiber analyzed for each group: sham AAV-GFP, 317 ± 62; sham AAV-Parkin, 300 ± 15; CLP AAV-GFP, 345 ± 30; CLP AAV-Parkin, 304 ± 46). Analyses were performed using ImageJ (NIH, Bethesda, MD, USA, https://imagej.nih.gov/ij/).

2.6. Transmission Electron Microscopy (TEM)

The samples for TEM were prepared as described in [34,36,37]. Briefly, small strips prepared from GAS were incubated in 2% glutaraldehyde buffer solution in 0.1 M cacodylate (pH 7.4) and were subsequently post-fixed in 1% osmium tetroxide in 0.1 M cacodylate buffer. Tissues were then dehydrated via increasing the concentrations of methanol to propylene oxide and infiltrated and embedded in EPON^{TM} resins at the Facility for Electron Microscopy Research (FEMR) of McGill University. Ultrathin sections (60 nm) were cut longitudinally using an ultramicrotome (Ultracut III, Reichert-Jung, Leica Biosystem Inc., Concord, ON, Canada) and mounted on nickel carbon-formvar-coated grids for electron microscopy. Uranyl acetate and lead citrate stained sections were then imaged using a FEI Tecnai 12 transmission electron microscope at 120 kV, and images were digitally captured using a XR80C CCD camera system (AMT, Woburn, MA, USA) at a magnification of 1400×. Individual intermyofibrillar (IMF) mitochondria from all groups were manually traced in longitudinal orientations using ImageJ 2.0.0 software (NIH, Bethesda, MD, USA, https://imagej.nih.gov/ij/) to measure the following morphological characteristics: area (in μm^2), perimeter (μm), circularity ($4\pi \cdot$(surface area/perimeter^2)), Feret's diameter (longest distance (μm) between any two points within a given mitochondrion), aspect ratio (major axis/minor axis)—a measure of the "length to width ratio" and form factor (perimeter/$4\pi \cdot$surface area)—a measure sensitive to the complexity and branching aspect of mitochondria [34,36,37]. An index of mitochondrial morphological complexity was finally calculated as follows: Mitochondrial complexity index = Aspect ratio × Form Factor. Details on the number of IMF mitochondria that were traced are available in the figure legends.

2.7. Immunoblotting

Frozen skeletal muscle tissues (15–30 mg) were homogenized in an ice-cold lysis buffer (50 mM Hepes, 150 mM NaCl, 100mM NaF, 5 mM EDTA, 0.5% Triton X-100, 0.1 mM DTT, 2 μg/mL leupeptin, 100 μg/mL PMSF, 2 μg/mL aprotinin, and 1 mg/100 mL pepstatin A, pH 7.2) using Mini-beadbeater (BioSpec Products) with a ceramic bead at 60 Hz. The muscle homogenates were kept on ice for 30 min with periodic agitation and were then centrifuged at 5000 g for 15 min at 4 °C, the supernatants were collected, and the pellets were discarded. The protein contents in each sample were determined using the Bradford method. The aliquots of crude muscle homogenates were mixed with Laemmli buffer (6×, reducing buffer, # BP111R, Boston BioProducts, Ashland, MA, USA) and subsequently denatured for 5 min at 95 °C. Equal amounts of protein extracts (30 μg per lanes) were separated by SDS-PAGE, and then transferred onto polyvinylidene difluoride (PVDF) membranes (Bio-Rad Laboratories, Saint-Laurent, QC, Canada) using a wet transfer technique. The total proteins on the membranes were detected with Ponceau-S solution (MilliporeSigma #P3504). The membranes were blocked in PBS + 1% Tween® 20 + 5% bovine serum albumin (BSA) for 1 h at room temperature and then incubated with the specific primary antibodies overnight at 4 °C. The complete list of antibodies used for immunoblots analysis can be found in Supplementary Table S1. Membranes were washed in PBST (3 × 5 min) and incubated with HRP-conjugated secondary anti-rabbit or anti-mouse secondary antibodies (Abcam, Toronto, ON, Canada, cat# Ab6728, Ab6721) for 1 h at room temperature, before further washing in PBST (3 × 5 min). Immunoreactivity was detected using an enhanced chemiluminescence substrate (Pierce™, Thermo Fisher Scientific, Saint-Laurent, QC, Canada) with the ChemiDoc™ XRS+ Imaging System. The optical densities (OD) of the protein bands were quantified using ImageLab software (Bio-Rad Laboratories) and normalized to loading control (Ponceau-stained PVDF membranes). Immunoblotting data are expressed as relative to Sham AAV-GFP.

2.8. Quantitative Real-Time PCR

Total RNA was extracted from frozen muscle samples using a PureLink™ RNA Mini Kit (Invitrogen Canada, Burlington, ON, Canada). The quantification and purity of RNA was assessed using the A260/A280 absorption method. Total RNA (2 μg) was reverse transcribed using a Superscript II® Reverse Transcriptase Kit and random primers (Invitrogen, Burlington, ON, Canada). The reactions were incubated at 42 °C for 50 min and at 90 °C for 5 min. The real-time PCR detection of mRNA expression was performed using a Prism® (Graphpad, San Diego, CA, USA) 7000 Sequence Detection System (Applied Biosystems, Foster, CA, USA). The cycle threshold (C_T) values were obtained for each target gene. The ΔC_T values (normalized gene expression) were calculated as C_T of target gene minus C_T of the geometric means of three housekeeping genes (*Cyclophilin B*, *β-Actin* and *18S*). The relative mRNA level quantifications of target genes were determined using the threshold cycle ($\Delta\Delta C_T$) method, as compared to sham AAV-GFP. The primer sequences for all genes are found in Supplementary Table S2.

2.9. Data Analysis and Statistics

All statistical analyses were performed using GraphPad Prism 8 (GraphPad, San Diego, CA, USA). Comparisons of initial body weight and body weight loss between sham-operated and CLP mice were performed using unpaired bilateral student t-tests (p-values < 0.05 were considered statistically significant). Comparisons of the effects of Parkin overexpression on parameters of interest were performed using two-way repeated measures analysis of variance (ANOVA) (except for comparisons of mitochondrial shape descriptors, as detailed below). Corrections for the multiple comparisons following two-way repeated measures ANOVA were performed with the two-stage step-up method of Benjamini and Krieger and Yekutieli (q < 0.1 was considered statistically significant). One-way ANOVA followed by the two-stage step-up method of Benjamini and Krieger and Yekutieli were used for the following comparisons: sham AAV-GFP vs. CLP AAV-GFP; sham AAV-GFP vs. CLP

AAV-Parkin; sham AAV-Parkin vs. CLP AAV-GFP; sham AAV-Parkin vs. CLP AAV-Parkin (except for comparisons of mitochondrial shape descriptors, as detailed below) ($q < 0.1$ was considered statistically significant). Differences for the median values of shape descriptors to assess mitochondrial morphology were assessed using a Kruskal–Wallis test followed by a Dunn's multiple comparisons test (adjusted p-values < 0.05 were considered statistically significant). The exact numbers of animals within each group in all figures are indicated in the figure legends.

3. Results

3.1. Successful Overexpression of Parkin in Skeletal Muscles of Sham and CLP Operated Mice

Four weeks after the intramuscular injections of AAVs, mice were subjected to cecal ligation and perforation (CLP) to induced polymicrobial sepsis. Sham-operated mice were used as control. At baseline (prior to sham and CLP procedures), body weight values were similar in the sham and CLP groups, as shown in Figure 1A. Body weight loss was more pronounced in the CLP group relative to the sham group ($-13.8 \pm 1.4\%$ vs. $-4.7\pm1.1\%$, respectively, $p < 0.05$), as shown in Figure 1B. As shown in Figure 1C,D, the intramuscular injection of AAV-Parkin significantly increased *Park2* mRNA expression and Parkin protein content, in the skeletal muscles of both Sham-operated and CLP mice. These results demonstrate that our approach was successful in overexpressing Parkin in mouse skeletal muscle.

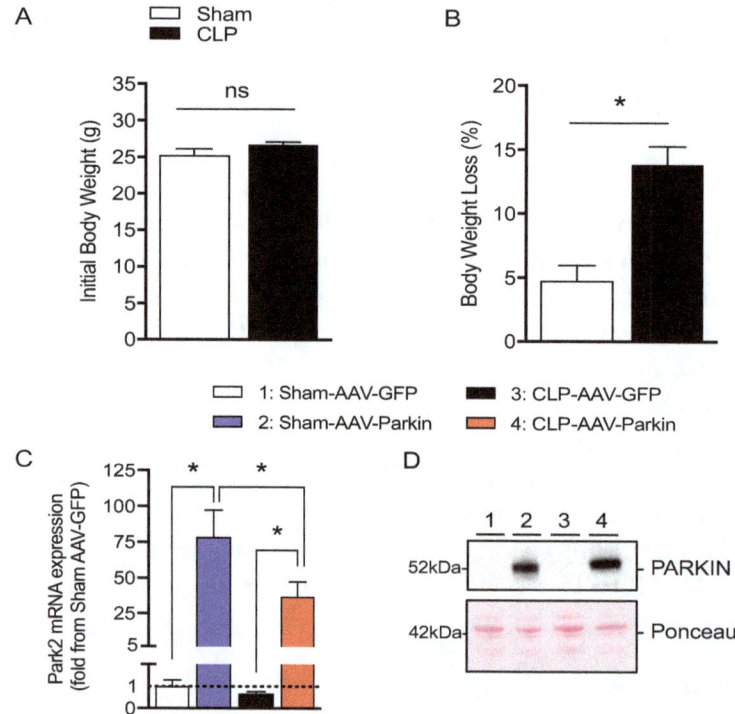

Figure 1. Effective Parkin overexpression in skeletal muscles of Sham and CLP operated mice. (**A**) Initial body weight and (**B**) percent of body weight loss in Sham-operated and or CLP mice. (**C**) qPCR analysis of *Park2* expression levels in the gastrocnemius muscles injected with either AAV-GFP or AAV-Parkin in Sham and CLP mice. (**D**) Representative Parkin immunoblots and its corresponding ponceau S stain performed on gastrocnemius samples of Sham and CLP mice injected with either AAV-GFP or AAV-Parkin. 1 = Sham-AAV-GFP; 2 = Sham-AAV-Parkin; 3 = CLP-AAV-GFP; 4 = CLP-AAV-Parkin. Data are presented as mean ± SEM ($n = 7$–9/group; * = statistically significant; ns = not statistically significant).

3.2. Parkin Overexpression Attenuates Sepsis-Induced Skeletal Muscle Atrophy

The effect of Parkin overexpression on muscle fiber size was evaluated 48 h after CLP, based on our previous reports which revealed that limb muscle atrophy develops at this time point [30,33]. In the sham group, Parkin expressing muscles had larger myofiber diameters relative to those expressing GFP, as shown in Figure 2B,C. This observation is in line with our previous report [32]. In the CLP group, GFP expressing muscles displayed a trend towards smaller myofiber diameters and a decreased proportion of large fibers relative to those expressing GFP in the sham group, as shown in Figure 2B,D, all of which are indicative of myofiber atrophy. As shown Figure 2B,E, no sign of atrophy was detected in the Parkin overexpressing muscles of CLP mice when compared to the Parkin expressing muscles of Sham-operated mice. In addition, the Parkin overexpressing muscles of CLP mice displayed larger myofibers vs. the GFP expressing muscles of CLP mice, as shown in Figure 2B,F. These results indicate that Parkin overexpression prevented the development of muscle atrophy in the CLP group and increased muscle fiber diameter in the sham group.

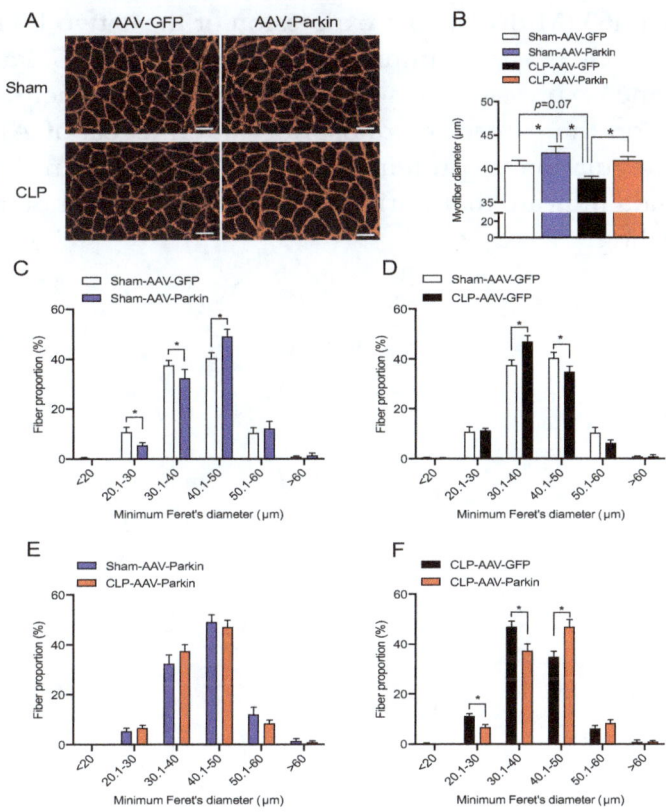

Figure 2. The impact of Parkin overexpression and sepsis on skeletal muscle fiber size. (**A**) Representative gastrocnemius (GAS) cryosections stained for laminin in all experimental groups. Scale bar: 50μm. (**B**) Quantification of minimum Ferret diameter of GAS myofibers of Sham and CLP animals injected with either AAV-GFP or AAV-Parkin. (**C**) Minimum Ferret distribution of the GAS myofibers of Sham AAV-GFP ($n = 8$ mice; 316 ± 21 fibers per GAS were traced) vs. Sham AAV-Parkin ($n = 8$ mice; 300 ± 5 fibers per GAS were traced). (**D**) Minimum Ferret distribution of the GAS myofibers of Sham AAV-GFP ($n = 8$ mice; 316 ± 21 fibers per GAS were traced) vs. CLP AAV-GFP ($n = 6$ mice; 345 ± fibers per GAS were traced). (**E**) Minimum Ferret distribution of the GAS myofibers of Sham AAV-Parkin ($n = 8$ mice; 300 ± 5 fibers per GAS were traced) vs. CLP AAV-Parkin ($n = 6$ mice; 304 ± 18 fibers per GAS were traced). (**F**) Minimum Ferret distribution of the GAS myofibers of CLP AAV-GFP ($n = 6$ mice; 345 ± fibers per GAS were traced) vs. CLP AAV-Parkin ($n = 6$ mice; 304 ± 18 fibers per GAS were traced). Data are presented as mean ± SEM. ($n = 6$–8/group; * = statistically significant).

3.3. The Impact of Parkin Overexpression and Sepsis on Skeletal Muscle Catabolic Signaling

We then investigated whether Parkin overexpression and sepsis affect the expression levels of apoptotic and autophagy-related genes. Neither Parkin overexpression nor sepsis affected the mRNA levels of pro-apoptotic *Bax*, *Bid*, *Bim*, and anti-apoptotic *Bcl2*, depicted in Figure 3A. As shown in Figure 3A, the expression level of BclXL was higher in septic animals. qPCR analyses revealed a significant increase in the mRNA levels of *Lc3b*, *Sqstm1*, *Gabarapl* and *Bnip3* in septic mice, shown in Figure 3B. The expression of *Gabarapl* was significantly higher in the Parkin overexpressing muscles of septic animals. No other impacts of Parkin overexpression on apoptotic and autophagy-related genes were observed. In line with our gene expression data, the protein contents of SQSTM1 (also known as p62) and BNIP3, two proteins regulating autophagy and mitophagy, were increased in septic animals, as shown in Figure 3C–E. The ratio of LC3-II to LC3-I was significantly increased in septic mice, suggesting an induction of autophagy, shown in Figure 3F. No impact of Parkin overexpression on the content of SQSTM1 and BNIP3 and the LC3-II to LC3-I ratio could be evidenced. We then assessed the expression levels of two key E3 ligases known to contribute to skeletal muscle atrophy [38,39], Fbxo32 (Atrogin-1) and Trim63 (MuRF1). The expression of these two E3 ligases was significantly increased in the skeletal muscle of septic animals, shown in Figure 3G. Parkin overexpression did not impact Fbxo32 and Trim63 expression. It is worth mentioning that neither Parkin overexpression nor sepsis had an impact on the content or phosphorylation levels of AKT and 4EBP1, two key proteins involved in the regulation of protein synthesis, as shown in Supplementary Figure S2. Taken altogether, these data indicate that Parkin overexpression did not attenuate sepsis-induced increases in catabolic signaling.

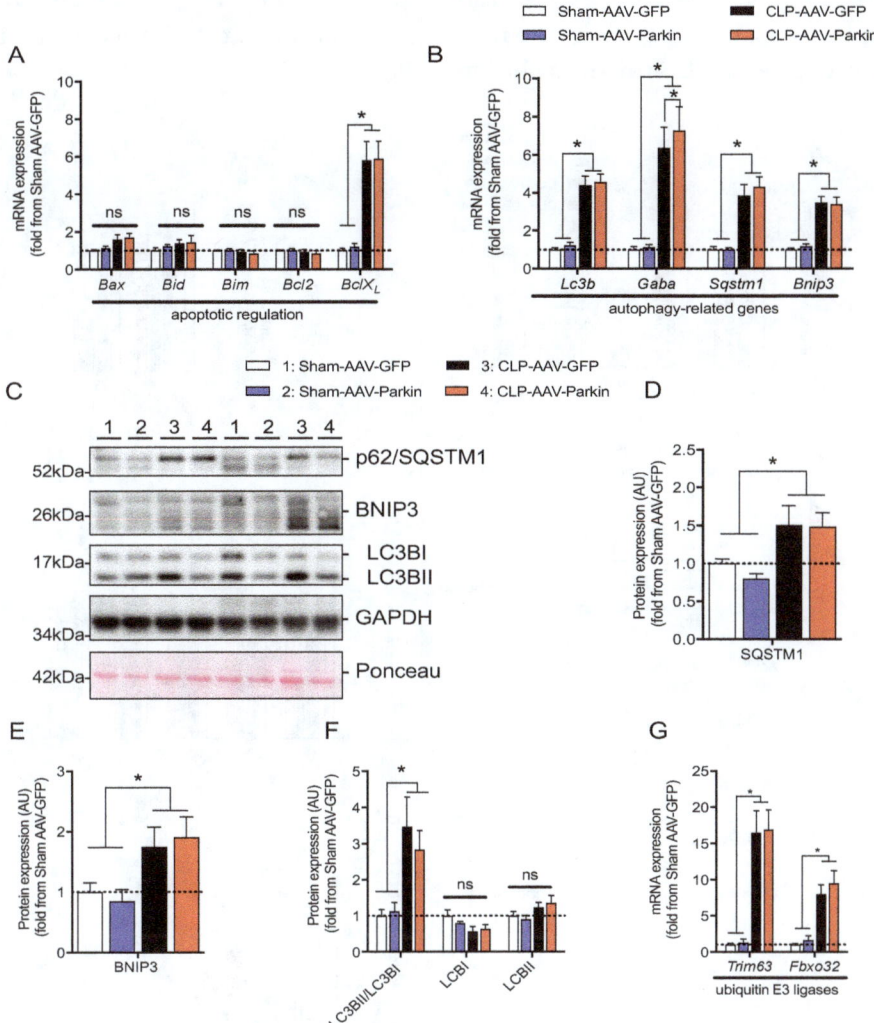

Figure 3. The impact of Parkin overexpression and sepsis on skeletal muscle catabolic signaling. (**A**) qPCR analysis of the mRNA expression of genes regulating apoptosis in the gastrocnemius (GAS) muscles of Sham and CLP animals injected with either AAV-GFP or AAV-Parkin. (**B**) qPCR analysis of autophagy-related gene expression in the gastrocnemius (GAS) muscles of Sham and CLP animals injected with either AAV-GFP or AAV-Parkin. *Gaba.* refers to *Gabarapl1*. (**C**) Immunoblot detection of SQSMT1(p62), BNIP3, LC3I/LC3II and GAPDH. (**D**) Quantification of SQSMT1 (p62) content. (**E**) Quantification of BNIP3 protein content. (**F**) Quantification of LC3I and LC3II protein content, as well as the LC3II to LC3I ratio. (**G**) qPCR analysis of *Fbxo32* (Atrogin-1) and *Trim63* (MuRF1) gene expression levels in the GAS muscles of Sham and CLP animals injected with either AAV-GFP or AAV-Parkin. 1 = Sham-AAV-GFP; 2 = Sham-AAV-Parkin; 3 = CLP-AAV-GFP; 4 = CLP-AAV-Parkin. Data are presented as mean ± SEM. (n = 6–9/group, * = statistically significant; ns = not statistically significant).

3.4. The Impact of Parkin Overexpression and Sepsis on the Expression of Genes and Proteins Regulating Mitochondrial Biology

Since Parkin plays a key role in mitochondrial quality control [23–26,40], and because sepsis is well known to impair mitochondrial function, we investigated whether Parkin overexpression could attenuate the impact of sepsis on skeletal muscle mitochondria. To this end, we first quantified the expression levels of the key transcriptional regulators of mitochondrial biology. As shown in Figure 4A,B, sepsis resulted in an increase in *Nrf1, Nrf2,* and *Sirt1* mRNA expression levels. In contrast, sepsis resulted in a decrease in the expression of *Pgc1-α, Tfam and Sirt3*, as shown in Figure 4A,B. In the skeletal muscles of both Sham-operated and CLP mice, Parkin overexpression resulted in a significant increase in *Nrf2* mRNA expression, depicted in Figure 4A. Parkin overexpression also led to an increased expression of *Sirt1* in the muscles of Sham-operated mice and an increase in *Tfam* expression in the muscles of CLP mice, as shown in Figure 4B.

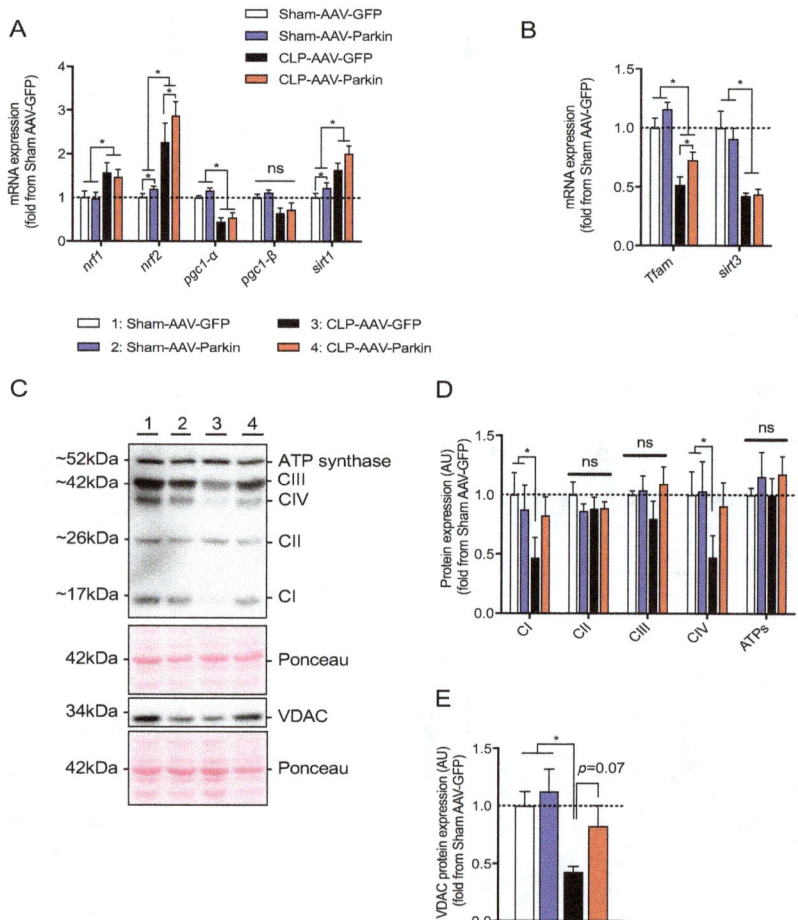

Figure 4. The impact of Parkin overexpression and sepsis in skeletal muscle on genes regulating mitochondrial biogenesis and on mitochondrial protein contents. (**A,B**) qPCR analysis of genes involved in mitochondrial biology. (**C**) Representative immunoblots performed with primary antibodies against representative subunits of the OXPHOS complexes and VDAC. Ponceau stains were used as loading controls. (**D,E**) Quantification of the contents of (**D**) representative subunits of the OXPHOS complexes and (**E**) VDAC. 1 = Sham-AAV-GFP; 2 = Sham-AAV-Parkin; 3 = CLP-AAV-GFP; 4 = CLP-AAV-Parkin. Data are presented as mean ± SEM. (n = 6–9/group, * = statistically significant; ns = not statistically significant).

We next assessed the impact of sepsis and Parkin overexpression on the content of proteins of the mitochondrial oxidative phosphorylation (OXPHOS) system. As shown in Figure 4D, sepsis significantly decreased the content of the representative subunits of Complex I and Complex IV. This finding is consistent with previous reports, which documented decreased mitochondrial contents in septic skeletal muscles [10,12–14]. Similarly, sepsis lowered VDAC protein content by 58% in the GFP expressing skeletal muscles, as shown in Figure 4E. Importantly, no impact of sepsis was observed on Complex I, Complex IV and VDAC contents in the Parkin overexpressing muscles, as shown in Figure 4D,E. Taken together, these data strongly suggest that Parkin overexpression prevented the inhibitory effect of sepsis on muscle mitochondrial content.

3.5. Effects of Parkin Overexpression and Sepsis on Mitochondrial Morphology and Dynamics

To analyze the impact of sepsis and Parkin overexpression on skeletal muscle mitochondrial morphology, we used TEM to evaluate the morphology of intermyofibrillar (IMF) mitochondria of the GAS of sham and CLP mice. Representative TEM images obtained from the GAS of sham and CLP mice are shown in Figure 5A–D and Supplemental Figure S3. In the CLP group, IMF mitochondria of GFP expressing muscles were larger, less circular and more complex (i.e., higher values of aspect ratio and form factor) than IMF mitochondria of GFP expressing muscles of the sham group, shown in Figure 5E–J. In the sham group, Parkin overexpressing muscles had larger, less circular and more complex IMF mitochondria compared to GFP expressing muscles, as shown in Figure 5E–J. In the CLP group, Parkin overexpressing muscles had smaller, more circular and simpler IMF mitochondria compared to GFP expressing counterparts, shown in Figure 5 E–J. Taken together, these results indicate that sepsis results in enlarged and more complex mitochondria, an impact that is abolished by Parkin overexpression.

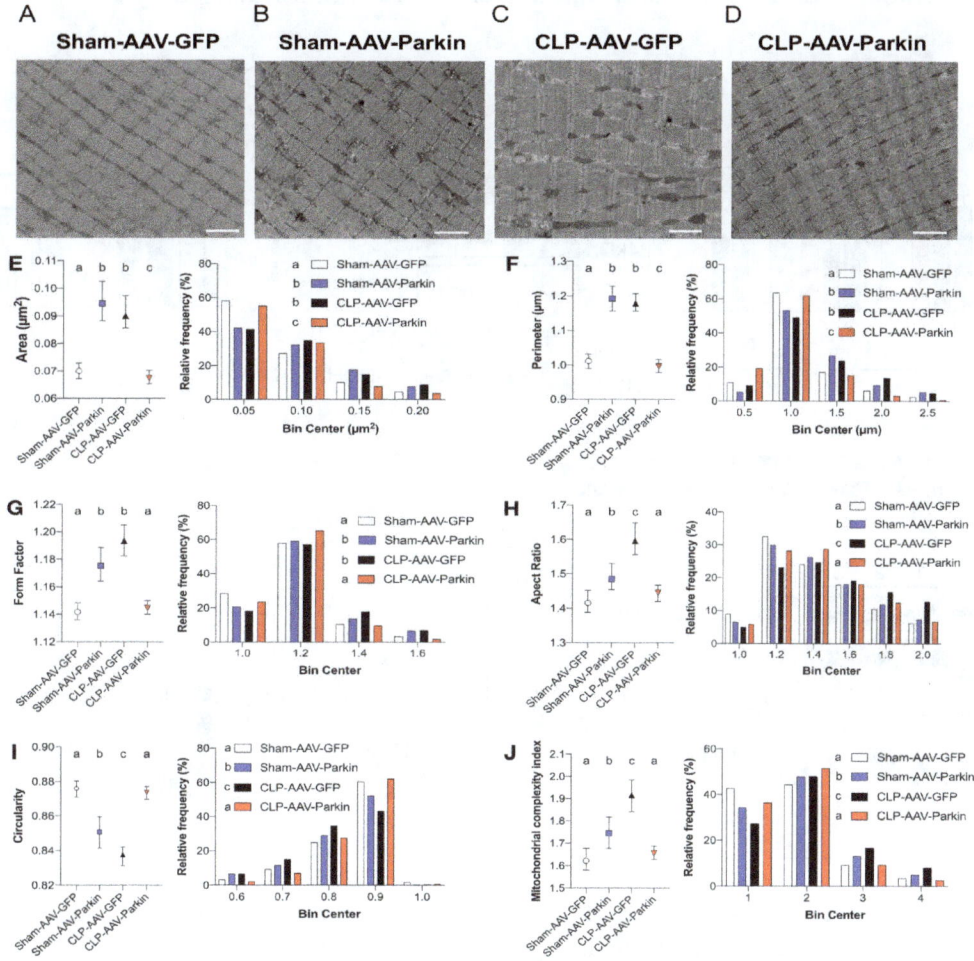

Figure 5. The impact of sepsis and Parkin overexpression on mitochondrial morphology in skeletal muscle. (**A–D**) Representative longitudinal TEM images from all groups that were used to assess mitochondrial morphology. Scale bar: 2μm. (**E–J**) Median values with 95% confidence interval (left) and relative frequencies (right) of multiple mitochondrial shape descriptors (Sham-AAV-GFP: $n = 1246$; Sham-AAV-Parkin: $n = 728$; CLP-AAV-GFP: $n = 1149$; CLP-AAV-Parkin: $n = 1206$). Groups not sharing a letter are significantly different (differences were tested using a Kruskal–Wallis test followed by a Dunn's multiple comparisons test; $p < 0.05$).

To gain better insights into the mechanisms underlying the impact of sepsis and Parkin overexpression on mitochondrial morphology, we next assessed the expression and content of major genes and proteins regulating mitochondrial dynamics. In the Sham-operated mice, Parkin overexpression had no impact on the mRNA expression and protein levels of *Mfn2*, *Opa1* and *Drp1*, as shown in Figure 6A–G. As shown in Figure 6A, sepsis in GFP expressing muscles resulted in a decrease in the mRNA levels of pro-fusion *Mfn2* and *Opa1* and pro-fission *Drp1*. In Parkin overexpressing muscles, CLP resulted in a significant decrease in the mRNA levels of Mfn2 and Drp1, while Opa1 expression remained unaffected, shown in Figure 6A. At the protein level, no impact of sepsis or Parkin overexpression could be evidenced on MFN2 and OPA1 protein content. Interestingly, DRP1 protein levels were lower in the GFP and Parkin expressing muscles of CLP mice, relative to the sham group, as shown in Figure 6D,E. Similarly, DRP1 phosphorylation on Ser[616], an activation site which triggers DRP1 translocation from the cytoplasm to mitochondria to promote mitochondrial fission [41], was also decreased in the GFP and Parkin expressing muscles of the CLP group, relative to the sham group, as shown in Figure 6D–G. These results indicate that sepsis seems to result in an inhibition of mitochondrial fission and that this effect was not influenced by Parkin overexpression.

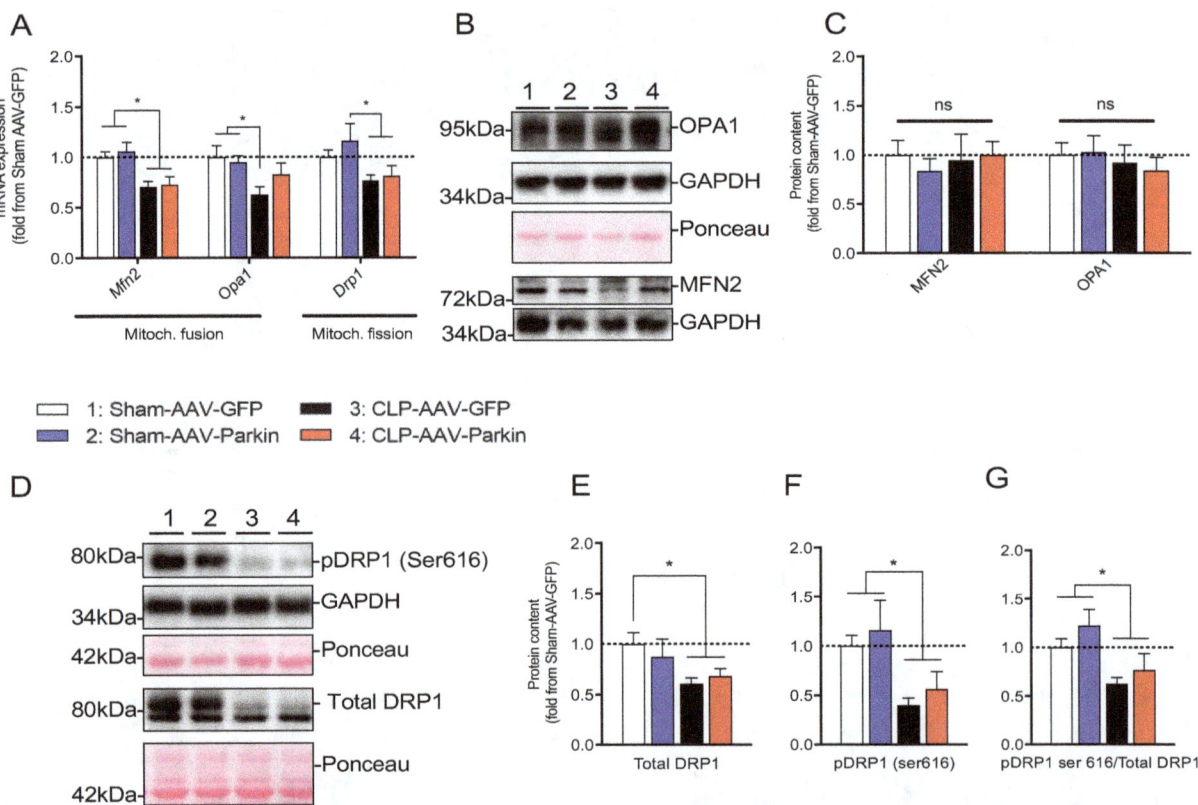

Figure 6. The impact of sepsis and Parkin overexpression on mitochondrial dynamics in skeletal muscle. (**A**) qPCR analysis of mitochondrial dynamic-related gene expression in the GAS muscles of Sham and CLP animals injected with either AAV-GFP or AAV-Parkin. (**B**) Representative immunoblots of OPA1, GADPH and MFN2. Ponceau stains or GAPDH immunoblots were used as loading controls. (**C**) Quantification of OPA1, GADPH and MFN2 content. (**D**) Representative immunoblots performed with primary antibodies against pDRP1(ser616) and total DRP1. Ponceau stains or GAPDH immunoblots were used as loading controls. (**E**) Quantification of DRP1 content. (**F**) Quantification of the contents of pDRP1(ser 616) content. (**G**) Quantification of the pDRP1(ser 616) to total DRP1 ratio. 1 = Sham-AAV-GFP; 2 = Sham-AAV-Parkin; 3 = CLP-AAV-GFP; 4 = CLP-AAV-Parkin. Data are presented as mean ± SEM. (*n* = 6–9/group; * = statistically significant; ns = not statistically significant).

4. Discussion

The accumulation of dysfunctional and injured mitochondria in skeletal muscles is believed to play a key role in the development of muscle weakness during sepsis [8,9]. In the current study, we investigated whether overexpressing Parkin, a key component of the PINK1-Parkin mitophagy pathway, could attenuate the negative impact of sepsis on skeletal muscles and their mitochondria. The current study indicates that Parkin overexpression prevented sepsis-induced accumulation of enlarged and complex mitochondria in the limb muscles of mice. Parkin overexpression also attenuated the sepsis-induced decrease in the content of complexes I and IV of the mitochondrial electron transfer system and prevented the development of limb muscle atrophy in septic mice. These results expand recent studies demonstrating that Parkin exerts protective effects on skeletal muscle health. Indeed, our group has recently reported that $Park2^{-/-}$ mice have decreased limb muscle contractility, depressed muscle mitochondrial respiration, increased mitochondrial uncoupling and enhanced susceptibility to the opening of mitochondrial permeability transition pore compared to wild-type (WT) mice [42]. $Park2^{-/-}$ mice also exhibit the impaired recovery of cardiac contractility and depressed cardiac mitochondrial functions in sepsis [29]. More recently, Peker et al. have reported that Parkin knockdown in C2C12 cells results in myotubular atrophy and that $Park2^{-/-}$ mice have decreased muscle mitochondrial respiration and increased levels of reactive oxygen species and fiber atrophy [43]. Parkin overexpression in the muscles of *Drosophila melanogaster* increased mitochondrial content, decreased proteotoxicity and extended lifespan [44]. Our finding that Parkin overexpression in the Sham group increased limb muscle fiber diameters is in accordance with our recent study documenting that Parkin overexpression for several months in young mice causes muscle hypertrophy, while in old mice, Parkin overexpression attenuates ageing-related loss of muscle mass and strength, increases mitochondrial content and enzymatic activities and protects from ageing-related oxidative stress, fibrosis and apoptosis [32]. Taken together, our current findings and published studies highlight the protective role that Parkin plays in skeletal muscle health.

Our findings that sepsis elicits distinct changes in skeletal muscle mitochondria, such as decreased VDAC level (a marker of mitochondrial content [45–47]), the downregulation of three mitochondrial biogenesis genes (*Pgc1-α*, *Tfam* and *Sirt3*) and decreased complexes I and IV levels, are in agreement with published studies on septic humans and experimental animals [10,12–14,20]. We report for the first time that Parkin overexpression in skeletal muscle prevents the inhibitory effects of sepsis on the expression of *Tfam* and on the content of complexes I and IV, as well as VDAC. Based on these results, we speculate that Parkin overexpression might have improved mitochondrial functions in septic muscles. This speculation is supported by the observation that Parkin overexpression increases mitochondrial content and enzymatic activities in normal skeletal muscles [32,44]. We should emphasize that, in the current study, Parkin overexpression increased *Nrf2* expression in the skeletal muscles of septic animals. Considering the role that this transcription factor has in the regulation of the expression of several anti-oxidant enzymes [48], we anticipate that increased *Nrf2* levels in muscles overexpressing Parkin might have contributed to the protection of mitochondrial morphology and contents in septic animals.

Mitochondria form a dynamic network constantly undergoing fusion and fission events that tightly regulate the shape (i.e., morphology), size and number of mitochondria [41,49]. In the present study, we show that sepsis significantly alters mitochondrial morphology by increasing the proportion of enlarged and more complex IMF mitochondria. These results extend previous observations, showing that sepsis causes major alterations of the mitochondrial ultrastructure in skeletal muscle [13,19–21]. This increase in mitochondrial size and complexity in septic muscles might have been caused by decreased DRP1 contents and activation [41], which are expected to alter the fusion/fission balance towards increased mitochondrial fusion. Since mitochondrial fission is required for mitochondrial degradation through mitophagy [50], it is possible that decreased DRP1 content and activation may play a role in the accumulation of damaged and dysfunctional mitochondria in septic muscles by impairing muscle capacity to recycle dysfunctional mitochondria through the mitophagy pathway.

It should also be noted that a decrease in DRP1 content per se might have also played a role in myofiber atrophy. Indeed, a recent study showed that muscle-specific DRP1 deletion results in severe muscle dysfunction, characterized by atrophy, weakness, fiber degeneration and mitochondrial dysfunction [51]. Importantly, we found that Parkin overexpression attenuated sepsis-induced changes in mitochondrial morphology and rendered muscle mitochondria to be smaller, more circular and simpler, relative to muscles expressing GFP. These findings are in agreement with previous reports, indicating that Parkin overexpression in skeletal muscles and neurons stimulates mitochondrial fragmentation [44,52]. We speculate that the decrease in mitochondrial size and complexity in septic muscles overexpressing Parkin might have facilitated the recycling of damaged/dysfunctional mitochondria.

A puzzling result of the present study is the increase in the proportion of enlarged and more complex mitochondria in the Parkin overexpressing muscles of sham-operated mice. The mechanisms behind the differences in the effects of Parkin on mitochondrial morphology in the sham and CLP groups remain unclear. We should point out, however, that although Parkin overexpression altered the mitochondrial morphology in skeletal muscles, none of the parameters related to mitochondrial dynamics that we investigated were affected by Parkin overexpression. Indeed, no significant impact of Parkin overexpression on the expression and protein content of MFN2, OPA1 and DRP1 was evident. Furthermore, Parkin overexpression had no effect on DRP1 phosphorylation on Ser^{616}, suggesting that there was no change in DRP1 activity. Further studies are therefore required to identify the mechanisms underlying the differential impact of Parkin overexpression on skeletal muscle mitochondrial morphology in healthy and septic animals.

In the current study, we report data indicating that autophagy was induced in septic skeletal muscles, as evidenced by the increased expression of several autophagy-related genes, including *Lc3b*, *Gabarapl1*, and *Sqstm1*, and by the increase in the LC3B-II/LC3B-I ratio in the muscles of CLP mice. These findings are in agreement with previous reports, which documented increased muscle autophagy in various models of sepsis [20,30,53]. An interesting finding in our study is that Parkin overexpression had no effects on the expression of autophagy-related genes and the LC3B-II/LC3B-I ratios in the sham and CLP groups. Given the key role that Parkin plays in the recycling of dysfunctional mitochondria by autophagosomes [23,50], our results indicate that basal and activated autophagy levels in normal and septic muscles, respectively, were sufficient to deal with increased mitophagy in muscles overexpressing Parkin. We also observed that BNIP3 mRNA and protein levels increased significantly in septic skeletal muscles, and that this induction was not influenced by Parkin overexpression. The BNIP3 protein localizes to the mitochondria and promotes PINK1-Parkin-independent mitophagy by interacting with the LC3 protein, resulting in the recruitment of autophagosomes to damaged mitochondria [54]. The lack of changes in BNIP3 levels in response to Parkin overexpression suggests that BNIP3-mediated mitophagy functions in an independent fashion to that of the PINK1-Parkin pathway. It is worth mentioning that the present study suffers from several limitations. First, we did not directly assess whether Parkin overexpression actually translates into increased mitophagic flux. Although it was recently reported that Parkin overexpression is sufficient to trigger higher mitochondrial clearance in cardiomyocytes [55], further studies should investigate whether Parkin overexpression is sufficient to increase mitophagy in healthy and septic skeletal muscles. Another important limitation arises from the fact that muscle contractility was not assessed in the present study. Further studies are therefore required to define whether Parkin overexpression can attenuate sepsis-induced skeletal muscle weakness.

5. Conclusions

The present study provides evidence that Parkin overexpression attenuates sepsis-induced myofiber atrophy and prevents sepsis-induced changes in mitochondrial morphology and protein contents. These findings suggest that targeting mitophagy may represent a promising therapeutic strategy to attenuate sepsis-induced skeletal muscle wasting.

Author Contributions: Designed and Conceived this Study, J.-P.L.-G., G.G. and S.N.A.H.; Collected, Analyzed and Interpreted the Data, Prepared all figures and tables and Wrote the first draft of the manuscript, J.-P.L.-G.; O.R., T.J.C., D.M. and F.E.B. were involved in data collection and analyses; G.G. and S.N.A.H. supervised the research, contributed to data analysis and interpretation and wrote the final version of the manuscript with J.-P.L.-G. Funding Acquisition: G.G. and S.N.A.H. All authors have read and approved the final version of the manuscript.

Acknowledgments: We thank Jeannie Mui from the Facility for Electron Microscopy Research (FEMR, McGill University, Montreal, QC, Canada) for her support and expertise. We are grateful for the technical support provided by Laurent Huck and the staff of the Meakins-Christie Laboratories at the Research Institute of the McGill University Health Center. We would like to thank Basil Petrof (McGill University and RI-MUHC) for his thoughtful discussions related to this study.

References

1. Angus, D.C.; van der Poll, T. Severe sepsis and septic shock. *N. Engl. J. Med.* **2013**, *369*, 840–851. [CrossRef] [PubMed]

2. Khan, J.; Harrison, T.B.; Rich, M.M.; Moss, M. Early development of critical illness myopathy and neuropathy in patients with severe sepsis. *Neurology* **2006**, *67*, 1421–1425. [CrossRef] [PubMed]

3. Tennila, A.; Salmi, T.; Pettila, V.; Roine, R.O.; Varpula, T.; Takkunen, O. Early signs of critical illness polyneuropathy in icu patients with systemic inflammatory response syndrome or sepsis. *Intensive Care Med.* **2000**, *26*, 1360–1363. [CrossRef] [PubMed]

4. Supinski, G.S.; Callahan, L.A. Diaphragm weakness in mechanically ventilated critically ill patients. *Crit. Care* **2013**, *17*, R120. [CrossRef] [PubMed]

5. De Jonghe, B.; Bastuji-Garin, S.; Durand, M.C.; Malissin, I.; Rodrigues, P.; Cerf, C.; Outin, H.; Sharshar, T. Respiratory weakness is associated with limb weakness and delayed weaning in critical illness. *Crit. Care Med.* **2007**, *35*, 2007–2015. [CrossRef]

6. Ali, N.A.; O'Brien, J.M., Jr.; Hoffmann, S.P.; Phillips, G.; Garland, A.; Finley, J.C.; Almoosa, K.; Hejal, R.; Wolf, K.M.; Lemeshow, S.; et al. Acquired weakness, handgrip strength, and mortality in critically ill patients. *Am. J. Respir. Crit. Care Med.* **2008**, *178*, 261–268. [CrossRef]

7. Iwashyna, T.J.; Ely, E.W.; Smith, D.M.; Langa, K.M. Long-term cognitive impairment and functional disability among survivors of severe sepsis. *JAMA* **2010**, *304*, 1787–1794. [CrossRef]

8. Friedrich, O.; Reid, M.; Van den Berghe, G.; Vanhorebeek, I.; Hermans, G.; Rich, M.; Larsson, L. The sick and the weak: Neuropathies/myopathies in the critically ill. *Physiol. Rev.* **2015**, *95*, 1025–1109. [CrossRef]

9. Callahan, L.A.; Supinski, G.S. Sepsis-induced myopathy. *Crit. Care Med.* **2009**, *37*, S354–S367. [CrossRef]

10. Brealey, D.; Brand, M.; Hargreaves, I.; Heales, S.; Land, J.; Smolenski, R.; Davies, N.A.; Cooper, C.E.; Singer, M. Association between mitochondrial dysfunction and severity and outcome of septic shock. *Lancet* **2002**, *360*, 219–223. [CrossRef]

11. Brealey, D.; Karyampudi, S.; Jacques, T.S.; Novelli, M.; Stidwill, R.; Taylor, V.; Smolenski, R.T.; Singer, M. Mitochondrial dysfunction in a long-term rodent model of sepsis and organ failure. *Am. J. Physiol. Regul. Integr. Comp. Physiol.* **2004**, *286*, R491–R497. [CrossRef] [PubMed]

12. Fredriksson, K.; Hammarqvist, F.; Strigard, K.; Hultenby, K.; Ljungqvist, O.; Wernerman, J.; Rooyackers, O. Derangements in mitochondrial metabolism in intercostal and leg muscle of critically ill patients with sepsis-induced multiple organ failure. *Am. J. Physiol. Endocrinol. Metab.* **2006**, *291*, E1044–E1050. [CrossRef] [PubMed]

13. Rooyackers, O.E.; Kersten, A.H.; Wagenmakers, A.J. Mitochondrial protein content and in vivo synthesis rates in skeletal muscle from critically ill rats. *Clin. Sci. (Lond.)* **1996**, *91*, 475–481. [CrossRef] [PubMed]

14. Callahan, L.A.; Supinski, G.S. Sepsis induces diaphragm electron transport chain dysfunction and protein depletion. *Am. J. Respir Crit. Care Med.* **2005**, *172*, 861–868. [CrossRef] [PubMed]

15. Crouser, E.D.; Julian, M.W.; Blaho, D.V.; Pfeiffer, D.R. Endotoxin-induced mitochondrial damage correlates with impaired respiratory activity. *Crit. Care Med.* **2002**, *30*, 276–284. [CrossRef]

16. Protti, A.; Carre, J.; Frost, M.T.; Taylor, V.; Stidwill, R.; Rudiger, A.; Singer, M. Succinate recovers mitochondrial oxygen consumption in septic rat skeletal muscle. *Crit. Care Med.* **2007**, *35*, 2150–2155. [CrossRef]

17. Alvarez, S.; Boveris, A. Mitochondrial nitric oxide metabolism in rat muscle during endotoxemia. *Free Radic Biol. Med.* **2004**, *37*, 1472–1478. [CrossRef]

18. Vanasco, V.; Cimolai, M.C.; Evelson, P.; Alvarez, S. The oxidative stress and the mitochondrial dysfunction caused by endotoxemia are prevented by alpha-lipoic acid. *Free Radic. Res.* **2008**, *42*, 815–823. [CrossRef]

19. Welty-Wolf, K.E.; Simonson, S.G.; Huang, Y.C.; Fracica, P.J.; Patterson, J.W.; Piantadosi, C.A. Ultrastructural changes in skeletal muscle mitochondria in gram-negative sepsis. *Shock* **1996**, *5*, 378–384. [CrossRef]

20. Mofarrahi, M.; Sigala, I.; Guo, Y.; Godin, R.; Davis, E.C.; Petrof, B.; Sandri, M.; Burelle, Y.; Hussain, S.N. Autophagy and skeletal muscles in sepsis. *PLoS ONE* **2012**, *7*, e47265. [CrossRef]

21. Owen, A.M.; Patel, S.P.; Smith, J.D.; Balasuriya, B.K.; Mori, S.F.; Hawk, G.S.; Stromberg, A.J.; Kuriyama, N.; Kaneki, M.; Rabchevsky, A.G.; et al. Chronic muscle weakness and mitochondrial dysfunction in the absence of sustained atrophy in a preclinical sepsis model. *eLife* **2019**, *8*. [CrossRef] [PubMed]

22. Jin, S.M.; Lazarou, M.; Wang, C.; Kane, L.A.; Narendra, D.P.; Youle, R.J. Mitochondrial membrane potential regulates pink1 import and proteolytic destabilization by parl. *J. Cell Biol.* **2010**, *191*, 933–942. [CrossRef] [PubMed]

23. Narendra, D.; Tanaka, A.; Suen, D.-F.; Youle, R.J. Parkin is recruited selectively to impaired mitochondria and promotes their autophagy. *J. Cell Biol.* **2008**, *183*, 795–803. [CrossRef] [PubMed]

24. Narendra, D.P.; Jin, S.M.; Tanaka, A.; Suen, D.-F.; Gautier, C.A.; Shen, J.; Cookson, M.R.; Youle, R.J. Pink1 is selectively stabilized on impaired mitochondria to activate parkin. *PLoS Biol.* **2010**, *8*, e1000298. [CrossRef]

25. Vives-Bauza, C.; Zhou, C.; Huang, Y.; Cui, M.; de Vries, R.L.; Kim, J.; May, J.; Tocilescu, M.A.; Liu, W.; Ko, H.S.; et al. Pink1-dependent recruitment of parkin to mitochondria in mitophagy. *Proc. Natl. Acad. Sci. USA* **2010**, *107*, 378–383. [CrossRef]

26. Matsuda, N.; Sato, S.; Shiba, K.; Okatsu, K.; Saisho, K.; Gautier, C.A.; Sou, Y.-S.; Saiki, S.; Kawajiri, S.; Sato, F. Pink1 stabilized by mitochondrial depolarization recruits parkin to damaged mitochondria and activates latent parkin for mitophagy. *J. Cell Biol.* **2010**, *189*, 211–221. [CrossRef]

27. Ni, H.-M.; Williams, J.A.; Ding, W.-X. Mitochondrial dynamics and mitochondrial quality control. *Redox Biol.* **2015**, *4*, 6–13. [CrossRef]

28. Tilokani, L.; Nagashima, S.; Paupe, V.; Prudent, J. Mitochondrial dynamics: Overview of molecular mechanisms. *Essays Biochem.* **2018**, *62*, 341–360.

29. Piquereau, J.; Godin, R.; Deschenes, S.; Bessi, V.L.; Mofarrahi, M.; Hussain, S.N.; Burelle, Y. Protective role of PARK2/Parkin in sepsis-induced cardiac contractile and mitochondrial dysfunction. *Autophagy* **2013**, *9*, 1837–1851. [CrossRef]

30. Stana, F.; Vujovic, M.; Mayaki, D.; Leduc-Gaudet, J.P.; Leblanc, P.; Huck, L.; Hussain, S.N.A. Differential regulation of the autophagy and proteasome pathways in skeletal muscles in sepsis. *Crit. Care Med.* **2017**, *45*, e971–e979. [CrossRef]

31. Buras, J.A.; Holzmann, B.; Sitkovsky, M. Animal models of sepsis: Setting the stage. *Nat. Rev. Drug Discov.* **2005**, *4*, 854–865. [CrossRef] [PubMed]

32. Leduc-Gaudet, J.P.; Reynaud, O.; Hussain, S.N.; Gouspillou, G. Parkin overexpression protects from ageing-related loss of muscle mass and strength. *J. Physiol.* **2019**, *597*, 1975–1991. [CrossRef] [PubMed]

33. Moarbes, V.; Mayaki, D.; Huck, L.; Leblanc, P.; Vassilakopoulos, T.; Petrof, B.J.; Hussain, S.N.A. Differential regulation of myofibrillar proteins in skeletal muscles of septic mice. *Physiol. Rep.* **2019**, *7*, e14248. [CrossRef] [PubMed]

34. Leduc-Gaudet, J.P.; Picard, M.; St-Jean Pelletier, F.; Sgarioto, N.; Auger, M.J.; Vallee, J.; Robitaille, R.; St-Pierre, D.H.; Gouspillou, G. Mitochondrial morphology is altered in atrophied skeletal muscle of aged mice. *Oncotarget* **2015**, *6*, 17923–17937. [CrossRef]

35. Briguet, A.; Courdier-Fruh, I.; Foster, M.; Meier, T.; Magyar, J.P. Histological parameters for the quantitative assessment of muscular dystrophy in the mdx-mouse. *Neuromuscul. Disord.* **2004**, *14*, 675–682. [CrossRef]

36. Picard, M.; Gentil, B.J.; McManus, M.J.; White, K.; St Louis, K.; Gartside, S.E.; Wallace, D.C.; Turnbull, D.M. Acute exercise remodels mitochondrial membrane interactions in mouse skeletal muscle. *J. Appl. Physiol.* **2013**, *115*, 1562–1571. [CrossRef]

37. Picard, M.; White, K.; Turnbull, D.M. Mitochondrial morphology, topology, and membrane interactions in skeletal muscle: A quantitative three-dimensional electron microscopy study. *J. Appl. Physiol.* **2013**, *114*, 161–171. [CrossRef]

38. Gomes, M.D.; Lecker, S.H.; Jagoe, R.T.; Navon, A.; Goldberg, A.L. Atrogin-1, a muscle-specific F-box protein highly expressed during muscle atrophy. *Proc. Natl. Acad. Sci. USA* **2001**, *98*, 14440–14445. [CrossRef]

39. Bodine, S.C.; Latres, E.; Baumhueter, S.; Lai, V.K.; Nunez, L.; Clarke, B.A.; Poueymirou, W.T.; Panaro, F.J.; Na, E.; Dharmarajan, K.; et al. Identification of ubiquitin ligases required for skeletal muscle atrophy. *Science* **2001**, *294*, 1704–1708. [CrossRef]

40. Kane, L.A.; Lazarou, M.; Fogel, A.I.; Li, Y.; Yamano, K.; Sarraf, S.A.; Banerjee, S.; Youle, R.J. Pink1 phosphorylates ubiquitin to activate parkin e3 ubiquitin ligase activity. *J. Cell Biol.* **2014**, *205*, 143–153. [CrossRef]

41. Chan, D.C. Fusion and fission: Interlinked processes critical for mitochondrial health. *Annu. Rev. Genet.* **2012**, *46*, 265–287. [CrossRef]

42. Gouspillou, G.; Godin, R.; Piquereau, J.; Picard, M.; Mofarrahi, M.; Mathew, J.; Purves-Smith, F.M.; Sgarioto, N.; Hepple, R.T.; Burelle, Y.; et al. Protective role of parkin in skeletal muscle contractile and mitochondrial function. *J. Physiol.* **2018**, *596*, 2565–2579. [CrossRef] [PubMed]

43. Peker, N.; Donipadi, V.; Sharma, M.; McFarlane, C.; Kambadur, R. Loss of parkin impairs mitochondrial function and leads to muscle atrophy. *Am. J. Physiol. Cell Physiol.* **2018**, *315*, C164–C185. [CrossRef]

44. Rana, A.; Rera, M.; Walker, D.W. Parkin overexpression during aging reduces proteotoxicity, alters mitochondrial dynamics, and extends lifespan. *Proc. Natl. Acad. Sci. USA* **2013**, *110*, 8638–8643. [CrossRef] [PubMed]

45. Gouspillou, G.; Sgarioto, N.; Norris, B.; Barbat-Artigas, S.; Aubertin-Leheudre, M.; Morais, J.A.; Burelle, Y.; Taivassalo, T.; Hepple, R.T. The relationship between muscle fiber type-specific pgc-1alpha content and mitochondrial content varies between rodent models and humans. *PLoS ONE* **2014**, *9*, e103044. [CrossRef] [PubMed]

46. Hernandez-Alvarez, M.I.; Thabit, H.; Burns, N.; Shah, S.; Brema, I.; Hatunic, M.; Finucane, F.; Liesa, M.; Chiellini, C.; Naon, D.; et al. Subjects with early-onset type 2 diabetes show defective activation of the skeletal muscle pgc-1{alpha}/mitofusin-2 regulatory pathway in response to physical activity. *Diabetes Care* **2010**, *33*, 645–651. [CrossRef] [PubMed]

47. Hanson, B.J.; Capaldi, R.A.; Marusich, M.F.; Sherwood, S.W. An immunocytochemical approach to detection of mitochondrial disorders. *J. Histochem. Cytochem.* **2002**, *50*, 1281–1288. [CrossRef]

48. Ma, Q. Role of nrf2 in oxidative stress and toxicity. *Annu. Rev. Pharm. Toxicol.* **2013**, *53*, 401–426. [CrossRef]

49. Suen, D.F.; Norris, K.L.; Youle, R.J. Mitochondrial dynamics and apoptosis. *Genes Dev.* **2008**, *22*, 1577–1590. [CrossRef]

50. Twig, G.; Shirihai, O.S. The interplay between mitochondrial dynamics and mitophagy. *Antioxid. Redox Signal.* **2011**, *14*, 1939–1951. [CrossRef]

51. Favaro, G.; Romanello, V.; Varanita, T.; Andrea Desbats, M.; Morbidoni, V.; Tezze, C.; Albiero, M.; Canato, M.; Gherardi, G.; De Stefani, D.; et al. Drp1-mediated mitochondrial shape controls calcium homeostasis and muscle mass. *Nat. Commun.* **2019**, *10*, 2576. [CrossRef] [PubMed]

52. Yu, W.; Sun, Y.; Guo, S.; Lu, B. The pink1/parkin pathway regulates mitochondrial dynamics and function in mammalian hippocampal and dopaminergic neurons. *Hum. Mol. Genet.* **2011**, *20*, 3227–3240. [CrossRef] [PubMed]

53. Kishta, O.A.; Guo, Y.; Mofarrahi, M.; Stana, F.; Lands, L.C.; Hussain, S.N.A. Pulmonary pseudomonas aeruginosa infection induces autophagy and proteasome proteolytic pathways in skeletal muscles: Effects of a pressurized whey protein-based diet in mice. *Food Nutr. Res.* **2017**, *61*, 1325309. [CrossRef] [PubMed]

54. Bellot, G.; Garcia-Medina, R.; Gounon, P.; Chiche, J.; Roux, D.; Pouysségur, J.; Mazure, N.M. Hypoxia-induced autophagy is mediated through hypoxia-inducible factor induction of bnip3 and bnip3l via their bh3 domains. *Mol. Cell. Biol.* **2009**, *29*, 2570–2581. [CrossRef]

55. Song, M.; Gong, G.; Burelle, Y.; Gustafsson, A.B.; Kitsis, R.N.; Matkovich, S.J.; Dorn, G.W., 2nd. Interdependence of parkin-mediated mitophagy and mitochondrial fission in adult mouse hearts. *Circ. Res.* **2015**, *117*, 346–351. [CrossRef]

8

The Transcription Factor Nfix Requires RhoA-ROCK1 Dependent Phagocytosis to Mediate Macrophage Skewing during Skeletal Muscle Regeneration

Marielle Saclier, Michela Lapi, Chiara Bonfanti, Giuliana Rossi [†], Stefania Antonini and Graziella Messina *

Department of Biosciences, University of Milan, via Celoria 26, 20133 Milan, Italy;
marielle.saclier@unimi.it (M.S.); michela.lapi@unimi.it (M.L.); chiara.bonfanti@unimi.it (C.B.);
giuliana.rossi@epfl.ch (G.R.); stefania.antonini@unimi.it (S.A.)
* Correspondence: graziella.messina@unimi.it;
† Current affiliation: Laboratory of Stem Cell Bioengineering, Institute of Bioengineering, School of Life Sciences and School of Engineering, École Polytechnique Fédérale de Lausanne (EPFL), 1015 Lausanne, Vaud, Switzerland.

Abstract: Macrophages (MPs) are immune cells which are crucial for tissue repair. In skeletal muscle regeneration, pro-inflammatory cells first infiltrate to promote myogenic cell proliferation, then they switch into an anti-inflammatory phenotype to sustain myogenic cells differentiation and myofiber formation. This phenotypical switch is induced by dead cell phagocytosis. We previously demonstrated that the transcription factor Nfix, a member of the nuclear factor I (Nfi) family, plays a pivotal role during muscle development, regeneration and in the progression of muscular dystrophies. Here, we show that Nfix is mainly expressed by anti-inflammatory macrophages. Upon acute injury, mice deleted for Nfix in myeloid line displayed a significant defect in the process of muscle regeneration. Indeed, Nfix is involved in the macrophage phenotypical switch and macrophages lacking Nfix failed to adopt an anti-inflammatory phenotype and interact with myogenic cells. Moreover, we demonstrated that phagocytosis induced by the inhibition of the RhoA-ROCK1 pathway leads to Nfix expression and, consequently, to acquisition of the anti-inflammatory phenotype. Our study identified Nfix as a link between RhoA-ROCK1-dependent phagocytosis and the MP phenotypical switch, thus establishing a new role for Nfix in macrophage biology for the resolution of inflammation and tissue repair.

Keywords: macrophages; Nfix; skeletal muscle; phagocytosis; RhoA-ROCK1

1. Introduction

During their lifetime, tissues encounter physiological and non-physiological damages and an effective regeneration is necessary to make these tissues able to continuously sustain their biological functions. Macrophage-mediated inflammation is a fundamental step for tissue recovery. Macrophages (MPs) are immune cells required for tissue regeneration, as their depletion prevents regeneration of different tissues/organs, such as liver [1], spinal cord [2] and skeletal muscle [3]. In several regenerative processes, two populations of MPs have been described. The first population reaching the damaged tissue is the pro-inflammatory population, also called M1 MPs. Pro-inflammatory MPs secrete pro-inflammatory molecules, being the main actors of dead cell clearance. The second population is composed of the anti-inflammatory MPs, named M2 MPs, that come from pro-inflammatory MPs and are involved in the resolution of the inflammation, wound healing and tissue regeneration or repair [4–7]. Several studies have shown that an impaired or a precocious phenotypical switch from M1 to M2 MPs results in defective tissue regeneration [1,8,9]. Interestingly, it has been observed that phagocytosis is at the basis of the pro to anti-inflammatory phenotypical switch in MPs [3,8,10–13]. Although the process of the induction of phagocytosis is well-known ("find-me", "eat-me" and "don't eat-me" signals), the molecular and transcriptional pathways between phagocytosis and the phenotypical switch are still unexplored [10,11,14,15].

Interestingly, the interplay between MPs and tissue regeneration has been widely documented in skeletal muscle [7,16–20]. In vertebrates, muscle progenitors originate from pre-somitic and cranial mesoderm. In pre-natal period, two myogenic waves are necessary for muscle establishment: the first forms the basic muscle pattern and is called primary or "embryonic" myogenesis, while the second or "fetal" myogenesis is characterized by muscle maturation and growth [21]. Adult skeletal muscle is able to regenerate thanks to resident stem cells called satellite cells (SCs), located under the basal lamina of myofibers [22]. Upon injury, SCs exit from quiescence, proliferate, differentiate in myoblasts and fuse to reform myofibers [23]. Nuclear factor I X (Nfix) is a transcription factor belonging to the highly conserved DNA-binding nuclear factor one family (Nfi) together with Nfia, Nfib and Nfic [24]. Nfix has a key role in prenatal myogenesis by driving the transcriptional switch from embryonic to fetal myogenesis [25,26]. Nfix is also required for adult myogenesis upon injury, since its absence leads to defect of SC differentiation [27]. Finally, we recently demonstrated that the deletion of Nfix in two mouse models of muscular dystrophy induces a significant morphological and functional amelioration of the pathology by slowing-down muscle regeneration and promoting a switch towards a more oxidative musculature [28].

During muscle regeneration, myogenic cells and MPs closely interact [7]. Soon after injury, activated SCs attract blood monocytes that infiltrate damaged muscle and differentiate in pro-inflammatory MPs that stimulate the proliferation of myoblasts. Then, by removing dead cells, MPs switch to an anti-inflammatory phenotype that sustains myogenic differentiation [3,29]. While MPs are required for muscle regeneration, preventing MPs infiltration in dystrophic disease decreases muscle damage [30]. Thus, depending on a context of acute or chronic injury, MPs adopt a complete opposite function toward muscle cells and environment [31,32].

In this study, we address the role of Nfix in MPs during skeletal muscle regeneration, by using a mouse model in which Nfix is deleted specifically in MPs. We report that mice lacking Nfix in myeloid lineages exhibit a delay of muscle regeneration upon acute injury. We demonstrated that the RhoA-ROCK1-dependent phagocytosis induces Nfix, whose expression is necessary for the acquisition of anti-inflammatory phenotype and thus pro-regenerative properties through myogenic cells. Indeed, during the process of muscle regeneration, in the absence of Nfix, MPs are able to phagocyte, but failed to adopt an anti-inflammatory phenotype necessary for the resolution of inflammation and muscle regeneration.

2. Materials and Methods

2.1. Animal Models and In Vivo Experimentations

WT, $Nfix^{fl/fl}$ and $LysM^{CRE}:Nfix^{fl/fl}$ mice were used in this study. $LysM^{CRE}:Nfix^{fl/fl}$ mice were generated, crossing $Nfix^{fl/fl}$ mice obtained from Prof. Richard M. Gronostajski [33] and $LysM^{CRE}$ mice obtained from Dr. Rémi Mounier [8]. All $LysM^{CRE}:Nfix^{fl/fl}$ mice analyzed were heterozygous for the $LysM^{CRE}$. Muscle regeneration was realized by the injection of 20 uL of 100 uM cardiotoxin (CTX, Latoxan, L8102) in the *Tibialis anterior* (TA) of 2-month-old mice. For the in vivo analysis of satellite cells and myoblasts proliferation, EdU (5-ethynyl-2'-deoxyuridine) was injected in $Nfix^{fl/fl}$ and $LysM^{CRE}:Nfix^{fl/fl}$ mice in intraperitoneal, 12 h before the sacrifice of the mice (100 µL of 6mg/mL EdU solution for 20 g of mouse weight) (Click-iT EdU Imaging Kits Alexa Fluor 594, Thermo Fisher A10044, Paisley, UK). Mice were kept in pathogen-free conditions and all procedures conformed to Italian law (D. Lgs n° 2014/26, implementation of the 2010/63/UE) and approved by the University of Milan Animal Welfare Body and by the Italian Minister of Health.

2.2. Isolation of MPs from Skeletal Muscle

Fascia of the TA muscles was removed. Muscles were dissociated and digested in RPMI medium containing 0.2% of collagenase B (Roche Diagnostics GmbH 11088815001) at 37 °C for 1 h and passed through a 70 μm and a 30 μm cell strainer. CD45$^+$ cells were isolated using magnetic beads (Miltenyi Biotec 130-052-301) and incubated with FcR blocking reagent (Miltenyi Biotec 130-059-901) for 20 min at 4 °C in PBS 2% FBS. Cells were then stained with Ly6C-PE (eBioscience 12-5932) and CD64-APC (BD Pharmingen 558539) antibodies for 30 min at 4 °C. MPs were analyzed or sorted using a FACS Aria III cell sorter (BD Biosciences) (gating strategy is shown Figure S1). In some experiments, Ly6C$^+$ and Ly6C$^-$ MPs were cytospined on starfrost (Knitterglaser, Bielefeld, Germany) slides and immunostained.

2.3. Histology and Immunofluorescence Analyses

The fascia of TA muscles was removed and the muscles were frozen in liquid nitrogen-cooled isopentane (VWR) and placed at −80 °C until cut. Then, 8 μm-thick cryosections were stained for hematoxylin-eosin (H&E) and immunofluorescence. H&E (Sigma-Aldrich, Saint-Louis, MO 63103, USA) staining was processed according to standard protocols. For immunofluorescence analysis, sections or cells were fixed for 15 min with 4% paraformaldehyde (except for F4/80 and eMyHC staining). Then, samples were permeabilized with 0.5% Triton X-100 (Sigma-Aldrich) in PBS for 10 min and blocked with 4% BSA (Sigma-Aldrich) in PBS at RT for 1 h. Primary antibodies were incubated O/N at 4 °C in PBS. After three washes of 5 min with PBS, samples were incubated with secondary antibodies (1:500, Jackson Laboratory. Fluorochromes used: 488, 594, 546 and 647) and Hoechst (1:500, Sigma-Aldrich) in PBS for 45 min at RT, then washed four times for 5 min with PBS and mounted with Fluorescence Mounting Medium (Dako). For Nfix-F4/80 double immunolabeling, cryosections were labelled with antibodies against F4/80 (1:400, Novus Biologicals NB300-605) overnight at 4 °C and Nfix labelling using (1:200, Novus Biologicals NBP2-15039) the antibody was performed for 2 h at 37 °C. For EdU-Pax7-laminin immunolabelling, after fixation and permeabilization of muscle sections, we followed the manufacturer's instructions of the Click-iT EdU Imaging Kits Alexa Fluor 594 (Thermo Fisher A10044) to reveal the DNA integrated EdU. Then, for Pax7 immunostaining, antigen retrieval was performed by incubating muscle sections in boiling 10 mM citrate buffer pH6 for 20 min. Muscle sections were then incubated O/N with Pax7 (1:2, Hybridoma, DSHB, Iowa City, IA 52242, USA) and laminin (1:200, Sigma L9393). The other antibodies used were eMyHC (1:2, Hybridome), MyoD (1:50, Santacruz Biotechnology sc-377460), TNFα (1:50, Abcam ab34839), CCL3 (1:500, Abcam ab32609, Cambridge, UK), iNOS (1:25, Novus Biologicals NB300-605, Centennial, CO 80112, USA), CD163 (1:50, Santacruz Biotechnology sc-33560), CD206 (1:50, Bio-Rad MCA2235GA), TGFβ (1:100, Abcam ab64715), Arginase I (1:100, Santacruz Biotechnology, Cambridge, UK).

2.4. Bone Marrow Derived MPs (BMDM) Culture

Total mouse bone marrow was obtained by flushing femur and tibiae with DMEM. Cells were cultured in DMEM containing 20% Fetal Bovine Serum (FBS) and 30% of L929 cell line-derived conditioned medium (enriched in CSF-1) for 6 to 7 days. MPs were polarized using 50 ng/mL IFNγ (for M1 polarization) (Peprotech #315-05), 10 ng/mL IL10 (for M2c polarization) (Peprotech #210-10), in DMEM (10% FBS) for 3 days. After washing three times, DMEM serum-free medium was added for 24 h, and supernatants were recovered and centrifuged to obtain macrophage-conditioned medium. For some experiments, cells were directly used for various analyses. In some experiments, DMSO or 10 μM of ROCK inhibitor Y27632 (Santacruz sc-3536) was added on MPs.

2.5. Myogenic Progenitor Cells (mpc) Culture

Murine WT myoblast progenitor cells (mpcs) were obtained from TA muscle and cultured in DMEM/F12 (Gibco, Paisley, UK), containing 20% FBS and 2.5 ng/mL of human FGF-basic (Peptrotech, 100-18B). For the proliferation assay, mpcs were seeded at 10 000 cell/cm^2 on Matrigel

(1/10) and incubated for 1 day with macrophage-conditioned medium + 2.5% FBS. Then, cells were incubated with the anti-Ki-67 antibody (1/50, BD Biosciences 550609). For differentiation assay, mpcs were seeded at 30 000 cell/cm^2 on Matrigel (diluted 1/10 in DMEM/F12) and incubated for 3 days with macrophage-conditioned medium containing 2% horse serum. Then, cells were incubated with a pan-myosin antibody (1:2, Hybridoma).

2.6. Phagocytosis Assay

Mpcs were labelled using the CellVue Claret Far Red kit (Sigma-Alrich MinClaret) by following the manufacturer's instructions (Sigma-Aldrich) and treated with staurosporin at 5 µM for 4 h, in order to induce apoptosis. M1 and M2c polarized MPs were incubated with apoptotic mpcs at a 1:3 ratio for 30 min at 4 °C or 6 h or 16 h at 37 °C. After three PBS washings, MPs were detached using trypsin and a cell scraper and cells were labelled with a CD64-APC (BD Pharmingen 558539) and analyzed by flow cytometry using a FACS Aria III cell sorter (BD Biosciences). The double-positive cells (CD64$^+$/Far Red$^+$ cells) were phagocytic MPs, whereas the CD64$^+$/Far Red$^-$ cells were nonphagocytic MPs. To exclude MPs that have bound, but not ingested, apoptotic cells, we subtracted the percentage of double-positive cells observed at 4 °C from the value observed at 37 °C. In some experiments, MPs were treated with 1 µg/mL of cytochalasin D (Sigma-Aldrich C8273), 45 min before adding apoptotic mpcs, and with the added mpcs.

2.7. Lentiviral Transduction

BMDM from WT mice were transduced with a lentivirus carrying a scrambled sequence or a shNfix [27]. Transduction was performed in suspension (in DMEM 20% FBS), at a MOI of 10 and in the presence of Polybrene (8 µg/mL, Sigma-Aldrich). After O/N incubation, the medium was changed and cells were treated with puromycin (2 µg/mL, Sigma-Aldrich).

2.8. RNA Extraction and qRT-PCR

RNA was isolated from the sorted apoptotic mpcs, non-phagocyted and phagocyted MPs, by using TRIzol Reagent (Invitrogen 15596026, Bleiswijk, Netherlands), according to the manufacturer's instructions. RNA was quantified using a NanoPhotoneter (Implen). For retro-transcription, 500 ng of RNA was used with the iScript Reverse Transcription Supermix for RT-quantitative qPCR (Bio-Rad 1708840). For qRT PCR, cDNA was diluted 1:10, and 5 µL of the diluted cDNA was loaded in a total volume of 20 µL (SYBR Green Supermix (Bio-Rad 172-5124) and run on the Bio-RAD CFX Connect Real-Time System. The relative quantification of gene expression was determined by the comparative CT method, and normalized to Cyclophiline A. Primers used were: Nfix for CTGGCTTACTTTGTCCACACTC; Nfix rev CCAGCTCTGTCACATTCCAGAC; Myogenin for CTGGGGACCCCTGAGCATTG; Myogenin rev ATCGCGCTCCTCCTGGTTGA; Cyclo A for GTGACTTTACACGCCATAATG; Cyclo A rev ACAAGATGCCAGGACCTGTAT.

2.9. Protein Extraction and Western Blot

Protein extracts were obtained from cultured MPs lysed using RIPA buffer (10 mM Tris-HCl pH 8.0, 1 mM EDTA, 1% Triton-X, 0.1% sodium deoxycholate, 0.1% sodium dodecylsulphate (SDS), 150 mM NaCl, in deionised water), plus protease and phosphatase inhibitors for 30 min on ice. Then, samples were centrifuged at 11.000× g for 10 min at 4 °C, and the supernatants collected for protein quantification (DC Protein Assays Bio-Rad 5000111). 40 µg protein of each sample were denatured at 95 °C for 5 min using SDS PAGE sample-loading buffer (100 mM Tris pH 6.8, 4% SDS, 0.2% bromophenol blue, 20% glycerol, 10 mM dithiothreitol) and loaded into 8% SDS acrylamide gels. After electrophoresis, the protein was blotted into nitrocellulose membranes (Protran nitrocellulose transfer membrane; Whatman) for 2 h at 70 V at 4 °C. Membranes were then blocked for 1 h with 5% milk in Tris-buffered saline, plus 0.02% Tween20 (Sigma-Aldrich). Membranes were incubated with the primary antibodies O/N at 4 °C, using the following antibodies: rabbit anti-Nfix (1:1000,

Novus Biologicals NBP2-15039), mouse anti-vinculin (1:2500, Sigma-Aldrich V9131), rabbit anti-MYPT1 phosphorylated in Thr696 (1:500, SantaCruz Biotechnology sc-17556-R), and rabbit anti-Tot MYPT1 (1:500; SantaCruz Biotechnology, H-130). After incubation with the primary antibodies, the membranes were washed 3 times for 5 min and incubated with the secondary antibodies (1:10,000, IgG-HRP, Bio-Rad) for 45 min at RT, and then washed again 5 times for 5 min. Bands were revealed using ECL detection reagent (ThermoFisher), with images acquired using the ChemiDoc MP system (Bio-Rad). The Image Lab software was used to measure and quantify the bands of at least three independent western blot experiments. The obtained absolute quantity was compared with the reference band (Vinculin) and expressed in the graphs as normalized volume (Norm. Vol. Int.).

2.10. Image Acquisition and Quantification

Images were acquired with an inverted microscope (Leica-DMI6000B) equipped with Leica DFC365FX and DFC400 cameras and 20× and 40× magnification objectives. Necrotic myofibers were defined as pink pale patchy fibers, and phagocyted myofibers were defined as pink pale fibers invaded by basophilic single cells (MPs). For the quantification of CSA, analyses were done on damaged TA, which presented at least 75% of injured muscle. At least 8 pictures in different fields were taken and at least 500 myofibers were analyzed. For each condition of each experiment, at least 8 fields chosen randomly were counted. The number of labelled MPs or mpcs was calculated using the cell tracker in ImageJ software and expressed as a percentage of total MPs or mpcs. Fusion index was the number of nuclei within myotubes divided by the total number of nuclei.

2.11. Statistical Analysis

All data shown in the graph are expressed as mean ± SEM. All experiments were performed using at least three different cultures or animals in independent experiments. A statistical analysis was performed using two-tailed unpaired Student's t-Test, one-way ANOVA or two-way ANOVA. * $p < 0.05$; ** $p < 0.01$; *** $p < 0.001$; confidence intervals 95%, alpha level 0.05.

3. Results

3.1. Nfix is Expressed by Anti-Inflammatory MPs

To understand if the transcription factor Nfix could be involved in MP function, we first analyzed Nfix expression in MPs during normal muscle regeneration in WT mice. We induced muscle injury by cardiotoxin (CTX) injection in the *Tibialis Anterior* (TA) and looked at the number of MPs (F4/80[+] cells) positive for Nfix (Figure 1a). While the number of Nfix-positive MPs was identical between day two (D2) and day four (D4) after injury, we observed an increase of MPs expressing Nfix at D7 after CTX injection (Figure 1a). During muscle regeneration, two populations of MPs are present in the damaged tissue. First, the Ly6C[+] pro-inflammatory MPs appear and then, they switch into Ly6C[−] anti-inflammatory population [3,9,29,34]. Thus, we asked if Nfix could be expressed by one subset of MPs. We sorted MPs after CTX injury at different time points and looked at Nfix expression by immunolabelling. We firstly enriched for CD45[+] cells (mainly composed of MPs and neutrophils) using magnetic beads and then we used the known markers CD64 and Ly6C to separate the pro-inflammatory (CD64[+]/Ly6C[+] cells) to the anti-inflammatory MPs (CD64[+]/Ly6C[−] cells) (Figure S1). We observed that the percentage of pro-inflammatory MPs expressing Nfix does not change over the time of the regeneration (Figure 1b). On the contrary, the percentage of CD64[+]/Ly6C[−] cells positive for Nfix always increased over time (Figure 1b). We also isolated BMDMs (bone marrow derived MPs) from WT mice and polarized them in pro- or anti-inflammatory phenotype. We observed that anti-inflammatory MPs express more Nfix compared to pro-inflammatory MPs (Figure 1c). Therefore, we can conclude that in both in vitro and in vivo analyses, Nfix is more expressed by anti-inflammatory MPs.

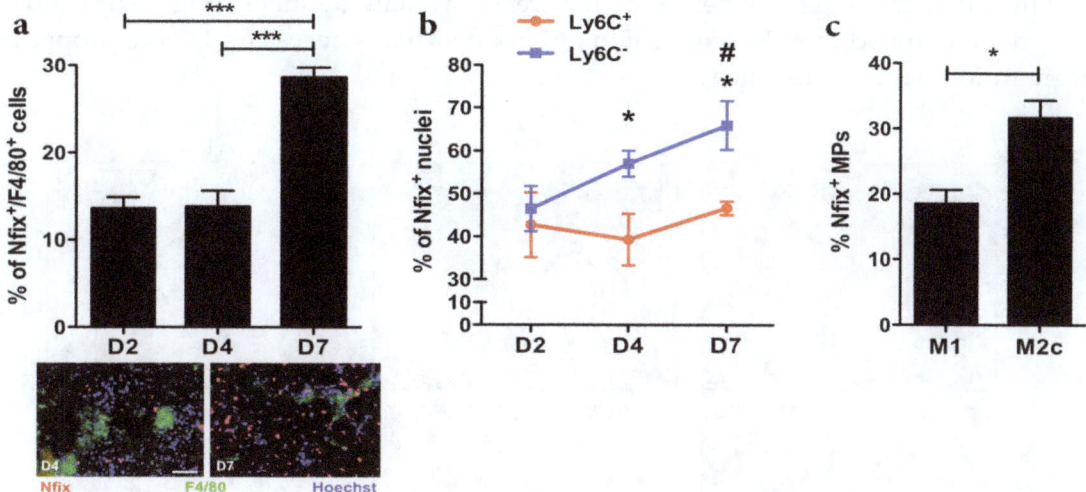

Figure 1. Nfix is mainly expressed by anti-inflammatory MPs. (**a**) Percentage of F4/80$^+$ MPs positive for Nfix in *Tibialis Anterior* muscles (TA) of WT mice injected by CTX at D2, D4 and D7, post-injury. Immunostaining for F4/80 (green), Nfix (red) and DAPI (blue) at D4 and D7 after CTX injection; (**b**) Percentage of Ly6C$^+$ and Ly6C$^-$ sorted MPs positive for Nfix in TA muscles of WT mice injected by CTX at D2, D4 and D7 post-injury; (**c**) Percentage of Nfix$^+$ MPs after M1 and M2c polarization (with IFNγ and IL10, respectively). * $p < 0.05$; *** $p < 0.001$; for (b) * $p < 0.05$ Ly6C+ vs. Ly6C$^+$ at D4 and D7; # $p < 0.05$ Ly6C$^-$ D7 vs. D2. Results are means ± SEM of at least three independent experiments. Scale bar = 50 μm.

3.2. Nfix Expression in MPs is Essential for Muscle Regeneration

We previously demonstrated that Nfix is necessary for the correct differentiation of SCs and, as a consequence, muscle regeneration [27]. In order to understand whether Nfix expression by anti-inflammatory MPs is required for this process, we generated the LysM^{CRE}:Nfix$^{fl/fl}$ mice to obtain an animal model deleted for Nfix only in the myeloid line. Once the proper deletion of Nfix in BMDM and CD45$^+$ infiltrated cells two days after muscle injury was verified (Figure S2a), we evaluated the overall phenotype of this new animal model, with particular interest in skeletal muscle morphology at one and two months of life (Figure S2b). No differences were observed between the Nfix$^{fl/fl}$ control and the LysM^{CRE}:Nfix$^{fl/fl}$ mice model in terms of general mouse growth, TA/mouse weight and myofiber size (CSA: Cross Sectional Area) (Figure S2b,c). Additionally, we did not observe significant differences in the number of resident MPs expressing Nfix between the Nfix$^{fl/fl}$ and the LysM^{CRE}: Nfix$^{fl/fl}$ mice (Figure S2d,e). Therefore, the specific deletion of Nfix in MPs in the LysM^{CRE}: Nfix$^{fl/fl}$ mice does not influence the general development of the mice. Notably, in the LysM^{CRE}: Nfix$^{fl/fl}$ animals resident MPs expressed Nfix similarly to control mice, meaning that the expression of LysM is not required for the establishment of resident MPs.

We then induced muscle injury in control and LysM^{CRE}: Nfix$^{fl/fl}$ mice by CTX injection in TA and we quantified the number of necrotic, phagocyted and regenerating myofibers (Figure 2a,b). Two days after injury, all the myofibers of Nfix$^{fl/fl}$ and LysM^{CRE}: Nfix$^{fl/fl}$ mice were in necrosis or phagocyted (Figure 2b). At D4 in the control mice, some necrotic and phagocyted myofibers were present, but already 60% of the fibers were centronucleated (Figure 2b). On the contrary, in the LysM^{CRE}:Nfix$^{fl/fl}$ mice, we observed a significant decrease in the percentage of centronucleated myofibers (−31%) (Figure 2b). While at D7, almost all myofibers were in regeneration in the control mice, the LysM^{CRE}:Nfix$^{fl/fl}$ mice still exhibited an increase of the percentage of necrotic and phagocyted myofibers and a decrease of centronucleated myofibers (+282%, +150% and −30% respectively), suggesting a delay in the process of muscle regeneration in the absence of Nfix (Figure 2b). We also quantified the CSA of myofibers at D14 and D28 after CTX injury and, in both cases, we observed a decrease of the caliber of myofibers in the LysM^{CRE}:Nfix$^{fl/fl}$ compared to the Nfix$^{fl/fl}$ mice, due to a decrease of the number of big myofibers and an increase of small myofibers (Figure S3a and Figure 2c). These results demonstrated that the expression of Nfix by MPs is necessary for the proper process of muscle regeneration upon acute injury.

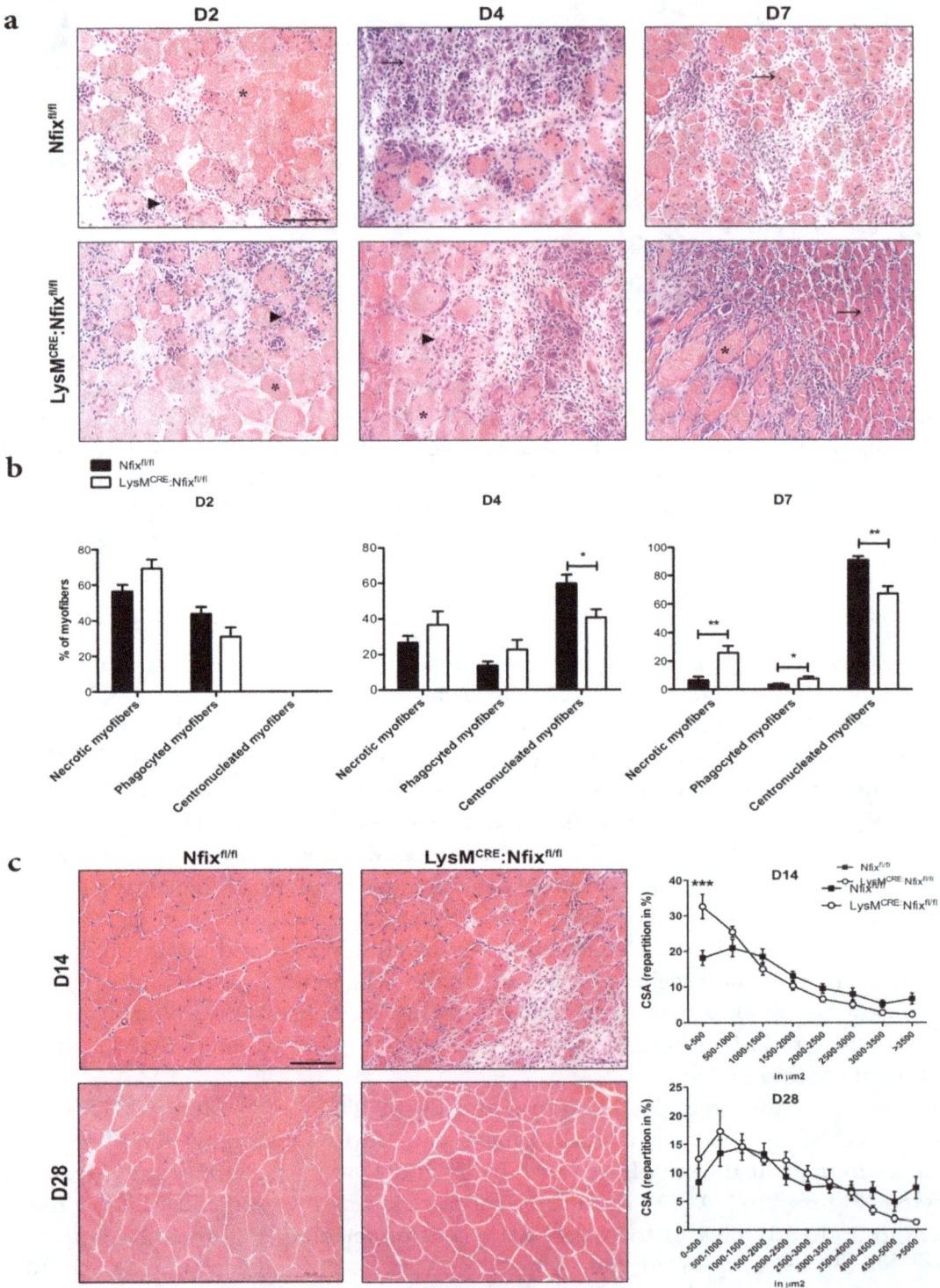

Figure 2. Lack of Nfix in MPs induces a delay of skeletal muscle regeneration. (**a**) Hematoxylin-eosin staining of Nfix[fl/fl] and LysM[CRE]:Nfix[fl/fl] TA muscles injected by CTX at D2, D4, D7 postinjury; (**b**) Quantification of necrotic (asterisk), phagocyted (arrowhead) and centrally-nucleated (arrow) myofibers, expressed as percentage out of total myofibers; (**c**) Hematoxylin-eosin staining of Nfix[fl/fl]

and LysM^{CRE}:Nfix$^{fl/fl}$ TA muscles injected by CTX at D14 and D28 postinjury and repartition in percentage of the cross-sectional area (CSA). * $p < 0.05$, ** $p < 0.01$, *** $p < 0.001$. Results are means ± SEM of at least three independent experiments. Scale bar = 100 μm.

3.3. Nfix is Required for MP Phenotypical Switch In Vivo and In Vitro

Defects of muscle regeneration due to MP dysfunction are usually linked to a defect of phenotype acquisition [8,9,35,36]. Thus, we looked at the switch from pro- to anti-inflammatory phenotype after CTX injury at different time points by FACS (Figure 3a). First, we did not observe any differences in neutrophils and MPs infiltration between the two mouse models at all time points analyzed (Figure S3b). At two days after injury, a majority of Ly6C$^+$ pro-inflammatory MPs was observed in the control Nfix$^{fl/fl}$ mice (Figure 3b). Then, at D4 and D7, the ratio between Ly6C$^+$/Ly6C$^-$ MPs decreased due to the switch from pro- to anti-inflammatory phenotype (Figure 3b). Interestingly, the ratio between Ly6C$^+$/Ly6C$^-$ in the LysM^{CRE}:Nfix$^{fl/fl}$ mice was always higher compared to the Nfix$^{fl/fl}$ control, meaning that Nfix is necessary for the switch from the pro- to anti-inflammatory phenotype (Figure 3b).

We also silenced Nfix in WT BMDM (Bone Marrow Derived MPs) by using a lentiviral vector carrying a small hairpin RNA targeting Nfix (shNfix), or a scrambled sequence as a control (shScramble) [27]. The decrease of Nfix expression in shNfix infected MPs was confirmed by qRT-PCR (Figure S3c). We polarized transduced MPs in pro-inflammatory (M1) and anti-inflammatory (M2c) phenotype (with IFN-γ and IL-10, respectively), and we looked at the expression of several pro- and anti-inflammatory markers by immunofluorescence. As expected, M1 shScramble MPs expressed significantly more TNFα, iNOS and CCl3 pro-inflammatory markers than M2c shScramble MPs (Figure 3c). Conversely, M2c shScramble MPs expressed more ArgI, TGFβ, CD163 and CD206 anti-inflammatory markers than M1 shScramble MPs (Figure 3c). Interestingly, in the absence of Nfix we observed an increase of pro-inflammatory markers (except for CCl3) in MPs polarized to M2c phenotype (Figure 3c). We also observed a decrease of MPs positive for anti-inflammatory markers in the polarized M2c MPs lacking Nfix (Figure 3b). These results clearly show that Nfix is necessary for the proper adoption of an anti-inflammatory phenotype and that, without Nfix, MPs remain in a pro-inflammatory status.

3.4. Nfix is Required for Macrophage Function on Mpcs In Vivo and In Vitro

Since depending on their phenotype MPs act differentially on WT myogenic progenitor cells (mpcs), we set experiments of conditioned medium (CM) coming from pro- or anti-inflammatory MPs [37]. We added CM coming from BMDM derived from Nfix$^{fl/fl}$ and LysM^{CRE}:Nfix$^{fl/fl}$ mice on proliferating or differentiating mpcs. We looked at mpc proliferation by mean of Ki67 staining and at their differentiation by the quantification of the fusion index. As expected, CM coming from M1 Nfix$^{fl/fl}$ MPs stimulated the proliferation of mpcs, while M2c CM had no effect (Figure 4a and Figure S4a). Similarly, CM coming from M1 LysM^{CRE}:Nfix$^{fl/fl}$ MPs stimulated at the same extent the proliferation of mpcs (Figure 4a and Figure S4a). Interestingly, CM from M2c LysM^{CRE}:Nfix$^{fl/fl}$ MPs stimulated the proliferation of mpcs as M1 CM does (Figure 4a and Figure S4b), whereas CM coming from both Nfix$^{fl/fl}$ and LysM^{CRE}:Nfix$^{fl/fl}$ M1 MPs had no effect on the fusion index of mpcs (Figure 4b and Figure S4b). While M2c Nfix$^{fl/fl}$ MPs CM increased the fusion of mpcs compared to M1 Nfix$^{fl/fl}$ CM, the CM from M2c LysM^{CRE}:Nfix$^{fl/fl}$ MPs lost its pro-fusion effect (Figure 4b and Figure S4b). We also investigated if the lack of Nfix in MPs affects myogenic cells in vivo. To quantify mpcs proliferation, we injured, using CTX, the TA of both Nfix$^{fl/fl}$ and LysM^{CRE}:Nfix$^{fl/fl}$ mice and we injected EdU 12 h before sacrifice. The proliferation of SCs (EdU$^+$/Pax7$^+$ cells) was identical between the two models at all the time points analyzed (Figure S4c). On the contrary, the percentage of EdU$^+$/MyoD$^+$ cells at D2 and D4 was higher in the LysM^{CRE}:Nfix$^{fl/fl}$ mice compared to Nfix$^{fl/fl}$ mice (Figure 4c). To quantify the number of newly formed myofibers, we performed an immunofluorescence for eMyHC (embryonic Myosin Heavy Chain) on both injured mouse models (Figure 4d). At D4, the percentage of myofibers positive for eMyHC was around 80%, meaning that almost all myofibers were formed de novo (Figure 4d). At D7, 20% of the Nfix$^{fl/fl}$ myofibers were positive for the eMyHC and only 6.5% at D14 (Figure 4d). On the contrary, at D7 and D14 we observed an increase in the number of eMyHC$^+$ myofibers in the LysM^{CRE}:Nfix$^{fl/fl}$ mice (34.7% and 15.8% respectively) (Figure 4d). To conclude, Nfix is necessary to MPs to adopt an anti-inflammatory phenotype and, consequently, function. The defect of the phenotypical switch due to the absence of Nfix results in a persistence of pro-inflammatory MPs in the injured muscle, leading to a continuous proliferation of MyoD$^+$ cells. The absence of anti-inflammatory MPs induces a delay in the differentiation of new myofibers and, therefore, in the proper muscle regeneration.

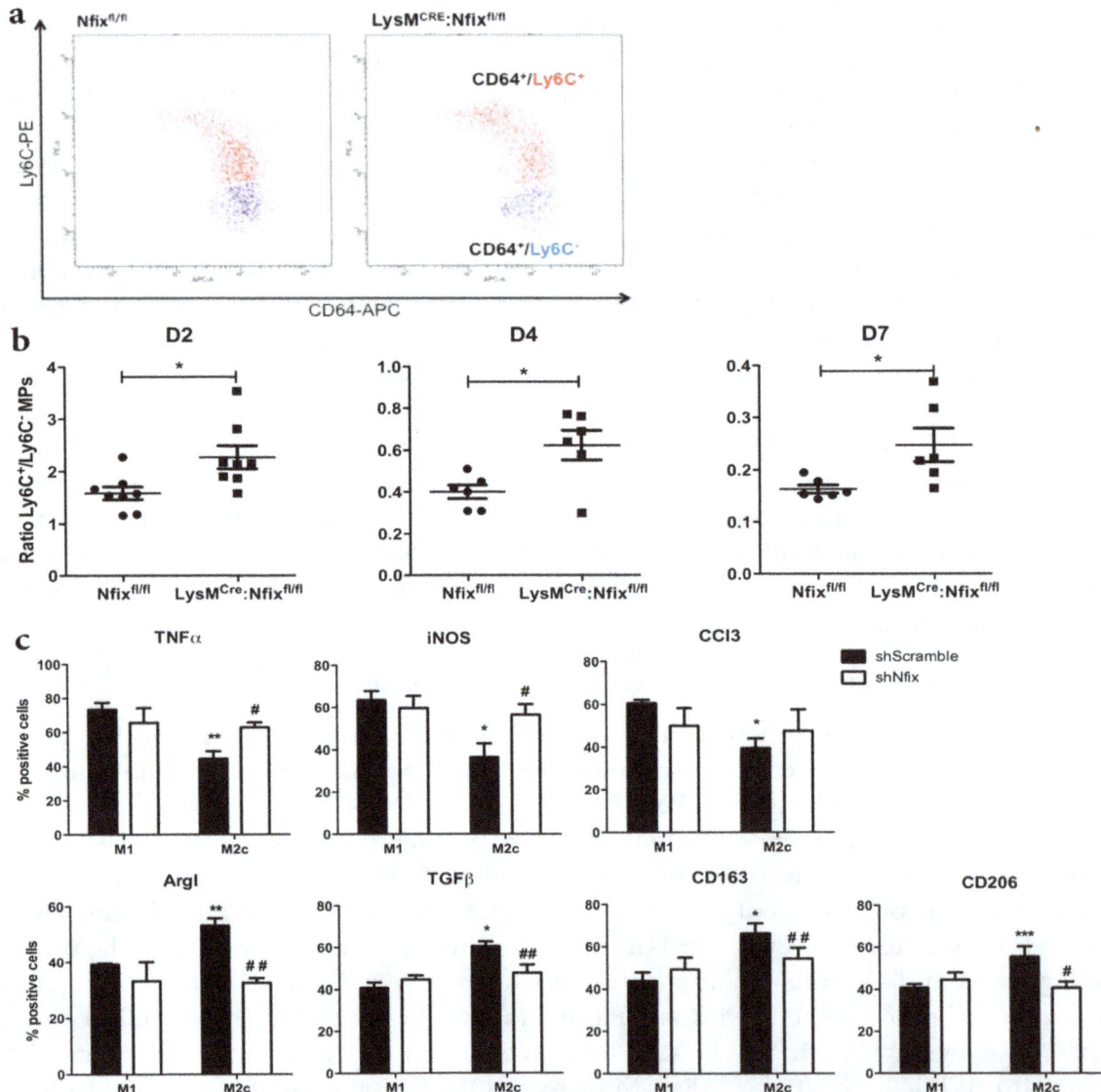

Figure 3. MPs lacking Nfix are unable to adopt an anti-inflammatory phenotype in vivo and in vitro. (a) Representative FACS (Fluorescence-Activated Cell Sorting) gate of pro- and anti-inflammatory CD64$^+$ MP populations in TA of Nfix$^{fl/fl}$ and LysM^{CRE}:Nfix$^{fl/fl}$ mice at D2 after CTX injection. (CD64$^+$/Ly6C$^+$ and CD64$^+$/Ly6C$^-$ respectively); (b) Ratio of Ly6C$^+$/Ly6C$^-$ MPs sorted from TA of Nfix$^{fl/fl}$ and LysM^{CRE}:Nfix$^{fl/fl}$ mice at D2, D4 and D7, after CTX injection; (c) WT BMDM (Bone Marrow Derived Macrophages) were transduced by shScramble and shNfix lentiviral vectors and then polarized into M1 and M2c MPs with IFNγ and IL10 treatment, respectively. MPs were immunolabeled for pro-inflammatory markers (TNFα, iNOS and CCl3) and anti-inflammatory markers (ArgI, TGFβ, CD163 and CD206). The number of positive cells is expressed as percentage out of total cells. * $p < 0.05$;

** $p < 0.01$; *** $p < 0.001$ vs. shScramble M1 MPs. # $p < 0.05$, ## $p < 0.01$, ### $p < 0.001$ vs. shScramble M2c MPs. Results are means ± SEM of at least three independent experiments.

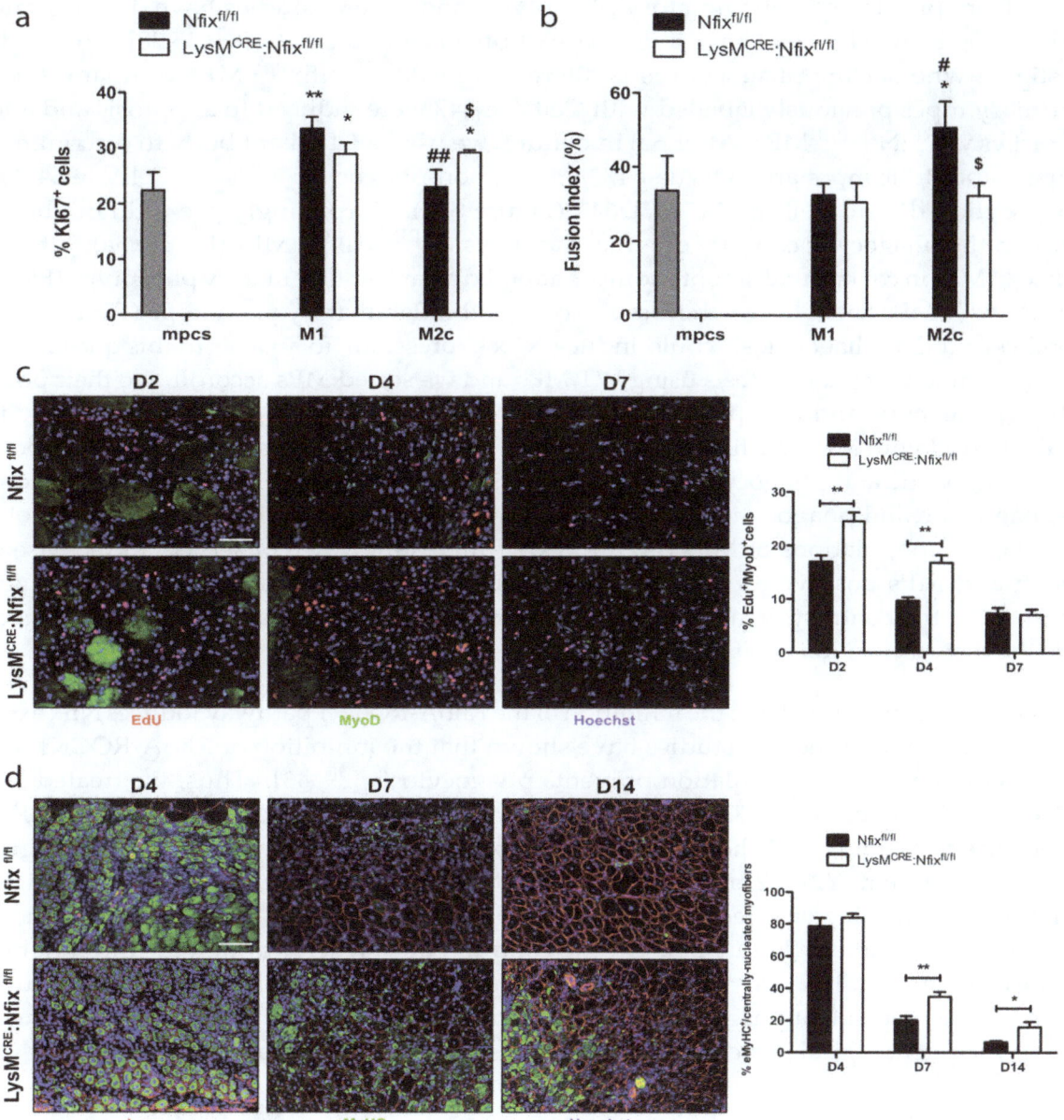

Figure 4. M2 MPs lacking Nfix display M1 MP features on myoblasts in vitro and in vivo. (**a**) Conditioned medium of M1 or M2c polarized Nfix$^{fl/fl}$ and LysM^{CRE}:Nfix$^{fl/fl}$ BMDM was added on mpcs, and after 24 h, mpc proliferation was measured as a percentage of Ki67^{+} cells; (**b**) Conditioned medium of M1 or M2c polarized Nfix$^{fl/fl}$ and LysM^{CRE}:Nfix$^{fl/fl}$ BMDM was added on mpcs and after 72 h, mpcs fusion index was calculated after sarcomeric MyHC staining (% of MyHC^{+}nuclei into myotubes out of the total nuclei). * $p < 0.05$, ** $p < 0.01$ vs. mpcs. # $p < 0.05$, ## $p < 0.01$ versus M1 Nfix$^{fl/fl}$. $ $p < 0.05$ versus same Nfix$^{fl/fl}$ polarization; (**c**) Immunostaining for EdU (red), MyoD (green) and Hoechst (blue) of Nfix$^{fl/fl}$ and LysM^{CRE}:Nfix$^{fl/fl}$ TA injected by CTX, at D2, D4 and D7 post-injury and quantification of EdU^{+}/MyoD^{+} cells. EdU was injected in Nfix$^{fl/fl}$ and LysM^{CRE}:Nfix$^{fl/fl}$ mice 8 h before sacrifice; (**d**) Immunostaining for Lam (red), eMyHC (green) and Hoechst (blue) of Nfix$^{fl/fl}$ and LysM^{CRE}:Nfix$^{fl/fl}$ TA injected by CTX, at D4, D7 and D14 post-injury and quantification of eMyHC^{+}/centrally-nucleated myofibers. * $p < 0.05$, ** $p < 0.01$ Results are means ± SEM of at least three independent experiments. Scale bar = 50 μm.

3.5. Phagocytosis Induces the Expression of Nfix

It has been shown in literature that the phagocytosis of apoptotic cells is the process driving the switch from pro- to anti-inflammatory phenotype, and several studies have demonstrated that MPs presenting a switch defect have a decrease of phagocytic capacity [8,9,35,38]. So, we decided to investigate whether the phagocytosis is altered in LysM^{CRE}:Nfix$^{fl/fl}$ MPs compared to Nfix$^{fl/fl}$ MPs. Primary mpcs previously labelled with CellVue-647 were induced to apoptosis and added on Nfix$^{fl/fl}$ or LysM^{CRE}:Nfix$^{fl/fl}$ MPs. After 6 h in culture, we used a CD64 antibody to discriminate MPs from mpcs: apoptotic mpcs are CellVue-647$^+$/CD64$^-$, non-phagocytic MPs are CellVue-647$^-$/CD64$^+$ and phagocytic MPs are CellVue-647$^+$/CD64$^+$ (Figure S5a). Surprisingly, we did not observe any difference in the phagocytic capacity of Nfix$^{fl/fl}$ and LysM^{CRE}:Nfix$^{fl/fl}$ MPs (Figure 5a). Interestingly, while Nfix$^{fl/fl}$ MPs in contact with apoptotic mpcs adopted an anti-inflammatory phenotype (Figure S5b), LysM^{CRE}:Nfix$^{fl/fl}$ MPs failed to switch from a pro- to anti-inflammatory phenotype (Figure S5c). Thus, we hypothesized that phagocytosis could induce Nfix expression. To answer to this question, we did the same experiment of phagocytosis using WT MPs and we sorted MPs according to their phagocytic capability (phagocytic and non-phagocytic WT MPs, respectively) (Figure 5b). To verify that no mpcs were sorted with MPs, we first analyzed the expression of myogenin in apoptotic mpcs and in both non-phagocytic and phagocytic MPs. Apoptotic mpcs highly expressed myogenin compared to non-phagocytic and phagocytic MPs and no differences in myogenin expression was observed between the two populations of MPs (Figure S5d). Interestingly, we observed an increase of Nfix expression and MPs positive for Nfix in phagocytic MPs compared to the non-phagocytic ones (Figure 5b). On the contrary, treatment of MPs with cytochalasin D (an inhibitor of phagocytosis) prevents the increase of Nfix positive MPs (Figure 5c and Figure S5e).

We recently demonstrated that the inhibition of the RhoA-ROCK1 pathway induces Nfix expression in fetal myoblasts and numerous studies have shown that the inhibition of RhoA-ROCK1 increases the phagocytosis, while its stimulation prevents phagocytosis [39–43]. Thus, we treated WT MPs with Y27632, an inhibitor of ROCK1, and after 1 h of treatment, the phosphorylation of ROCK1-target Mypt decreased, meaning that the inhibition of RhoA-ROCK1 pathway was effective (Figure S5e). After 16 h of treatment, Y27632-treated WT MPs exhibited an increase of Nfix protein (Figure 5d); most importantly, this increase led to a reduction of pro-inflammatory markers and an increase of anti-inflammatory markers (Figure 5e). On the contrary, this switch through an anti-inflammation phenotype did not occur in LysM^{CRE}:Nfix$^{fl/fl}$ MPs treated with Y27632 (Figure 5f). These results show that RhoA-ROCK-dependent phagocytosis induces the expression of Nfix, which in turn is necessary to promote the phenotypical switch of MPs from pro- to anti-inflammatory.

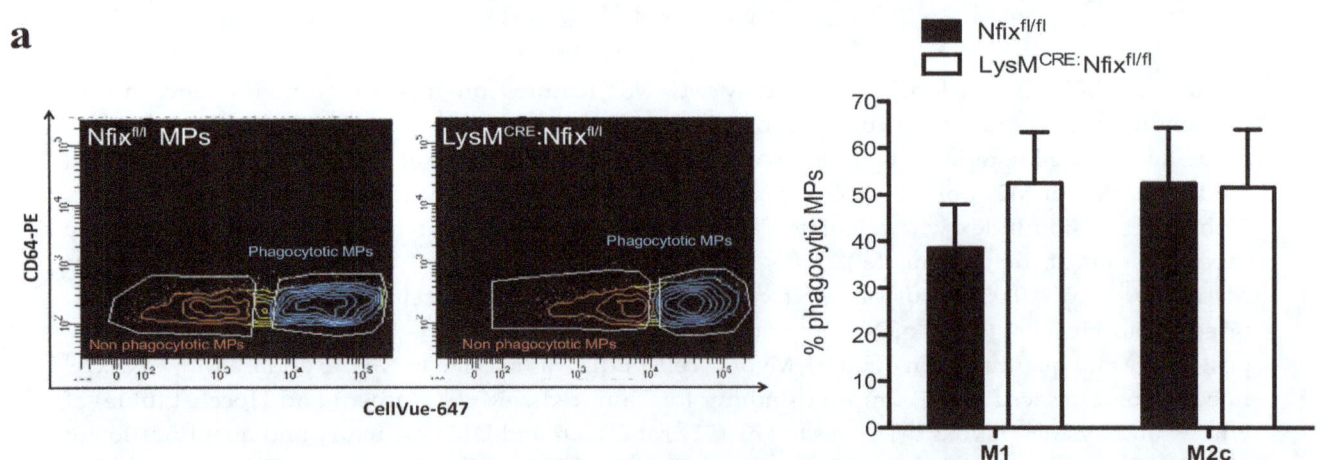

Figure 5. *Cont.*

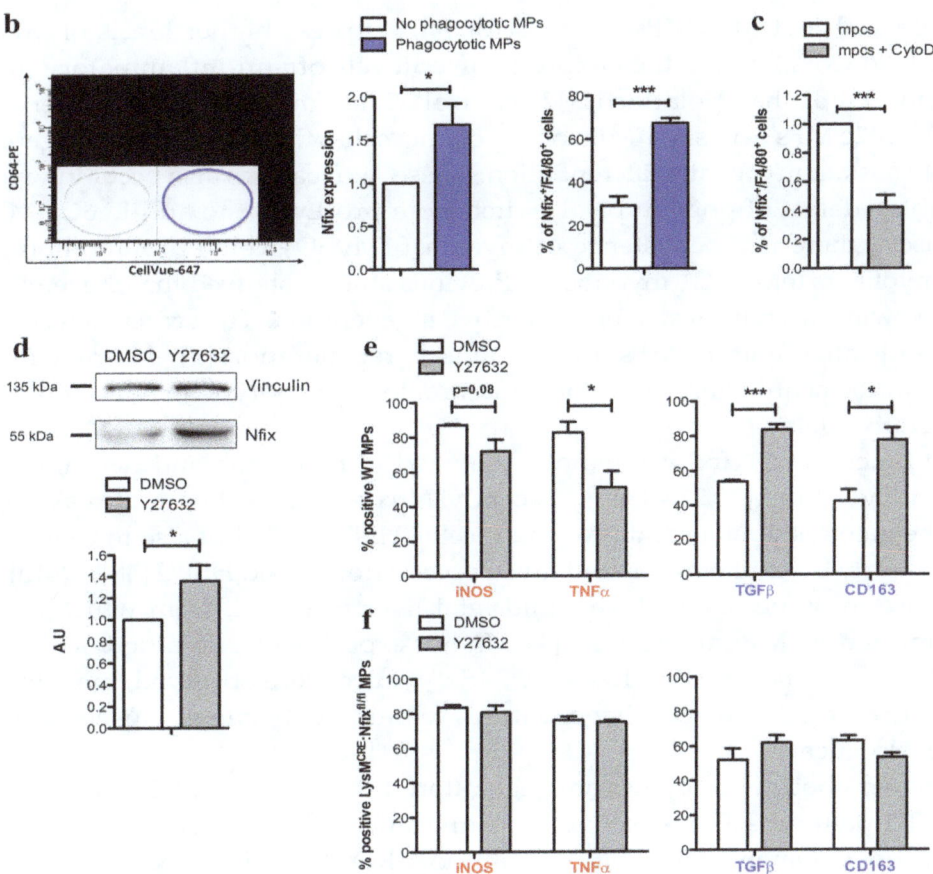

Figure 5. Nfix is expressed after phagocytosis and drive MP phenotypical switch. (**a**) Phagocytosis assay of M1 and M2c Nfix$^{fl/fl}$ and LysM^{CRE}:Nfix$^{fl/fl}$ MPs cocultured 8h with apoptotic mpc. Representative FACS gate of phagocytotic M2c Nfix$^{fl/fl}$ and LysM^{CRE}:Nfix$^{fl/fl}$ MPs (CD64$^+$CellVue$^+$) and percentage of phagocytotic M1 and M2c MPs coming from Nfix$^{fl/fl}$ and LysM^{CRE}:Nfix$^{fl/fl}$ BMDM; (**b**) WT MPs were cocultured 16h with apoptotic mpcs. Representative FACS gate of non-phagocytotic (CD64$^+$CellVue$^-$) and phagocytotic (CD64$^+$CellVue$^+$) WT MPs. Quantification of Nfix expression realized by RT-qPCR on sorted non-phagocytotic and phagocytotic WT MPs and quantification of MPs positive for Nfix (Nfix$^+$/F4/80$^+$) realized by IF on non-phagocytotic and phagocytotic WT MPs; (**c**) WT MPs were cocultured for 16 h with apoptotic mpcs, with or without addition of Cytochalasin D. Quantification of F4/80$^+$ MPs were positive for Nfix on a total of F4/80$^+$ MPs; (**d**) Western blot of Nfix expression in WT MPs treated with DMSO (Dimethyl sulfoxide) or Y27632 for 16 h and quantification. Vinculin was used to normalize; (**e**) WT MPs were treated with DMSO or Y27632 for 16 h and were immunolabeled for pro-inflammatory markers (iNOS and TNFα) and anti-inflammatory markers (TGFβ and CD163). The number of positive cells is expressed as percentage out of total cells; (**f**) LysM^{CRE}:Nfix$^{fl/fl}$ MPs were treated with DMSO or Y27632 for 16 h and were immunolabeled for pro-inflammatory markers (iNOS and TNFα) and anti-inflammatory markers (TGFβ and CD163). The number of positive cells is expressed as percentage out of total cells. * $p < 0.05$, *** $p < 0.001$. Results are means ± SEM of at least three independent experiments.

4. Discussion

Skeletal muscle regeneration requires specific temporal steps for the efficacious tissue reconstruction and MPs are the immune cells that are necessary to this process [3,29]. Previous work from our group demonstrated that *Nfix* null mice exhibit a delay of muscle regeneration, due to a defect of SC differentiation [27]. In this study, we show that the transcription factor Nfix is also expressed by MPs and that mice lacking Nfix in the myeloid lineage have defects in muscle regeneration upon acute injury. We observed that Nfix is preferentially expressed by anti-Ly6C$^-$ MPs and that its expression increases in time with the progression of the regenerative process. Using an shNfix strategy, we observed that M2c MPs silenced for Nfix express higher levels of pro-inflammatory markers (TNFα and Cox2), while they express lower levels of anti-inflammatory markers (CD163, CD206, ArgI and TGFβ) than polarized M2c control MPs. Importantly, we observed in vitro that LysM^{CRE}:Nfixf$^{l/fl}$ M2c MPs act as M1 MPs on myogenic cells: they stimulate myogenic proliferation and are unable to sustain myogenic differentiation. These two features also occur in vivo since without Nfix, MPs exhibit a defect of phenotypical switch from pro-Ly6C$^+$ to anti-Ly6C$^-$ MPs, and within the injured muscle, there is a persistence of myoblast (MyoD$^+$ cells) proliferation and a delay of newly formed myofibers (eMyHC$^+$ myofibers). Previous studies showed that the temporal window of the phenotype skewing is a critical step of an effective regeneration. The switch defect [8,35,36] or early appearance of anti-inflammatory MPs impairs muscle regeneration [9]. In line with this evidence, the impairment in the acquisition of an anti-inflammatory phenotype in MPs lacking Nfix leads to a muscle regenerative delay.

So far, the function of Nfix was mainly analyzed in myogenic and neural cells during both development and adult life [25,27,44–46]. Recently, Nfix was also shown to play a positive role in the survival of hematopoietic stem and progenitor cells (HSPC) [47], but also to be involved in the fate decision between early B lymphopoiesis and myelopoiesis from blood HSPC [48]. During development, yolk sac gives rise to tissue resident MPs and fetal liver to HSPC, from which blood monocytes and damaged-infiltrating MPs are derived [49]. In our experiments, no differences in the number of infiltrating MPs between control and LysM^{CRE}:Nfix$^{fl/fl}$ mice were observed, meaning that the delay observed is due to a defect of macrophage features within the damaged muscle, but not in terms of failed HSPC development.

Little is known about Nfix up-stream regulation, but recently our laboratory identified ERK and RhoA-ROCK1 pathways as, respectively, positive and negative regulators of Nfix expression in pre-natal muscle development. The inhibition of RhoA-ROCK1 induces Nfix expression, promoting myoblasts fusion which is a reflect of myogenesis progression [39]. In MPs, the inhibition of the RhoA-ROCK1 pathway increases the clearance of dead cell phagocytosis, while the constitutive activation of RhoA reduces their phagocytic capacity [40,41]. Importantly, phagocytosis is the process responsible for the induction of the pro- to anti-phenotypical switch in MPs. While numerous studies investigated the mechanisms involved in the progression or inhibition of phagocytosis, how apoptotic cells attract MPs and how MPs recognize them is still unknown [10,14,15,50,51]. In our study, phagocytosis of LysM^{CRE}:Nfix$^{fl/fl}$ MPs was not impaired compared to control cells. We observed that upon phagocytosis, MPs exhibit an increase in Nfix expression and, conversely, the inhibition of phagocytosis, by using the inhibitor of actin polymerization cytochalasin D, prevents Nfix expression. The stimulation of phagocytosis using the ROCK1 inhibitor Y27632 increases Nfix protein, therefore decreasing pro-inflammatory markers and increasing anti-inflammatory markers in WT MPs. On the contrary, either after phagocytosis or after ROCK1 inhibitor treatment, we observed that MPs lacking Nfix do not have a decrease of pro-inflammatory markers and an increase of anti-inflammatory markers. Thus, the inhibition of the RhoA-ROCK1 pathway induces phagocytosis, leading to Nfix expression that, in turn, drives the MP phenotypical switch.

This study is particularly relevant in light of the recent role for Nfix in muscular dystrophies (MDs)[28]. We indeed demonstrated that the lack of Nfix in two different dystrophic animal models improves both morphological and functional parameters associated to the disease, by promoting a more oxidative musculature and by slowing down muscle regeneration [28]. Different studies have shown that the improvement of dystrophies correlates with a decrease of MPs infiltration [30,32]. While MPs are necessary for muscle regeneration upon acute injury, they are deleterious in the case of chronic injury. Indeed, in muscle myopathies, as in several chronic injured pathologies, MPs are at the origin of fibrosis [4,32,52,53]. In the context of acute injury regeneration, pro-inflammatory MPs secrete TNFα that stimulates myoblast proliferation and fibroblast apoptosis, whereas anti-inflammatory MPs secrete TGFβ that promotes myoblast fusion, but also fibroblast proliferation [29,54]. In muscular dystrophies, numerous studies demonstrated that the fibrosis establishment is linked to an over-activation of the TGFβ pathway that stimulates collagen expression by fibroblasts, and in a dystrophic context, more than 75% of MPs express TGFβ [54–62]. Thus, in muscle tissue, MPs closely interact with fibroblasts, promoting normal matrix reformation upon acute injury and fibrosis in chronic injury. With this study, we identified Nfix as a new actor of MPs, demonstrating that Nfix is the link between phagocytosis and the phenotypical switch, a necessary step for the resolution of inflammation and tissue repair. Increasing knowledge about signals and factors controlling MP phenotype and, consequently, functions, will help us to understand and control their function in fibrotic pathologies.

Supplementary Materials:
Figure S1: Gating strategy to isolate MPs from CTX-injured muscles. Figure S2: Characterization of the LysM^{CRE}:Nfix$^{fl/fl}$ mice. Figure S3: CSA quantification, NT and MPs infiltration in Nfix$^{fl/fl}$ and LysM^{CRE}:Nfix$^{fl/fl}$ mice after CTX injury and Nfix silencing in WT BMDM. Figure S4: In vitro proliferation and differentiation assay. Proliferation of Pax7$^+$ cells after CTX injury. Figure S5: Phagocytosis strategy, inhibition and stimulation.

Author Contributions: Conceptualization, M.S. and G.M.; methodology, M.S., M.L., C.B. and S.A.; validation, M.S., M.L., C.B. and S.A.; formal analysis, M.S.; investigation, M.S., M.L., C.B, G.R. and S.A.; resources, G.M.; data curation, M.S.; writing—original draft preparation, M.S.; writing—review and editing, G.M.; visualization, M.S.; supervision, G.M.; project administration, G.M.; funding acquisition, G.M. All authors have read and agreed to the published version of the manuscript.

Acknowledgments: We thank Richard Gronostajski for the kind exchange of information and animal models. We are also grateful to Bénédicte Chazaud and Rémi Mounier for helpful discussions and the exchange of animal models.

References

1.   Duffield, J.S.; Forbes, S.J.; Constandinou, C.M.; Clay, S.; Partolina, M.; Vuthoori, S.; Wu, S.; Lang, R.; Iredale, J.P. Selective depletion of macrophages reveals distinct, opposing roles during liver injury and repair. *J. Clin. Invest.* **2005**, *115*, 56–65. [CrossRef] [PubMed]

2.   Shechter, R.; Miller, O.; Yovel, G.; Rosenzweig, N.; London, A.; Ruckh, J.; Kim, K.W.; Klein, E.; Kalchenko, V.; Bendel, P.; et al. Recruitment of Beneficial M2 Macrophages to Injured Spinal Cord Is Orchestrated by Remote Brain Choroid Plexus. *Immunity* **2013**, *38*, 555–569. [CrossRef] [PubMed]

3.   Arnold, L.; Henry, A.; Poron, F.; Baba-Amer, Y.; Van Rooijen, N.; Plonquet, A.; Gherardi, R.K.; Chazaud, B. Inflammatory monocytes recruited after skeletal muscle injury switch into antiinflammatory macrophages to support myogenesis. *J. Exp. Med.* **2007**, *204*, 1057–1069. [CrossRef] [PubMed]

4.   Wynn, T.A.; Vannella, K.M. Macrophages in Tissue Repair, Regeneration, and Fibrosis. *Immunity* **2016**, *44*, 450–462. [CrossRef]

5.   Vannella, K.M.; Wynn, T.A. Mechanisms of Organ Injury and Repair by Macrophages. *Annu. Rev. Physiol.* **2017**, *79*, 593–617. [CrossRef]

6.   Chazaud, B. Macrophages: Supportive cells for tissue repair and regeneration. *Immunobiology* **2014**, *219* 172–178. [CrossRef]

7.   Saclier, M.; Cuvellier, S.; Magnan, M.; Mounier, R.; Chazaud, B. Monocyte/macrophage interactions with myogenic precursor cells during skeletal muscle regeneration. *FEBS J.* **2013**, *280*, 4118–4130. [CrossRef]

8.   Mounier, R.; Théret, M.; Arnold, L.; Cuvellier, S.; Bultot, L.; Göransson, O.; Sanz, N.; Ferry, A.; Sakamoto, K.; Foretz, M.; et al. AMPKα1 regulates macrophage skewing at the time of resolution of inflammation during skeletal muscle regeneration. *Cell Metab.* **2013**, *18*, 251–264. [CrossRef]

9.   Perdiguero, E.; Sousa-Victor, P.; Ruiz-Bonilla, V.; Jardí, M.; Caelles, C.; Serrano, A.L.; Muñoz-Cánoves, P. p38/MKP-1-regulated AKT coordinates macrophage transitions and resolution of inflammation during tissue repair. *J. Cell Biol.* **2011**, *195*, 307–322. [CrossRef]

10.   Lemke, G. How macrophages deal with death. *Nat. Rev. Immunol.* **2019**, *19*, 539–549. [CrossRef]

11.   Elliott, M.R.; Ravichandran, K.S. The Dynamics of Apoptotic Cell Clearance. *Dev. Cell* **2016**, *38*, 147–160. [CrossRef] [PubMed]

12.   Xiao, Y.Q.; Freire-de-Lima, C.G.; Schiemann, W.P.; Bratton, D.L.; Vandivier, R.W.; Henson, P.M. Transcriptional and Translational Regulation of TGF-β Production in Response to Apoptotic Cells. *J. Immunol.* **2008**, *181*, 3575–3585. [CrossRef] [PubMed]

13. Johann, A.M.; Barra, V.; Kuhn, A.M.; Weigert, A.; Von Knethen, A.; Brüne, B. Apoptotic cells induce arginase II in macrophages, thereby attenuating NO production. *FASEB J.* **2007**, *21*, 2704–2712. [CrossRef] [PubMed]

14. Hochreiter-Hufford, A.; Ravichandran, K.S. Clearing the dead: Apoptotic cell sensing, recognition, engulfment, and digestion. *Cold Spring Harb. Perspect. Biol.* **2013**, *5*. [CrossRef]

15. Freeman, S.A.; Grinstein, S. Phagocytosis: Receptors, signal integration, and the cytoskeleton. *Immunol. Rev.* **2014**, *262*, 193–215. [CrossRef]

16. Tidball, J.G.; Wehling-Henricks, M. Damage and inflammation in muscular dystrophy: Potential implications and relationships with autoimmune myositis. *Curr. Opin. Rheumatol.* **2005**, *17*, 707–713. [CrossRef]

17. Dort, J.; Fabre, P.; Molina, T.; Dumont, N.A. Macrophages Are Key Regulators of Stem Cells during Skeletal Muscle Regeneration and Diseases. *Stem Cells Int.* **2019**, *2019*. [CrossRef]

18. Farup, J.; Madaro, L.; Puri, P.L.; Mikkelsen, U.R. Interactions between muscle stem cells, mesenchymal-derived cells and immune cells in muscle homeostasis, regeneration and disease. *Cell Death Dis.* **2015**, *6*, e1830. [CrossRef]

19. Chazaud, B.; Brigitte, M.; Yacoub-Youssef, H.; Arnold, L.; Gherardi, R.; Sonnet, C.; Lafuste, P.; Chretien, F. Dual and beneficial roles of macrophages during skeletal muscle regeneration. *Exerc. Sport Sci. Rev.* **2009**, *37*, 18–22. [CrossRef]

20. Rigamonti, E.; Zordan, P.; Sciorati, C.; Rovere-Querini, P.; Brunelli, S. Macrophage plasticity in skeletal muscle repair. *Biomed Res. Int.* **2014**, *2014*. [CrossRef]

21. Biressi, S.; Molinaro, M.; Cossu, G. Cellular heterogeneity during vertebrate skeletal muscle development. *Dev. Biol.* **2007**, *308*, 281–293. [CrossRef] [PubMed]

22. Mauro, A. Satellite Cell of Skeletal Muscle Fibers. *J. Biophys Biochem Cytol* **1961**, *9*, 493–498. [CrossRef] [PubMed]

23. Dumont, N.A.; Bentzinger, C.F.; Sincennes, M.C.; Rudnicki, M.A. Satellite cells and skeletal muscle regeneration. *Compr. Physiol.* **2015**, *5*, 1027–1059. [PubMed]

24. Gronostajski, R.M. Roles of the NFI/CTF gene family in transcription and development. *Gene* **2000**, *249*, 31–45. [CrossRef]

25. Messina, G.; Biressi, S.; Monteverde, S.; Magli, A.; Cassano, M.; Perani, L.; Roncaglia, E.; Tagliafico, E.; Starnes, L.; Campbell, C.E.; et al. Nfix Regulates Fetal-Specific Transcription in Developing Skeletal Muscle. *Cell* **2010**, *140*, 554–566. [CrossRef] [PubMed]

26. Pistocchi, A.; Gaudenzi, G.; Foglia, E.; Monteverde, S.; Moreno-Fortuny, A.; Pianca, A.; Cossu, G.; Cotelli, F.; Messina, G. Conserved and divergent functions of Nfix in skeletal muscle development during vertebrate evolution. *Development* **2013**, *140*, 2443. [CrossRef]

27. Rossi, G.; Antonini, S.; Bonfanti, C.; Monteverde, S.; Vezzali, C.; Tajbakhsh, S.; Cossu, G.; Messina, G. Nfix Regulates Temporal Progression of Muscle Regeneration through Modulation of Myostatin Expression. *Cell Rep.* **2016**, *14*, 2238–2249. [CrossRef]

28. Rossi, G.; Bonfanti, C.; Antonini, S.; Bastoni, M.; Monteverde, S.; Innocenzi, A.; Saclier, M.; Taglietti, V.; Messina, G. Silencing Nfix rescues muscular dystrophy by delaying muscle regeneration. *Nat. Commun.* **2017**, *8*. [CrossRef]

29. Saclier, M.; Yacoub-Youssef, H.; Mackey, A.L.; Arnold, L.; Ardjoune, H.; Magnan, M.; Sailhan, F.; Chelly, J.; Pavlath, G.K.; Mounier, R.; et al. Differentially activated macrophages orchestrate myogenic precursor cell fate during human skeletal muscle regeneration. *Stem Cells* **2013**, *31*, 384–396. [CrossRef]

30. Wehling, M.; Spencer, M.J.; Tidball, J.G. A nitric oxide synthase transgene ameliorates muscular dystrophy in mdx mice. *J. Cell Biol.* **2001**, *155*, 123–131. [CrossRef]

31. Kharraz, Y.; Guerra, J.; Mann, C.J.; Serrano, A.L.; Muñoz-Cánoves, P. Macrophage plasticity and the role of inflammation in skeletal muscle repair. *Mediators Inflamm.* **2013**, *2013*. [CrossRef] [PubMed]

32. Muñoz-Cánoves, P.; Serrano, A.L. Macrophages decide between regeneration and fibrosis in muscle. *Trends Endocrinol. Metab.* **2015**, *26*, 449–450. [CrossRef] [PubMed]

33. Campbell, C.E.; Piper, M.; Plachez, C.; Yeh, Y.-T.; Baizer, J.S.; Osinski, J.M.; Litwack, E.D.; Richards, L.J.; Gronostajski, R.M. The transcription factor Nfix is essential for normal brain development. *BMC Dev. Biol.* **2008**, *8*, 52. [CrossRef] [PubMed]

34. Varga, T.; Mounier, R.; Horvath, A.; Cuvellier, S.; Dumont, F.; Poliska, S.; Ardjoune, H.; Juban, G.; Nagy, L.; Chazaud, B. Highly Dynamic Transcriptional Signature of Distinct Macrophage Subsets during Sterile Inflammation, Resolution, and Tissue Repair. *J. Immunol.* **2016**, *196*, 4771–4782. [CrossRef] [PubMed]

35. Ruffell, D.; Mourkioti, F.; Gambardella, A.; Kirstetter, P.; Lopez, R.G.; Rosenthal, N.; Nerlov, C. A CREB-C/EBPbeta cascade induces M2 macrophage-specific gene expression and promotes muscle injury repair. *Proc. Natl. Acad. Sci. USA* **2009**, *106*, 17475–17480. [CrossRef] [PubMed]

36. Nie, M.; Liu, J.; Yang, Q.; Seok, H.Y.; Hu, X.; Deng, Z.-L.; Wang, D.-Z. MicroRNA-155 facilitates skeletal muscle regeneration by balancing pro- and anti-inflammatory macrophages. *Cell Death Dis.* **2016**, *7*, e2261. [CrossRef]

37. Saclier, M.; Theret, M.; Mounier, R.; Chazaud, B. Effects of macrophage conditioned-medium on murine and human muscle cells: Analysis of proliferation, differentiation, and fusion. *Proc. Natl. Acad. Sci. USA* **2009**, *106*, 17475–17480.

38. Arnold, L.; Perrin, H.; de Chanville, C.B.; Saclier, M.; Hermand, P.; Poupel, L.; Guyon, E.; Licata, F.; Carpentier, W.; Vilar, J.; et al. CX3CR1 deficiency promotes muscle repair and regeneration by enhancing macrophage ApoE production. *Nat. Commun.* **2015**, *6*, 8972. [CrossRef]

39. Taglietti, V.; Angelini, G.; Mura, G.; Bonfanti, C.; Caruso, E.; Monteverde, S.; Le Carrou, G.; Tajbakhsh, S.; Relaix, F.; Messina, G. RhoA and ERK signalling regulate the expression of the transcription factor Nfix in myogenic cells. *Development* **2018**, *145*. [CrossRef]

40. Bros, M.; Haas, K.; Moll, L. Grabbe RhoA as a Key Regulator of Innate and Adaptive Immunity. *Cells* **2019**, *8*, 733. [CrossRef]

41. Nakaya, M.; Tanaka, M.; Okabe, Y.; Hanayama, R.; Nagata, S. Opposite effects of Rho family GTPases on engulfment of apoptotic cells by macrophages. *J. Biol. Chem.* **2006**, *281*, 8836–8842. [CrossRef] [PubMed]

42. Königs, V.; Jennings, R.; Vogl, T.; Horsthemke, M.; Bachg, A.C.; Xu, Y.; Grobe, K.; Brakebusch, C.; Schwab, A.; Bähler, M.; et al. Mouse Macrophages completely lacking Rho subfamily GTPases (RhoA, RhoB, and RhoC) have severe lamellipodial retraction defects, but robust chemotactic navigation and altered motility. *J. Biol. Chem.* **2014**, *289*, 30772–30784. [CrossRef] [PubMed]

43. Kim, S.Y.; Kim, S.; Bae, D.J.; Park, S.Y.; Lee, G.Y.; Park, G.M.; Kim, I.S. Coordinated balance of Rac1 and RhoA plays key roles in determining phagocytic appetite. *PLoS ONE* **2017**, *12*. [CrossRef] [PubMed]

44. Harris, L.; Zalucki, O.; Gobius, I.; McDonald, H.; Osinki, J.; Harvey, T.J.; Essebier, A.; Vidovic, D.; Gladwyn-Ng, I.; Burne, T.H.; et al. Transcriptional regulation of intermediate progenitor cell generation during hippocampal development. *Development* **2016**, *143*, 4620–4630. [CrossRef]

45. Harris, L.; Dixon, C.; Cato, K.; Heng, Y.H.E.; Kurniawan, N.D.; Ullmann, J.F.P.; Janke, A.L.; Gronostajski, R.M.; Richards, L.J.; Burne, T.H.J.; et al. Heterozygosity for Nuclear Factor One X Affects Hippocampal-Dependent Behaviour in Mice. *PLoS ONE* **2013**, *8*. [CrossRef]

46. Fraser, J.; Essebier, A.; Gronostajski, R.M.; Boden, M.; Wainwright, B.J.; Harvey, T.J.; Piper, M. Cell-type-specific expression of NFIX in the developing and adult cerebellum. *Brain Struct. Funct.* **2017**, *222*, 2251–2270. [CrossRef]

47. Holmfeldt, P.; Pardieck, J.; Saulsberry, A.C.; Nandakumar, S.K.; Finkelstein, D.; Gray, J.T.; Persons, D.A.; Mckinney-freeman, S. Nfix is a novel regulator of murine hematopoietic stem and progenitor cell survival. *Blood* **2015**, *122*, 2987–2997. [CrossRef]

48. O'Connor, C.; Campos, J.; Osinski, J.M.; Gronostajski, R.M.; Michie, A.M.; Keeshan, K. Nfix expression critically modulates early B lymphopoiesis and myelopoiesis. *PLoS ONE* **2015**, *10*, 1–15. [CrossRef]

49. Gomez Perdiguero, E.; Klapproth, K.; Schulz, C.; Busch, K.; de Bruijn, M.; Rodewald, H.R.; Geissmann, F. The Origin of Tissue-Resident Macrophages: When an Erythro-myeloid Progenitor Is an Erythro-myeloid Progenitor. *Immunity* **2015**, *43*, 1023–1024. [CrossRef]

50. Park, S.Y.; Kim, I.S. Engulfment signals and the phagocytic machinery for apoptotic cell clearance. *Exp. Mol. Med.* **2017**, *49*. [CrossRef]

51. Haney, M.S.; Bohlen, C.J.; Morgens, D.W.; Ousey, J.A.; Barkal, A.A.; Tsui, C.K.; Ego, B.K.; Levin, R.; Kamber, R.A.; Collins, H.; et al. Identification of phagocytosis regulators using magnetic genome-wide CRISPR screens. *Nat. Genet.* **2018**, *50*, 1716–1727. [CrossRef] [PubMed]

52. Ngambenjawong, C.; Gustafson, H.H.; Pun, S.H. Progress in tumor-associated macrophage (TAM)-targeted therapeutics. *Adv. Drug Deliv. Rev.* **2017**, *114*, 206–221. [CrossRef]

53. Tang, P.M.K.; Nikolic-Paterson, D.J.; Lan, H.Y. Macrophages: Versatile players in renal inflammation and fibrosis. *Nat. Rev. Nephrol.* **2019**, *15*, 144–158. [CrossRef] [PubMed]

54. Lemos, D.R.; Babaeijandaghi, F.; Low, M.; Chang, C.-K.; Lee, S.T.; Fiore, D.; Zhang, R.-H.; Natarajan, A.; Nedospasov, S.A.; Rossi, F.M. V Nilotinib reduces muscle fibrosis in chronic muscle injury by promoting TNF-mediated apoptosis of fibro/adipogenic progenitors. *Nat. Med.* **2015**, *21*, 786–794. [CrossRef]

55. Ueha, S.; Shand, F.H.W.; Matsushima, K. Cellular and molecular mechanisms of chronic inflammation-associated organ fibrosis. *Front. Immunol.* **2012**, *3*, 1–6. [CrossRef]

56. Tan, R.J.; Liu, Y. Macrophage-derived TGF-beta in renal fibrosis: Not a macro- impact after all. *Am. J. Physiol. Renal Physiol.* **2013**, 1–7.

57. Mann, C.J.; Perdiguero, E.; Kharraz, Y.; Aguilar, S.; Pessina, P.; Serrano, A.L.; Muñoz-Cánoves, P. Aberrant repair and fibrosis development in skeletal muscle. *Skelet. Muscle* **2011**, *1*, 21. [CrossRef]

58. Vidal, B.; Serrano, A.L.; Tjwa, M.; Suelves, M.; Ardite, E.; De Mori, R.; Baeza-Raja, B.; De Lagrán, M.M.; Lafuste, P.; Ruiz-Bonilla, V.; et al. Fibrinogen drives dystrophic muscle fibrosis via a TGFβ/alternative macrophage activation pathway. *Genes Dev.* **2008**, *22*, 1747–1752. [CrossRef] [PubMed]

59. Tidball, J.G.; Wehling-Henricks, M. Shifts in macrophage cytokine production drive muscle fibrosis. *Nat. Med.* **2015**, *21*, 665–666. [CrossRef]

60. Pakshir, P.; Hinz, B. The big five in fibrosis: Macrophages, myofibroblasts, matrix, mechanics, and miscommunication. *Matrix Biol.* **2018**, *68–69*, 81–93. [CrossRef]

61. Smith, L.R.; Barton, E.R. Regulation of fibrosis in muscular dystrophy. *Matrix Biol.* **2018**, *68–69*, 602–615. [CrossRef] [PubMed]

62. Biernacka, A.; Dobaczewski, M.; Frangogiannis, N.G. TGF-β signaling in fibrosis. *Growth Factors* **2011**, *29*, 196–202. [CrossRef] [PubMed]

9

Older Adults with Physical Frailty and Sarcopenia Show Increased Levels of Circulating Small Extracellular Vesicles with a Specific Mitochondrial Signature

Anna Picca [1,†], Raffaella Beli [2,†], Riccardo Calvani [1,*], Hélio José Coelho-Júnior [3], Francesco Landi [1,3], Roberto Bernabei [1,3], Cecilia Bucci [2], Flora Guerra [2,*] and Emanuele Marzetti [1,3]

1   Fondazione Policlinico Universitario "Agostino Gemelli" IRCCS, 00168 Rome, Italy; anna.picca@guest.policlinicogemelli.it (A.P.); francesco.landi@unicatt.it (F.L.); roberto.bernabei@unicatt.it (R.B.); emanuele.marzetti@policlinicogemelli.it (E.M.)
2   Department of Biological and Environmental Sciences and Technologies, Università del Salento, 73100 Lecce, Italy; raffaella.beli@unisalento.it (R.B.); cecilia.bucci@unisalento.it (C.B.)
3   Università Cattolica del Sacro Cuore, 00168 Rome, Italy; coelhojunior@hotmail.com.br
*   Correspondence: riccardo.calvani@guest.policlinicogemelli.it (R.C.); guerraflora@gmail.com (F.G.);
†   These authors contributed equally.

Abstract: Mitochondrial dysfunction and systemic inflammation are major factors in the development of sarcopenia, but the molecular determinants linking the two mechanisms are only partially understood. The study of extracellular vesicle (EV) trafficking may provide insights into this relationship. Circulating small EVs (sEVs) from serum of 11 older adults with physical frailty and sarcopenia (PF&S) and 10 controls were purified and characterized. Protein levels of three tetraspanins (CD9, CD63, and CD81) and selected mitochondrial markers, including adenosine triphosphate 5A (ATP5A), mitochondrial cytochrome C oxidase subunit I (MTCOI), nicotinamide adenine dinucleotide reduced form (NADH):ubiquinone oxidoreductase subunit B8 (NDUFB8), NADH:ubiquinone oxidoreductase subunit S3 (NDUFS3), succinate dehydrogenase complex iron sulfur subunit B (SDHB), and ubiquinol-cytochrome C reductase core protein 2 (UQCRC2) were quantified by Western immunoblotting. Participants with PF&S showed higher levels of circulating sEVs relative to controls. Protein levels of CD9 and CD63 were lower in the sEV fraction of PF&S older adults, while CD81 was unvaried between groups. In addition, circulating sEVs from PF&S participants had lower amounts of ATP5A, NDUFS3, and SDHB. No signal was detected for MTCOI, NDUFB8, or UQCRC2 in either participant group. Our findings indicate that, in spite of increased sEV secretion, lower amounts of mitochondrial components are discarded through EV in older adults with PF&S. In-depth analysis of EV trafficking might open new venues for biomarker discovery and treatment development for PF&S.

Keywords: aging; biomarkers; mitophagy; mitochondrial dynamics; mitochondrial quality control; mitochondrial-derived vesicles (MDVs); exosomes; mitochondrial-lysosomal axis

1. Introduction

Advancing age is associated with declining muscle mass, function, and strength, a condition referred to as sarcopenia which increases the risk of incurring negative health-related outcomes (e.g., disability, loss of independence, institutionalization, death) [1]. Hence, sarcopenia and its clinical correlates are major public health priorities. Physical activity, nutritional interventions, and multi-component programs have proven to be valuable strategies for managing sarcopenia [2–4]. Yet, no effective pharmacological treatments are currently available to prevent, delay, or treat sarcopenia, which is mostly due to the incomplete knowledge of the underlying pathophysiology [2]. To further complicate the matter, at the clinical level, sarcopenia shows remarkable overlap with frailty, a "multidimensional syndrome characterized by a decrease in physiological reserve and reduced resistance to stressors", often envisioned as a pre-disability condition [5]. Hence, the two conditions have been merged into a new entity, referred to as physical frailty and sarcopenia (PF&S) [6].

Mitochondrial dysfunction and sterile inflammation are invoked among the pathogenic factors of PF&S [7,8]. Derangements at different levels of the mitochondrial quality control (MQC) machinery have been reported in older adults with PF&S [7]. However, whether and how cell-based alterations may spread at the systemic level and impact muscle homeostasis is presently unknown.

One of the mechanisms by which cells communicate with each other involves a conserved delivery system based on the generation and release of extracellular vesicles (EVs) [9]. These vesicles transfer information between cells through several categories of cargo-enriched biomolecules (i.e., proteins, lipids, nucleic acids, and sugars), each of them selectively influencing different cellular domains [10]. This shuttle system also contributes to degradative pathways responsible for eliminating oxidized cell components, including mitochondria, by establishing inter-organelle contact sites [11]. In particular, in the setting of incomplete mitochondrial depolarization, cells may either delay autophagy to remove mildly damaged organelles or shift from mitophagy to the extrusion of mitochondrial components within EVs [12,13]. As such, the generation and release of mitochondrial-derived vesicles (MDVs) may represent a complement to MQC systems before whole-sale organelle is triggered [13,14].

Cell-free mitochondrial DNA (mtDNA) has been identified among the molecules released within exosomes that may act as damage-associated molecular patterns (DAMPs) [15]. One of the biological roles for these molecules is the activation of innate immunity through binding of their hypomethylated CpG motifs, resembling those of bacterial DNA, to membrane- or cytoplasmic-pattern recognition receptors (PRRs), including Toll-like receptor (TLR), nucleotide-binding oligomerization domain (NOD)-like receptor (NLR) [16], and cytosolic cyclic GMP-AMP synthase (cGAS)-stimulator of interferon genes (STING) DNA sensing system-mediated pathways [17]. However, mtDNA is not the only mitochondrial constituent that may be displaced via MDVs and trigger these responses. Recently, the extrusion of mitochondrial components other than mtDNA has been reported within small EVs (sEVs) purified from the serum of older adults with Parkinson's disease (PD) [14]. However, whether and how this mechanism is in place in the setting of PF&S is unexplored.

In the present study, we purified sEVs from older adults with and without PF&S, quantified their amount, and characterized their content for the presence of mitochondrial components. The identification of specific derangements in sEVs in PF&S may shed light on its pathophysiology as well as suggest new biomarkers and possible biological targets for drug development.

2. Materials and Methods

2.1. Participants

Older adults aged 70+ with and without PF&S were recruited among the participants of the "BIOmarkers associated with Sarcopenia and Physical frailty in EldeRly pErsons" (BIOSPHERE) study [18]. BIOSPHERE was designed to determine and validate a panel of PF&S biomarkers through multivariate statistical modeling of biomolecules pertaining to inflammation, redox homeostasis, amino acid metabolism, neuromuscular junction dysfunction, and muscle remodeling pathways [18–20].

The operational definition used in the "Sarcopenia and Physical fRailty IN older people: multi-componenT Treatment strategies" (SPRINTT) project [21,22] was applied to diagnose PF&S: (a) physical frailty, based on a summary score on the Short Physical Performance Battery (SPPB) [23] between 3 and 9, (b) low appendicular muscle mass (aLM), according to the cut-points proposed by the Foundation for the National Institutes of Health (FNIH) sarcopenia project [24], and (c) absence of mobility disability (i.e., inability to complete the 400-m walk test) [25]. The present investigation involved a convenience sample of 21 participants, 11 older adults with PF&S and 10 non-sarcopenic non-frail (non-PF&S) controls. Participants were randomly chosen from the cohort of the BIOSPHERE study [18], among those from whom serum was available for vesicle purification.

The study was approved by the Ethics Committee of the Università Cattolica del Sacro Cuore (Rome, Italy; protocol number BIOSPHERE: 8498/15) and all participants signed an informed consent prior to inclusion. Study procedures and criteria for participant selection were described thoroughly elsewhere [18].

2.2. Measurement of Appendicular Lean Mass by Dual X-Ray Absorptiometry

Appendicular lean mass was quantified through whole-body Dual X-Ray Absorptiometry (DXA) scans on a Hologic Discovery A densitometer (Hologic, Inc., Bedford, MA, USA) according to the manufacturer's procedures. Criteria for low aLM were as follows: (a) aLM to body mass index (BMI) ratio (aLM$_{BMI}$) < 0.789 in men and <0.512 in women, or (b) crude aLM < 19.75 kg in men and <15.02 kg in women [24].

2.3. Blood Sampling

Blood samples were collected in the morning by venipuncture of the median cubital vein after overnight fasting, using commercial collection tubes (BD Vacutainer®; Becton, Dickinson and Co., Franklin Lakes, NJ, USA). One blood tube was delivered to the centralized diagnostic laboratory of the Fondazione Policlinico Universitario "Agostino Gemelli" IRCCS (Rome, Italy) for standard blood biochemistry. The remaining tubes were processed for serum collection in the Biogerontology lab of the Università Cattolica del Sacro Cuore (Rome, Italy). Serum separation was obtained after 30 min of clotting at room temperature and subsequent centrifugation at 1000× g for 15 min at 4 °C. The upper clear fraction (serum) was collected in 0.5-mL aliquots and stored at −80 °C until analysis.

2.4. Small Extracellular Vesicles Isolation and Characterization

2.4.1. Purification of Small Extracellular Vesicles by Differential Ultracentrifugation

Small EVs/exosomes were purified through differential centrifugation as previously described [14,26]. Briefly, serum samples were diluted with equal volumes of phosphate-buffered saline (PBS) to reduce fluid viscosity. Diluted samples were centrifuged at 2000× g at 4 °C for 30 min and pellets were discarded to remove cell contaminants. Subsequently, supernatants were centrifuged at 12,000× g at 4 °C for 45 min to remove apoptotic bodies, mitochondrial fragments, cell debris, and large vesicles (mean size > 200 nm). Supernatants were collected and ultracentrifuged at 110,000× g at 4 °C for 2 h. Pellets were recovered and resuspended in PBS, filtered through a 0.22-μm filter, and ultracentrifuged at 110,000× g at 4 °C for 70 min to eliminate contaminant proteins. Pellets enriched in purified sEVs were finally resuspended in 100 μL of PBS. To quantify sEVs, total protein concentration was measured using the Bradford assay [27].

2.4.2. Western Immunoblot Analysis of Small Extracellular Vesicles

Western immunoblot analysis was performed to assess the purity of sEV isolation, to determine the type of sEVs on the basis of the expressed tetraspanins, and to characterize their protein cargo as previously described [14,28]. Briefly, equal amounts (1.25 μg) of sEV proteins were separated by sodium dodecyl sulphate polyacrylamide gel electrophoresis (SDS-PAGE) and subsequently electroblotted onto polyvinylidenefluoride (PVDF) Immobilon-P (Millipore, Burlington, MA, USA). Membranes were probed with primary antibodies against tetraspanins CD63 (1:200), CD9 (1:200), CD81 (1:200), a specific cocktail of antibodies (1:250) targeting mitochondrial markers (Table 1), flotilin (1:200), and heterogeneous nuclear ribonucleoprotein A1 (HNRNPA1; 1:1000). Technical specifications of primary antibodies used for Western immunoblotting are detailed in Supplementary Table S1.

Table 1. Mitochondrial components and related electron transport chain complexes assayed in purified small extracellular vesicles by Western immunoblotting.

Mitochondrial Marker	ETC Complex
ATP5A	V
MTCOI	IV
NDUFB8	I
NDUFS3	I
SDHB	II
UQCRC2	III

Abbreviations: ATP5A, adenosine triphosphate 5A; ETC, electron transport chain; MTCOI, mitochondrial cytochrome C oxidase subunit I; NDUFB8, nicotinamide adenine dinucleotide reduced form (NADH):ubiquinone oxidoreductase subunit B8; NDUFS3, NADH:ubiquinone oxidoreductase subunit S3; SDHB, succinate dehydrogenase complex iron sulfur subunit B; UQCRC2, ubiquinol-cytochrome C reductase core protein 2.

The following day, membranes were incubated for 1 h at room temperature with anti-mouse peroxidase-conjugated secondary antibodies (1:2000) (Bio-Rad Laboratories, Inc., Hercules, CA, USA). Blots were visualized using the Clarity Max ECL Western Blotting Substrate (Bio-Rad Laboratories) and images were acquired by the ChemiDoc MP Imaging System and analyzed by Image Lab ™ software version 6.0.1 (Bio-Rad Laboratories). Values of optical density (OD) units of each protein band immunodetected were normalized for the amount of sEV total proteins, as determined by the Bradford assay, and related to the control group, whose OD was set at 100%.

2.4.3. Analysis of Small Extracellular Vesicles by Scanning Electron Microscopy Imaging

Small EVs were fixed in a solution of 3.7% glutaraldehyde (Sigma–Aldrich, St. Luis, MO, USA) in PBS for 15 min, washed twice with PBS, and dehydrated through a series of ascending grades of ethanol (i.e., 40%, 60%, 80%, 96%–98%). Subsequently, samples were mounted on carbon adhesive stubs (Agar Scientifics, Stansted, UK) and left at room temperature for 24 h to obtain complete ethanol evaporation. Samples were gold-coated with a Balzers SCD 040 sputter coater (BAL–TEC AG, Balzers, Lichtenstein, Germany; thickness of gold layer: 40 nm) and analyzed at 132.21 K× magnification by a ZEISS EVO HD 15 Scanning Electron Microscope (Carl Zeiss Microscopy GmbH, Oberkochen, Germany) operating under high-vacuum at an accelerating voltage of 5 kV.

2.5. Statistical Analysis

Descriptive statistics were run on all data. Differences in demographic, anthropometric, and clinical parameters between PF&S and control participants were assessed via t-test statistics and χ^{-2} or Fisher exact tests, for continuous and categorical variables, respectively. All tests were two-sided, with statistical significance set at $p < 0.05$. Analyses were performed using the GraphPrism 5.03 software (GraphPad Software, Inc., San Diego, CA, USA).

3. Results

3.1. Characteristics of the Study Participants

The subset of participants included in the present study was representative of the whole BIOSPHERE cohort in terms of age, sex distribution, clinical characteristics, and body composition and functional parameters [8]. The main characteristics of study participants are presented in Table 2. Sex distribution, BMI, number of comorbid conditions and medications, total serum protein concentrations, and albumin levels did not differ between older adults with and without PF&S. PF&S participants tended to be older than controls, but the difference did not reach statistical significance. As per the selection criteria, SPPB scores and aLM either crude or adjusted by BMI were lower in older adults with PF&S relative to non-PF&S participants.

Table 2. Participant characteristics according to the presence of physical frailty and sarcopenia.

Characteristic	Non-PF&S (n = 10)	PF&S (n = 11)	p-Value
Age (years), mean ± SD	73.9 ± 2.7	77.7 ± 5.4	0.0557
Gender (female), n (%)	5 (50)	8 (73)	0.5344
BMI (kg/m^2), mean ± SD	28.1 ± 2.8	30.3 ± 4.3	0.1891
SPPB summary score, mean ± SD	12.0 ± 1.0	7.0 ± 0.3	<0.0001
aLM (kg), mean ± SD	20.21 ± 4.10	15.84 ± 3.63	0.0390
aLM$_{BMI}$, mean ± SD	0.81 ± 0.32	0.51 ± 0.11	0.0118
Albumin (g/L), mean ± SD	45.4 ± 12.7	39.8 ± 1.2	0.1536
Total serum protein concentration (g/L), mean ± SD	71.8 ± 4.6	75.5 ± 3.1	0.0914
Number of diseases $^{¥}$, mean	3.2 ± 1.6	3.1 ± 1.2	0.8647
Number of medications $^{#}$, mean ± SD	2.9 ± 1.6	3.2 ± 1.8	0.7061

Abbreviations: aLM, appendicular lean mass; aLM$_{BMI}$, aLM adjusted by body mass index (BMI); non-PF&S, non-physically frail non-sarcopenic; PF&S: physical frailty & sarcopenia; SD: standard deviation; SPPB: short physical performance battery. $^{¥}$ includes hypertension, coronary artery disease, prior stroke, peripheral vascular disease, diabetes, chronic obstructive pulmonary disease, and osteoarthritis. $^{#}$ includes prescription and over-the-counter drugs

3.2. Characterization of Small Extracellular Vesicles from the Serum of Participants with and without Physical Frailty and Sarcopenia

3.2.1. Verification of the Purity of Serum Small Extracellular Vesicles

The purity of sEVs obtained by serum ultracentrifugation was ascertained according to the guidelines of the International Society of Extracellular Vesicles [29]. In particular, the presence of the cytosolic protein flotilin (positive control) and the absence of the non-sEV component HNRNPA1 (negative control) were verified (Figure 1A). The purified biospecimen was also analyzed by scanning electron microscopy (SEM) to confirm enrichment in sEVs. Small EVs appear in the scanning electron micrographs as objects of spherical shape and less than 100 nm in size (Figure 1B).

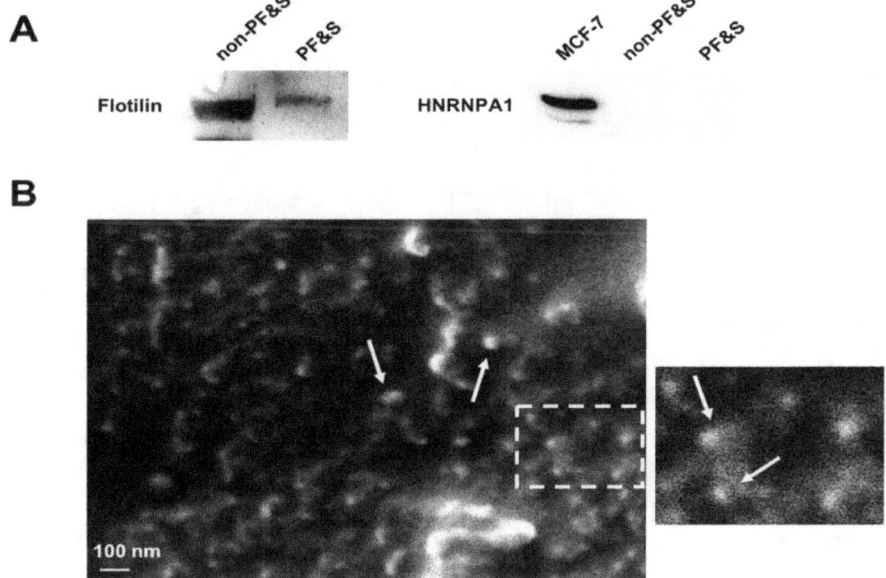

Figure 1. (**A**) Blots of the cytosolic protein flotilin and heterogeneous nuclear ribonucleoprotein A1 (HNRNPA1) as positive and negative markers respectively, in purified small extracellular vesicles (sEVs) obtained by serum ultracentrifugation from participants with physical frailty and sarcopenia (PF&S) and non-physically frail non-sarcopenic (non-PF&S) controls. The Michigan Cancer Foundation-7 (MCF-7) cell extract was used as the positive control for the anti-HNRNPA1 antibody. (**B**) Scanning electron micrographs of purified sEVs. The white-dashed box delimitates the area zoomed on the right. White arrows indicate some of the sEVs found in the observation field. Scale bar: 100 nm.

3.2.2. Quantification of the Amount of Circulating Small Extracellular Vesicles

The total amount of sEVs purified from the serum of PF&S participants was significantly greater than in non-PF&S controls ($p < 0.0001$, Figure 2).

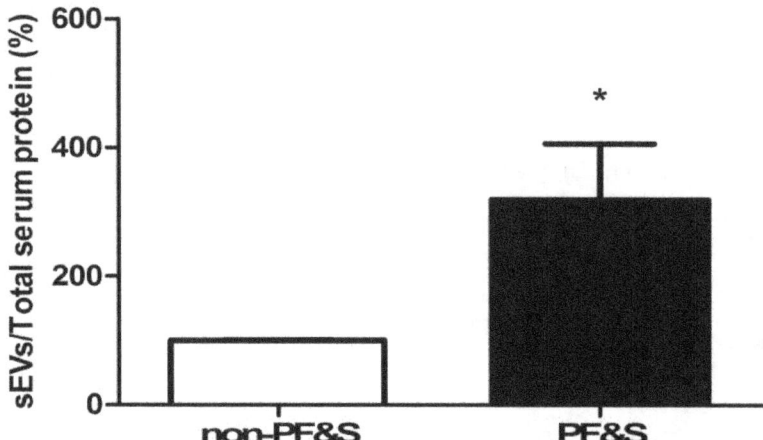

Figure 2. Serum levels of small extracellular vesicles (sEVs) in non-physically frail non-sarcopenic (non-PF&S) controls (n = 10) and participants with physical frailty and sarcopenia (PF&S; n = 11). Data were normalized for the amount of total serum proteins and are shown as percentage of the control group set at 100%. Bars represent mean values (±standard error of the mean). * $p < 0.05$ versus non-PF&S.

3.2.3. Characterization of the Origin and Cargo of Small Extracellular Vesicles

Protein levels of the two tetraspanins, CD9 and CD63, were lower in participants with PF&S than in non-PF&S controls (Figure 3A,B), while CD81 content was unvaried between groups (Figure 3C).

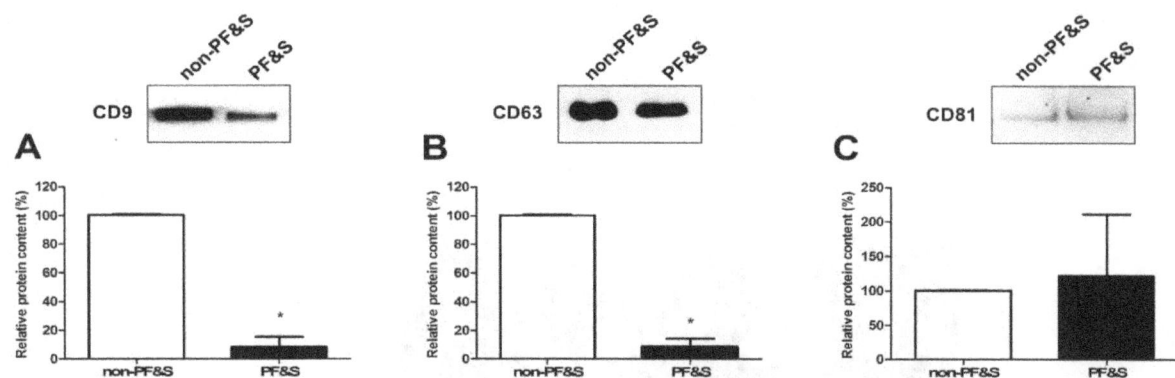

Figure 3. Protein expression of (**A**) CD9, (**B**) CD63, and (**C**) CD81 in purified small extracellular vesicles (sEVs) from non-physically frail non-sarcopenic (non-PF&S) controls (n = 10) and participants with physical frailty and sarcopenia (PF&S; n = 11). Data were normalized for the amount of sEV total proteins and are shown as percentage of the control group set at 100%. Bars represent mean values (±standard error of the mean). * $p < 0.0001$ versus non-PF&S.

As for sEV cargo characterization, protein levels of adenosine triphosphate 5A (ATP5A; complex V), nicotinamide adenine dinucleotide reduced form (NADH):ubiquinone oxidoreductase subunit S3 (NDUFS3; complex I), and succinate dehydrogenase complex iron sulfur subunit B (SDHB; complex II) were lower in participants with PF&S than in non-PF&S controls (Figure 4A–C). No signal was detected for mitochondrial cytochrome C oxidase subunit I (MTCOI, complex IV), NADH:ubiquinone oxidoreductase subunit B8 (NDUFB8; complex I), or ubiquinol-cytochrome C reductase core protein 2 (UQCRC2; complex III) in either participant group.

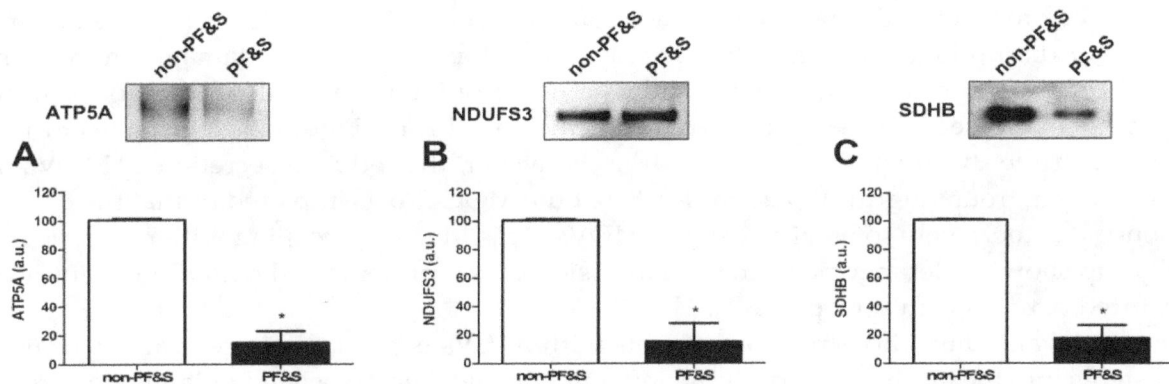

Figure 4. Protein expression of (**A**) adenosine triphosphate 5A (ATP5A), (**B**) nicotinamide adenine dinucleotide reduced form (NADH):ubiquinone oxidoreductase subunit S3 (NDUFS3), and (**C**) succinate dehydrogenase complex iron sulfur subunit (SDHB) in purified small extracellular vesicles (sEVs) from non-physically frail non-sarcopenic (non-PF&S) controls (n = 10) and participants with physical frailty and sarcopenia (PF&S; n = 11). Data were normalized for the amount of sEV total proteins and are shown as percentage of the control group set at 100%. Bars represent mean values (±standard error of the mean). * $p < 0.0001$ versus non-PF&S.

4. Discussion

Among the factors involved in muscle degeneration associated with PF&S, mitochondrial dysfunction and the accrual of abnormal organelles have been indicated as relevant players [30]. However, the exact mechanisms underlying mitochondrial decay are not completely deciphered.

Derangements in MQC processes have been reported in older adults with PF&S [7,31,32]. Nevertheless, alterations in sEV trafficking, which might contribute to MQC dyshomeostasis in muscle [33], have remained largely unexplored. To start filling this gap in knowledge, we purified sEVs from the serum of older adults with and without PF&S and, after ascertaining purity of the preparation, we determined the overall quantity of the mixed sEV population. Our results show a greater amount of sEVs in serum of PF&S participants compared with non-PF&S controls (Figure 2). The verification of the three tetraspanins, CD9, CD63, and CD81, in purified sEVs allowed these vesicles to be identified as a fraction of endosome-derived vesicles, referred to as exosomes, originating from the fusion of multivesicular bodies with the plasma membrane [28]. A lower protein expression of CD9 and CD63 was found in the exosome fraction purified from participants with PF&S (Figure 3), while levels of CD81 were comparable between groups. These observations are in keeping with the heterogenous composition of exosomes themselves, likely reflecting a different vesicle trafficking regulation [34]. Indeed, RAB27A, a guanosine triphosphatase (GTPase) that modulates exosome secretion, has been shown to regulate the secretion of CD63-positive exosomes, but not of those positive for CD9 [35]. Notably, exosomes derived by B-cells are characterized by the tetraspanin markers CD9 and CD81, while CD63 is absent [36]. A previous report by our group showed that RAB7A, a small GTPase and a master regulator of the late endocytic pathway, was able to modulate secretion of CD9- and CD81-positive exosomes [37]. The decreased expression of tetraspanin CD63 found in the present study may therefore be indicative of an altered late endocytic pathway [38], possibly suggesting disarrangements in late endocytic trafficking in PF&S.

The identification of mitochondrial components within the purified material allowed for classification of MDVs among sEVs. In particular, lower levels of the mitochondrial components ATP5A (complex V), NDUFS3 (complex I), and SDHB (complex II) were found in participants with PF&S (Figure 4). With the intent of preserving mitochondrial homeostasis, mitochondrial hyper-fission segregates severely damaged or unnecessary organelles [39,40] that are subsequently disposed via mitophagy [41]. However, mitochondrial-lysosomal crosstalk may dispose mildly oxidized mitochondria via MDV release [42]. Such a mechanism may therefore restore mitochondrial homeostasis before whole-sale organelle degradation is triggered [42]. Though, in the case of defective mitophagy or disruption of the mitochondrial-lysosomal axis, accrual of damaged mitochondria, misfolded proteins, and lipofuscin may occur as a result of inefficient cellular quality control [43]. Therefore, the increased sEV secretion in participants with PF&S (Figure 2) might reflect the cell's attempt to extrude dysfunctional mitochondria. However, the reduced secretion of MDVs in the same participant group (Figure 4) may indicate that the MQC flux is impaired or that the damage to mitochondria is too severe to be disposed via MDVs. This idea is in keeping with previous reports by our group showing derangements in the expression of key proteins of the MQC machinery in old hip-fractured patients with sarcopenia [7,31].

The retrieval of mitochondrial components within sEVs is particularly relevant as it provides novel insights into the mechanisms of sterile inflammation, an age-associated inflammatory response mounted in the absence of infections [44]. This process is framed within the innate immune response and has been included as part of the "danger theory" of inflammation [45]. According to this view, misplaced noxious material from injured cells (i.e., damage-associated molecular patterns (DAMPs)) triggers caspase-1 activation and the secretion of pro-inflammatory cytokines [46]. The release of MDV content (e.g., mitochondrial proteins, mtDNA) can activate inflammatory pathways by interacting with several receptors/systems including TLRs, family pyrin domain-containing 3 (NLRP3) inflammasome, and cGAS-STING DNA sensing system [47].

Recently, we described the existence of a frailty "cytokinome" in older adults with PF&S defined by higher levels of P-selectin, C-reactive protein, and interferon-γ-induced protein 10, and lower levels of myeloperoxidase, interleukin 8, monocyte chemoattractant protein-1, macrophage inflammatory protein 1-α, and platelet-derived growth factor BB [8]. Pro-sarcopenic/pro-disability effects have traditionally been attributed to inflammation [48,49] as much as to dysfunction of anti-inflammatory pathways [49,50]. Furthermore, circulating MDVs have been identified in serum of older adults with PD and associated with a specific inflammatory profile [14]. However, the liaison among failing mitochondrial fidelity pathways, MDV secretion, and systemic inflammation may not be exclusive of neurodegeneration. Indeed, other conditions, such as HIV infection, a model of accelerated and accentuated aging [51], are characterized by pyroptotic bystander cell death and release of DAMPs that may trigger the same pathways as those identified in PD and inflamm-aging [52]. In addition, a massive release of DAMPs is acknowledged as a factor in the development of multiorgan failure in patients with severe injuries or during hemorrhagic shock [53]. Although the pathophysiology of multiple organ failure syndrome, neurodegeneration, and PF&S is heterogeneous, the release of mitochondrial DAMPs might be a converging mechanism shared by all of them. Should this assumption hold true, the scavenging of circulating mitochondrial DAMPs might represent a yet unexplored therapeutic option for the management of age-associated disarrangements, including PF&S. From this perspective, our findings are in line with the geroscience hypothesis, according to which the roots of most chronic diseases may reside in perturbations of a set of basic mechanisms (i.e., hallmarks of aging), including mitochondrial dysfunction [54].

Albeit presenting novel and promising findings, our work has limitations that need to be discussed. First of all, the cross-sectional design of the study precludes establishing cause–effect or temporal relationships between the analyzed pathways and PF&S pathophysiology. Also, although participants were carefully selected and thoroughly characterized, we cannot rule out the possibility that unknown comorbidities may have affected our results. In addition, our study provides an initial characterization of the heterogeneous population of circulating sEVs. Indeed, the analysis of the MDV cargo was limited to selected components/subunits of the mitochondrial electron transport chain. Hence, we cannot exclude that the analysis of other biomolecules, including mtDNA, that may be transported along the same road could provide additional insights into the relationship between sEV trafficking and PF&S. Finally, a deeper characterization of sEVs for their structure and content by means of transmission electron microscopy analysis is needed to confirm and expand our findings as well as to gain further information into the dynamic regulation of vesicle trafficking in PF&S.

Author Contributions: Conceptualization, A.P., C.B., E.M., F.G., and R.C.; Data curation, A.P., F.G., and R.B. (Raffaella Beli); Methodology, A.P., F.G., H.J.C.-J., and R.B. (Raffaella Beli); Writing—original draft preparation, A.P., E.M., and R.C.; Writing—review and editing, C.B., F.G., F.L., and R.B. (Raffaella Beli); Supervision, F.L., and R.B. (Roberto Bernabei); Funding acquisition, C.B. and R.B. (Roberto Bernabei). All authors have read and agreed to the published version of the manuscript.

References

1. Landi, F.; Calvani, R.; Cesari, M.; Tosato, M.; Martone, A.M.; Ortolani, E.; Savera, G.; Salini, S.; Sisto, A.; Picca, A.; et al. Sarcopenia: An overview on current definitions, diagnosis and treatment. *Curr. Protein Pept. Sci.* **2018**, *19*, 633–638. [CrossRef] [PubMed]

2. Calvani, R.; Miccheli, A.; Landi, F.; Bossola, M.; Cesari, M.; Leeuwenburgh, C.; Sieber, C.C.; Bernabei, R.; Marzetti, E. Current nutritional recommendations and novel dietary strategies to manage sarcopenia. *J. Frailty Aging* **2013**, *2*, 38–53. [CrossRef] [PubMed]

3. Chan, D.C.D.; Tsou, H.H.; Chang, C.B.; Yang, R.S.; Tsauo, J.Y.; Chen, C.Y.; Hsiao, C.F.; Hsu, Y.T.; Chen, C.H.; Chang, S.F.; et al. Integrated care for geriatric frailty and sarcopenia: A randomized control trial. *J. Cachexia Sarcopenia Muscle* **2017**, *8*, 78–88. [CrossRef] [PubMed]

4. Bauer, J.M.; Verlaan, S.; Bautmans, I.; Brandt, K.; Donini, L.M.; Maggio, M.; McMurdo, M.E.T.; Mets, T.; Seal, C.; Wijers, S.L.; et al. Effects of a vitamin D and leucine-enriched whey protein nutritional supplement on measures of sarcopenia in older adults, the PROVIDE study: A randomized, double-blind, placebo-controlled trial. *J. Am. Med. Dir. Assoc.* **2015**, *16*, 740–747. [CrossRef] [PubMed]

5. Cesari, M.; Calvani, R.; Marzetti, E. Frailty in older persons. *Clin. Geriatr. Med.* **2017**, *33*, 293–303. [CrossRef] [PubMed]

6. Cesari, M.; Landi, F.; Calvani, R.; Cherubini, A.; Di Bari, M.; Kortebein, P.; Del Signore, S.; Le Lain, R.; Vellas, B.; Pahor, M.; et al. Rationale for a preliminary operational definition of physical frailty and sarcopenia in the SPRINTT trial. *Aging Clin. Exp. Res.* **2017**, *29*, 81–88. [CrossRef]

7. Marzetti, E.; Calvani, R.; Lorenzi, M.; Tanganelli, F.; Picca, A.; Bossola, M.; Menghi, A.; Bernabei, R.; Landi, F. Association between myocyte quality control signaling and sarcopenia in old hip-fractured patients: Results from the Sarcopenia in HIp FracTure (SHIFT) exploratory study. *Exp. Gerontol.* **2016**, *80*, 1–5. [CrossRef]

8. Marzetti, E.; Picca, A.; Marini, F.; Biancolillo, A.; Coelho-Junior, H.J.; Gervasoni, J.; Bossola, M.; Cesari, M.; Onder, G.; Landi, F.; et al. Inflammatory signatures in older persons with physical frailty and sarcopenia: The frailty "cytokinome" at its core. *Exp. Gerontol.* **2019**, *122*, 129–138. [CrossRef] [PubMed]

9. Stahl, P.D.; Raposo, G. Extracellular vesicles: Exosomes and microvesicles, integrators of homeostasis. *Physiology* **2019**, *34*, 169–177. [CrossRef] [PubMed]

10. Maas, S.L.N.; Breakefield, X.O.; Weaver, A.M. Extracellular vesicles: Unique intercellular delivery vehicles. *Trends Cell Biol.* **2017**, *27*, 172–188. [CrossRef] [PubMed]

11. Picca, A.; Calvani, R.; Coelho-Junior, H.J.; Landi, F.; Bernabei, R.; Marzetti, E. Inter-organelle membrane contact sites and mitochondrial quality control during aging: A geroscience view. *Cells* **2020**, *9*, 598. [CrossRef] [PubMed]

12. Bowling, J.L.; Skolfield, M.C.; Riley, W.A.; Nolin, A.P.; Wolf, L.C.; Nelson, D.E. Temporal integration of mitochondrial stress signals by the PINK1:Parkin pathway. *BMC Mol. Cell Biol.* **2019**, *20*, 33. [CrossRef] [PubMed]

13. Soubannier, V.; McLelland, G.-L.; Zunino, R.; Braschi, E.; Rippstein, P.; Fon, E.A.; McBride, H.M. A vesicular transport pathway shuttles cargo from mitochondria to lysosomes. *Curr. Biol.* **2012**, *22*, 135–141. [CrossRef] [PubMed]

14. Picca, A.; Guerra, F.; Calvani, R.; Marini, F.; Biancolillo, A.; Landi, G.; Beli, R.; Landi, F.; Bernabei, R.; Bentivoglio, A.R.; et al. Mitochondrial signatures in circulating extracellular vesicles of older adults with Parkinson's disease: Results from the EXosomes in PArkiNson's Disease (EXPAND) study. *J. Clin. Med.* **2020**, *9*, 504. [CrossRef]

15. Picca, A.; Lezza, A.M.S.; Leeuwenburgh, C.; Pesce, V.; Calvani, R.; Landi, F.; Bernabei, R.; Marzetti, E. Fueling inflamm-aging through mitochondrial dysfunction: Mechanisms and molecular targets. *Int. J. Mol. Sci.* **2017**, *18*, 933. [CrossRef]

16. Collins, L.V.; Hajizadeh, S.; Holme, E.; Jonsson, I.-M.; Tarkowski, A. Endogenously oxidized mitochondrial DNA induces in vivo and in vitro inflammatory responses. *J. Leukoc. Biol.* **2004**, *75*, 995–1000. [CrossRef]

17. Cai, X.; Chiu, Y.H.; Chen, Z.J. The cGAS-cGAMP-STING pathway of cytosolic DNA sensing and signaling. *Mol. Cell* **2014**, *54*, 289–296. [CrossRef]

18. Calvani, R.; Picca, A.; Marini, F.; Biancolillo, A.; Cesari, M.; Pesce, V.; Lezza, A.M.S.; Bossola, M.; Leeuwenburgh, C.; Bernabei, R.; et al. The "BIOmarkers associated with Sarcopenia and PHysical frailty in EldeRly pErsons" (BIOSPHERE) study: Rationale, design and methods. *Eur. J. Intern. Med.* **2018**, *56*, 19–25. [CrossRef]

19. Calvani, R.; Picca, A.; Marini, F.; Biancolillo, A.; Gervasoni, J.; Persichilli, S.; Primiano, A.; Coelho-Junior, H.J.; Bossola, M.; Urbani, A.; et al. A distinct pattern of circulating amino acids characterizes older persons with physical frailty and sarcopenia: Results from the BIOSPHERE study. *Nutrients* **2018**, *10*, 1691. [CrossRef]

20. Picca, A.; Ponziani, F.R.; Calvani, R.; Marini, F.; Biancolillo, A.; Coelho-Junior, H.J.; Gervasoni, J.; Primiano, A.; Putignani, L.; Del Chierico, F.; et al. Gut microbial, inflammatory and metabolic signatures in older people with physical frailty and sarcopenia: Results from the BIOSPHERE study. *Nutrients* **2019**, *12*, 65. [CrossRef]

21. Marzetti, E.; Calvani, R.; Landi, F.; Hoogendijk, E.; Fougère, B.; Vellas, B.; Pahor, M.; Bernabei, R.; Cesari, M. Innovative medicines initiative: The SPRINTT project. *J. Frailty Aging* **2015**, *4*, 207–208. [CrossRef] [PubMed]

22. Marzetti, E.; Cesari, M.; Calvani, R.; Msihid, J.; Tosato, M.; Rodriguez-Mañas, L.; Lattanzio, F.; Cherubini, A.; Bejuit, R.; Di Bari, M.; et al. The "Sarcopenia and Physical fRailty IN older people: Multi-componenT Treatment strategies" (SPRINTT) randomized controlled trial: Case finding, screening and characteristics of eligible participants. *Exp. Gerontol.* **2018**, *113*, 48–57. [CrossRef] [PubMed]

23. Guralnik, J.M.; Simonsick, E.M.; Ferrucci, L.; Glynn, R.J.; Berkman, L.F.; Blazer, D.G.; Scherr, P.A.; Wallace, R.B. A short physical performance battery assessing lower extremity function: Association with self-reported disability and prediction of mortality and nursing home admission. *J. Gerontol.* **1994**, *49*, M85–M94. [CrossRef] [PubMed]

24. Studenski, S.A.; Peters, K.W.; Alley, D.E.; Cawthon, P.M.; McLean, R.R.; Harris, T.B.; Ferrucci, L.; Guralnik, J.M.; Fragala, M.S.; Kenny, A.M.; et al. The FNIH sarcopenia project: Rationale, study description, conference recommendations, and final estimates. *J. Gerontol. A Biol. Sci. Med. Sci.* **2014**, *69*, 547–558. [CrossRef]

25. Newman, A.B.; Simonsick, E.M.; Naydeck, B.L.; Boudreau, R.M.; Kritchevsky, S.B.; Nevitt, M.C.; Pahor, M.; Satterfield, S.; Brach, J.S.; Studenski, S.A.; et al. Association of long-distance corridor walk performance with mortality, cardiovascular disease, mobility limitation, and disability. *J. Am. Med. Assoc.* **2006**, *295*, 2018–2026. [CrossRef]

26. Picca, A.; Guerra, F.; Calvani, R.; Bucci, C.; Lo Monaco, M.R.; Bentivoglio, A.R.; Landi, F.; Bernabei, R.; Marzetti, E. Mitochondrial-derived vesicles as candidate biomarkers in Parkinson's disease: Rationale, design and methods of the exosomes in PArkiNson Disease (EXPAND) Study. *Int. J. Mol. Sci.* **2019**, *20*, 2373. [CrossRef]

27. Théry, C.; Amigorena, S.; Raposo, G.; Clayton, A. Isolation and characterization of exosomes from cell culture supernatants and biological fluids. *Curr. Protoc. Cell Biol.* **2006**, *30*. [CrossRef]

28. Kowal, E.J.K.; Ter-Ovanesyan, D.; Regev, A.; Church, G.M. Extracellular vesicle isolation and analysis by Western blotting. *Methods Mol. Biol.* **2017**, *1660*, 143–152. [CrossRef]

29. Théry, C.; Witwer, K.W.; Aikawa, E.; Alcaraz, M.J.; Anderson, J.D.; Andriantsitohaina, R.; Antoniou, A.; Arab, T.; Archer, F.; Atkin-Smith, G.K.; et al. Minimal information for studies of extracellular vesicles 2018 (MISEV2018): A position statement of the International Society for Extracellular Vesicles and update of the MISEV2014 guidelines. *J. Extracell. Vesicles* **2018**, *7*, 1535750. [CrossRef]

30. Picca, A.; Calvani, R.; Bossola, M.; Allocca, E.; Menghi, A.; Pesce, V.; Lezza, A.M.S.; Bernabei, R.; Landi, F.; Marzetti, E. Update on mitochondria and muscle aging: All wrong roads lead to sarcopenia. *Biol. Chem.* **2018**, *399*, 421–436. [CrossRef]

31. Picca, A.; Calvani, R.; Lorenzi, M.; Menghi, A.; Galli, M.; Vitiello, R.; Randisi, F.; Bernabei, R.; Landi, F.; Marzetti, E. Mitochondrial dynamics signaling is shifted toward fusion in muscles of very old hip-fractured patients: Results from the Sarcopenia in HIp FracTure (SHIFT) exploratory study. *Exp. Gerontol.* **2017**, *96*, 63–67. [CrossRef] [PubMed]

32. Romanello, V.; Sandri, M. Mitochondrial quality control and muscle mass maintenance. *Front. Physiol.* **2016**, *6*, 422. [CrossRef] [PubMed]

33. Picca, A.; Guerra, F.; Calvani, R.; Bucci, C.; Lo Monaco, M.R.; Bentivoglio, A.R.; Coelho-Júnior, H.J.; Landi, F.; Bernabei, R.; Marzetti, E. Mitochondrial dysfunction and aging: Insights from the analysis of extracellular vesicles. *Int. J. Mol. Sci.* **2019**, *20*, 805. [CrossRef]

34. Andreu, Z.; Yáñez-Mó, M. Tetraspanins in extracellular vesicle formation and function. *Front. Immunol.* **2014**, *5*, 442. [CrossRef] [PubMed]

35. Ostrowski, M.; Carmo, N.B.; Krumeich, S.; Fanget, I.; Raposo, G.; Savina, A.; Moita, C.F.; Schauer, K.; Hume, A.N.; Freitas, R.P.; et al. Rab27a and Rab27b control different steps of the exosome secretion pathway. *Nat. Cell Biol.* **2010**, *12*, 19–30. [CrossRef]

36. Saunderson, S.C.; Schuberth, P.C.; Dunn, A.C.; Miller, L.; Hock, B.D.; MacKay, P.A.; Koch, N.; Jack, R.W.; McLellan, A.D. Induction of exosome release in primary B cells stimulated via CD40 and the IL-4 Receptor. *J. Immunol.* **2008**, *180*, 8146–8152. [CrossRef]

37. Guerra, F.; Paiano, A.; Migoni, D.; Girolimetti, G.; Perrone, A.M.; De Iaco, P.; Fanizzi, F.P.; Gasparre, G.; Bucci, C. Modulation of RAB7A protein expression determines resistance to cisplatin through late endocytic pathway impairment and extracellular vesicular secretion. *Cancers* **2019**, *11*, 52. [CrossRef]

38. Guerra, F.; Bucci, C. Role of the RAB7 protein in tumor progression and cisplatin chemoresistance. *Cancers* **2019**, *11*, 1096. [CrossRef]

39. Twig, G.; Hyde, B.; Shirihai, O.S. Mitochondrial fusion, fission and autophagy as a quality control axis: The bioenergetic view. *Biochim. Biophys. Acta* **2008**, *1777*, 1092–1097. [CrossRef]

40. Marzetti, E.; Calvani, R.; Cesari, M.; Buford, T.W.; Lorenzi, M.; Behnke, B.J.; Leeuwenburgh, C. Mitochondrial dysfunction and sarcopenia of aging: From signaling pathways to clinical trials. *Int. J. Biochem. Cell Biol.* **2013**, *45*, 2288–2301. [CrossRef]

41. Youle, R.J.; Narendra, D.P. Mechanisms of mitophagy. *Nat. Rev. Mol. Cell Biol.* **2011**, *12*, 9–14. [CrossRef] [PubMed]

42. Miyamoto, Y.; Kitamura, N.; Nakamura, Y.; Futamura, M.; Miyamoto, T.; Yoshida, M.; Ono, M.; Ichinose, S.; Arakawa, H. Possible existence of lysosome-like organella within mitochondria and its role in mitochondrial quality control. *PLoS ONE* **2011**, *6*, e16054. [CrossRef] [PubMed]

43. Terman, A.; Kurz, T.; Navratil, M.; Arriaga, E.A.; Brunk, U.T. Mitochondrial turnover and aging of long-lived postmitotic cells: The mitochondrial-lysosomal axis theory of aging. *Antioxid. Redox Signal.* **2010**, *12*, 503–535. [CrossRef] [PubMed]

44. Chen, G.Y.; Nuñez, G. Sterile inflammation: Sensing and reacting to damage. *Nat. Rev. Immunol.* **2010**, *10*, 826–837. [CrossRef] [PubMed]

45. Zhang, Q.; Raoof, M.; Chen, Y.; Sumi, Y.; Sursal, T.; Junger, W.; Brohi, K.; Itagaki, K.; Hauser, C.J. Circulating mitochondrial DAMPs cause inflammatory responses to injury. *Nature* **2010**, *464*, 104–107. [CrossRef] [PubMed]

46. Krysko, D.V.; Agostinis, P.; Krysko, O.; Garg, A.D.; Bachert, C.; Lambrecht, B.N.; Vandenabeele, P. Emerging role DAMPs derived from mitochondria in inflammation. *Trends Immunol.* **2011**, *32*, 157–164. [CrossRef] [PubMed]

47. Picca, A.; Lezza, A.M.S.; Leeuwenburgh, C.; Pesce, V.; Calvani, R.; Bossola, M.; Manes-Gravina, E.; Landi, F.; Bernabei, R.; Marzetti, E. Circulating mitochondrial DNA at the crossroads of mitochondrial dysfunction and inflammation during aging and muscle wasting disorders. *Rejuvenation Res.* **2018**, *21*, 350–359. [CrossRef]

48. Franceschi, C.; Garagnani, P.; Parini, P.; Giuliani, C.; Santoro, A. Inflammaging: A new immune–metabolic viewpoint for age-related diseases. *Nat. Rev. Endocrinol.* **2018**, *14*, 576–590. [CrossRef]

49. Furman, D.; Campisi, J.; Verdin, E.; Carrera-Bastos, P.; Targ, S.; Franceschi, C.; Ferrucci, L.; Gilroy, D.W.; Fasano, A.; Miller, G.W.; et al. Chronic inflammation in the etiology of disease across the life span. *Nat. Med.* **2019**, *25*, 1822–1832. [CrossRef]

50. Wilson, D.; Jackson, T.; Sapey, E.; Lord, J.M. Frailty and sarcopenia: The potential role of an aged immune system. *Ageing Res. Rev.* **2017**, *36*, 1–10. [CrossRef]

51. Cesari, M.; Marzetti, E.; Canevelli, M.; Guaraldi, G. Geriatric syndromes: How to treat. *Virulence* **2017**, *8*, 577–585. [CrossRef] [PubMed]

52. Heil, M.; Brockmeyer, N.H. Self-DNA sensing fuels HIV-1-associated inflammation. *Trends Mol. Med.* **2019**, *25*, 941–954. [CrossRef] [PubMed]

53. Aswani, A.; Manson, J.; Itagaki, K.; Chiazza, F.; Collino, M.; Wupeng, W.L.; Chan, T.K.; Wong, W.S.F.; Hauser, C.J.; Thiemermann, C.; et al. Scavenging circulating mitochondrial DNA as a potential therapeutic option for multiple organ dysfunction in trauma hemorrhage. *Front. Immunol.* **2018**, *9*, 891. [CrossRef] [PubMed]

10

Transthyretin Maintains Muscle Homeostasis through the Novel Shuttle Pathway of Thyroid Hormones during Myoblast Differentiation

Eun Ju Lee [1,†], Sibhghatulla Shaikh [1,†], Dukhwan Choi [1], Khurshid Ahmad [1], Mohammad Hassan Baig [1], Jeong Ho Lim [1], Yong-Ho Lee [2], Sang Joon Park [3], Yong-Woon Kim [4], So-Young Park [4] and Inho Choi [1,*]

[1] Department of Medical Biotechnology, Yeungnam University, Gyeongsan 38541, Korea;
     gorapadoc0315@hanmail.net (E.J.L.); sibhghat.88@gmail.com (S.S.); apdltkd@naver.com (D.C.);
     ahmadkhursheed2008@gmail.com (K.A.); mohdhassanbaig@gmail.com (M.H.B.);
     lim2249@kitech.re.kr (J.H.L.)
[2] Department of Biomedical Science, Daegu Catholic University, Gyeongsan 38430, Korea; ylee325@cu.ac.kr
[3] College of Veterinary Medicine, Kyungpook National University, Daegu 41566, Korea; psj26@knu.ac.kr
[4] Department of Physiology, College of Medicine, Yeungnam University, Daegu 42415, Korea;
     ywkim@yumail.ac.kr (Y.-W.K.); sypark@med.yu.ac.kr (S.-Y.P.)
*   Correspondence: inhochoi@ynu.ac.kr;
†   These two authors contributed equally to this work.

Abstract: Skeletal muscle, the largest part of the total body mass, influences energy and protein metabolism as well as maintaining homeostasis. Herein, we demonstrate that during murine muscle satellite cell and myoblast differentiation, transthyretin (TTR) can exocytose via exosomes and enter cells as TTR- thyroxine (T_4) complex, which consecutively induces the intracellular triiodothyronine (T_3) level, followed by T_3 secretion out of the cell through the exosomes. The decrease in T_3 with the TTR level in 26-week-old mouse muscle, compared to that in 16-week-old muscle, suggests an association of TTR with old muscle. Subsequent studies, including microarray analysis, demonstrated that T_3-regulated genes, such as FNDC5 (Fibronectin type III domain containing 5, irisin) and RXRγ (Retinoid X receptor gamma), are influenced by TTR knockdown, implying that thyroid hormones and TTR coordinate with each other with respect to muscle growth and development. These results suggest that, in addition to utilizing T_4, skeletal muscle also distributes generated T_3 to other tissues and has a vital role in sensing the intracellular T_4 level. Furthermore, the results of TTR function with T_4 in differentiation will be highly useful in the strategic development of novel therapeutics related to muscle homeostasis and regeneration.

Keywords: muscle satellite cell; transthyretin; thyroid hormone; myogenesis; exosomes; skeletal muscle

1. Introduction

Skeletal muscle is comprised of multinucleated myofibers and has excellent regeneration capability, which deteriorates progressively with age, restraining the voluntary functions of daily life. The regenerative capacity is mostly facilitated by muscle satellite or stem cells (MSCs) that reside between the basal lamina and sarcolemma, a distinct 'niche' in the muscle fibers [1,2]. MSCs vigorously regulate myofiber growth, and MSC progression is typically regulated by the expression of myogenic transcription factors (Pax3, Pax7, myoblast determination protein; MYOD, and myogenin; MYOG) [3]. After injury, quiescent Pax7[+] MSCs are triggered to undergo sequential activation, proliferation and differentiation involving MYOD, Myf5 and MYOG to generate multinucleated myotubes [4].

MSC differentiation is indispensable in the regeneration of skeletal muscle and is typically regulated by multiple signaling pathways and by the interaction of several extracellular matrix components with MSCs. Fibromodulin was reported to have a robust role in muscle regeneration by enhancing the recruitment of MSCs to injury sites [5].

Thyroid hormones (THs, thyroxin; T_4 and triiodothyronine; T_3) have vital roles in the development of various tissues, as well as in postnatal life, by modulating gene expressions [6,7]. THs regulate the expression of various proteins crucial for muscle development and contractility [8–10]. Indeed, the foremost targets of THs are muscles, as they regulate the expression of several genes at the transcriptional level [11,12]. The effects of TH signaling in the development and function of skeletal muscle are the result of a remarkably complex mechanism [11]. Generally, to retain homeostasis, regeneration capability, and development, binding of T_3 to thyroid hormone receptors (TR) is essential [13]. TRs are encoded by two genes (THRA and THRB), and alternate splicing of each gene produces TRα1, TRβ1, and TRβ2 receptor subtypes. TRα is the predominant subtype in cardiac and skeletal muscle [14]. TRα has a key role in regulation of heart rate and basal metabolism [15]. Transcription of MYOD is directly regulated by T_3 [16]. Therefore, TH signaling can control several events during myogenesis via direct and/or indirect regulation of myogenic gene expression.

Retinoids (synthetic vitamin A derivatives) can influence development and metabolism through nuclear hormone receptors (retinoic acid receptor and retinoid X receptor, RXR). RXR forms heterodimers with retinoic acid, TH, and vitamin D receptors, enhancing transcriptional function on their respective response elements [17]. Three different RXR isoforms (RXRα, β and γ) have been characterized. RXRγ is the dominant isoform in adult heart and skeletal muscle [18].

Exosomes are small (40–100 nm) membrane vesicles of endocytic origin that are released from most cell types into the extracellular environment [19]. Exosomes were first defined in 1983, and interest in these vesicles increased markedly after finding that they contain mRNA and microRNA [20]. Exosomes have been shown to facilitate cellular communication by transporting proteins, cytokines, and nucleic acids and to sustain the normal physiological function of cells [21].

Transthyretin (TTR) is a 55-kDa homotetrameric transporter protein for T_4 and retinol-binding protein in the blood [22,23]. The liver is the main contributing organ for TTR synthesis in plasma. TTR null (TTR$^{-/-}$) mice exhibit a delayed suckling-to-weaning transition, delayed growth, reduced muscle mass, and stunted longitudinal bone growth [24]. Among the transporters existing in blood, thyroxine-binding globulin (TBG) has the highest affinity for T_4 and T_3 (1.0×10^{10} and 4.6×10^8 M^{-1}, respectively), followed by TTR (7.0×10^7 and 1.4×10^7 M^{-1}) and albumin (7.0×10^5 and 1.0×10^5 M^{-1}) [25]. The binding efficacy of TH distributor proteins determines the transportation times for distribution of THs to tissues, thus, TTR (with transitional affinity), more than TBG, is responsible for instant delivery of THs to tissues [6,25].

Though it is known that human placenta, trophoblasts, JEG-3 and HepG2 cells secrete and internalize TTR [26–28], its cellular uptake in skeletal muscle has not been fully described. We have demonstrated that TTR initiates myoblast differentiation by inducing the expression of myogenic genes involved in the early phase of myogenesis and the associated calcium channels [6], and we have elucidated its functional role in maintaining the cellular T_4 level. Furthermore, we reported that TTR enhances recruitment of MSCs to the site of injury, thereby regulating muscle regeneration [29]. However, the detailed mechanism of TTR with T_4 in MSCs differentiation into muscle cells is unclear. In the current work, we have confirmed TTR secretion and internalization in myoblast cell. We found that TTR uptake and internalization by myoblast cells is increased by T_4. By using microarray analysis and other studies, we have elucidated that TTR and TH coordinate with each other to modulate gene expression in muscle growth, development, and homeostasis.

2. Materials and Methods

2.1. Animal Experiments

C57BL/6 male mice were obtained from Daehan Biolink (Dae-Jeon, South Korea) and housed at four per cage in a temperature controlled room under a 12 h light/12 h dark cycle. In the period mice (six weeks) were fed a normal diet containing 4.0% (w/w) total fat (Rodent NIH-31 Open Formula Auto; Zeigler Bros., Inc., Gardners, PA, USA). Gastrocnemius muscle tissues were collected after 10 or 20 weeks. After collection, muscle tissues were fixed and stored at -80 °C until required for RNA and protein extraction or fixed overnight at 4 °C for paraffin-embedded tissue blocks to be used in immunohistochemistry. All experimental were done by following the guidelines issued by the Institutional Animal Care and Use Committees of the Catholic University of Daegu (IACUC-2017-051).

2.2. C2C12 Cell Culture

C2C12 cells (murine myoblast, Korean Cell Line Bank, Seoul, Korea) were cultured in DMEM (HyClone Laboratories, Logan, UT, USA) supplemented with 10% FBS (fetal bovine serum, HyClone Laboratories) and 1% P/S (penicillin/streptomycin, Thermo Fisher Scientific, Waltham, MA, USA) in a humidified 5% CO_2 incubator at 37 °C. For differentiation, cells were cultured for two or three days in DMEM + 2% FBS + 1% P/S (serum (+) differentiation media) or DMEM + 1% P/S (serum (−) differentiation media). T_4 (50 ng/mL, Sigma Aldrich, St. Louis, MO, USA), I-850 (5 ug/mL, Sigma Aldrich), TTR (0.1 ug/mL, Sigma Aldrich) or bovine serum albumin (BSA, 1 mg/mL, Sigma Aldrich) was added to the indicated differentiation medium after two or three days.

2.3. Mouse MSCs Culture

Gastrocnemius and cranial thigh muscles were collected from C57BL male mice (six weeks) and minced, digested with 1% pronase (Roche, Mannheim, Germany) for 1 h at 37 °C, and then centrifuged at 1000× g for 3 min followed by passage of the digested tissue phase through a 100 mm syringe filter (Millipore, Darmstadt, Germany). After centrifugation of the filtrate at 1000× g for 5 min, the pellets were suspended in DMEM + 20% FBS + 1% P/S + 5 ng/mL FGF2 (fibroblast growth factor 2, Miltenyi Biotec GmbH, Auburn, CA, USA), seeded on collagen-coated plates (Corning, Brooklyn, NY, USA), and incubated in a humidified 5% CO_2 atmosphere at 37 °C. The medium was changed every day. For induction of MSC differentiation into muscle cells, media were switched to DMEM + 2% FBS + 1% P/S or DMEM + 1% P/S followed by incubation for two days. MSC purity was confirmed with Pax7 protein expression (Santa Cruz Biotechnology, Paso Robles, CA, USA) using immunocytochemistry.

2.4. MTT Assay

C2C12 cells were cultured with DMEM + 10% FBS + 1% P/S for two days for analysis of cell viability. The cells were washed with DMEM and then incubated with 0.5 mg/mL MTT reagent (Sigma Aldrich) for 1 h. After dissolving the formazan crystals with DMSO (Sigma Aldrich), absorbance was measured at 540 nm (Tecan Group Ltd., Männedorf, Switzerland).

2.5. Immunoneutralization

TTR protein neutralization was carried out with TTR-specific antibodies (5 μg/mL, Santa Cruz Biotechnology) for two or three days in DMEM + 2% FBS + 1% P/S or DMEM + 1% P/S differentiation media.

2.6. Exosomes Isolation

Cells were cultured with DMEM + 1% P/S differentiation media. The cells were incubated for two or three days and the media were then collected, centrifuged at 2000× g for 30 min, and the upper phase collected for exosomes isolation. Using a total exosomes isolation reagent (Thermo Fisher Scientific, MA, USA), the exosomes from the upper phase were isolated according to the manufacturer's protocol. In brief, the media were incubated with the total exosomes isolation reagent at 4 °C overnight and centrifuged at 10,000× g for 60 min. After discarding the supernatant, the pellet was dried at room temperature and suspended in PBS.

Mouse plasma (4 mL) was filtered with a 0.8 um syringe filter (Sartorius, Goettingen, Germany), and the exosomes were then isolated according to the manufacturer's protocol (exoEasy Maxi Kit, Qiagen, Germantown, MD, USA).

2.7. T_4 and T_3 Concentration Measurement

An ELISA kit (DRG International, Marburg, Germany) was used to measure the concentration of T_4 or T_3 hormones. In brief, cell lysates or cultured media with T_4 or T_3 enzyme conjugate reagent were homogenized and added to specific antibody-coated microtiter plates and then incubated for 60 min at room temperature. After discarding the mixtures, the unbound materials were removed by washing the plates. Substrate solution was added followed by incubation for 20 min. Stop solution was then applied to terminate the reaction. Color intensities were then measured at 450 nm by using a spectrophotometer (Tecan Group Ltd., Switzerland).

2.8. Gene Knockdown

When C2C12 cells confluency reached 30%, 1 ng TTR, TR-α, RXRγ, or fibronectin type III domain containing 5 (FNDC5) shRNA vector (Santa Cruz Biotechnology) and scrambled vector (empty vector as negative control, Santa Cruz Biotechnology) were transfected using plasmid transfection reagent and transfection medium according to the manufacturer's protocol (Santa Cruz Biotechnology). After three days, transfected cells were selected with puromycin (2 ug/mL, shRNA or scrambled vector is a puromycin selection vector, Santa Cruz Biotechnology). Selected cells were grown to 70% confluence before switching to differentiation media. Knockdown efficiencies were determined by analyzing the expressions of control (scrambled vector transfected cell) and knockdown cells. Supplementary Table S1 shows the sequences of the shRNA constructs.

2.9. RNA Isolation, cDNA Synthesis and RealTime RT-PCR

Trizol reagent (Thermo Fisher Scientific) was used following the manufacturer's instructions to extract total RNA from cells. Two micrograms of RNA in 20 μL of reaction mixture was employed for the synthesis of 1st strand cDNA with random hexamer and reverse transcriptase at 25 °C for 10 min, 37 °C for 120 min, and 85 °C for 5 min. The cDNA product (2 μL) and gene-specific primers (10 pmole, 2 μL) were used for analysis of real-time RT-PCR (40 cycles), which was performed using a 7500 real-time PCR system with power SYBR Green PCR Master Mix (Thermo Fisher Scientific) as the fluorescence source. Glyceraldehyde 3-phosphate dehydrogenase (GAPDH) was used as the reference gene. Primer information is presented in Supplementary Table S2.

2.10. RT-PCR

Exosomes RNA was synthesized into cDNA and 2 μL cDNA and gene-specific primers (10 pmole, 2 μL) were used for PCR, which was performed using a 2720 Thermal Cycler PCR machine with PCR Master mix (Genetbio, Daejeon, Korea). The PCR conditions were as follow; denaturation 95 °C for 30 s, annealing at 59 °C for 30 s, extension at 72 °C, post-extension 72 °C for 5 min followed by holding (40 cycles). The PCR product was examined by performing electrophoresis on agarose gel.

2.11. Protein Isolation from Culture Media

The cells were cultured with DMEM + 1% P/S differentiation media for two days, centrifuged at $5000\times g$ for 5 min, and the supernatant was then incubated with 1.3% potassium acetate (Sigma Aldrich) for 1 h at 4 °C. The mixture was centrifuged at $1500\times g$ for 10 min, the supernatant was discarded, and the pellet washed with 100% acetone (Merck, Darmstadt, Germany). The isolated proteins were then dried, and Western blot analysis was performed by adding buffer with protease inhibitor cocktail (Thermo Fisher Scientific).

2.12. Western Blot

After washing the cells with PBS, they were lysed with RIPA buffer supplemented with protease inhibitor cocktail (Thermo Fisher Scientific). The Bradford assay was used to estimate the total protein concentration. Proteins (60 μg) were electrophoresed in 10% or 12% SDS-polyacrylamide gel and then transferred to PVDF membrane (EMS–Millipore, Billerica, MA, USA). The blots were then blocked with 3% skim milk or BSA in Tris-buffered saline (TBS)-Tween 20 for 1 h, incubated overnight with protein-specific primary antibodies [TTR (1:400), MYOD (1:500), MYOG (1:500), D2 (iodothyronine deiodinase type 2; 1:500), RXRγ (1:500) (Santa Cruz Biotechnology) or β-actin (1:2000) antibody (Santa Cruz Biotechnology), TR-α (1:500, Thermo Fisher Scientific), MYL2 (myosin light chain 2, 1:1000, Abcam, Cambridge, MA, USA) or FNDC5 (1:500, Bioss Antibodies, Woburn, MA, USA)] in 1% skim milk or BSA in TBS at 4 °C. The blots were then washed and incubated with horse radish peroxidase (HRP)-conjugated secondary antibody (Santa Cruz Biotechnology) for 1 h at room temperature and then developed with Super Signal West Pico Chemiluminescent Substrate (Thermo Fisher Scientific). Supplementary Table S3 shows the molecular weight of protein.

2.13. Fusion Index

After washing with PBS, cells were fixed with methanol and then stained with 0.04% Giemsa G250 (Sigma Aldrich). Images were taken randomly of three different sections per dish. The number of nuclei in myotubes and the total number of nuclei in the cells were counted in each field. Fusion indices were calculated by expressing the number of nuclei in the myotubes as percentages of the total numbers of nuclei.

2.14. TTR Protein Labeling with Fluorescence

TTR protein and BSA were labeled with the Alexa Fluor 594 protein labeling kit (Thermo Fisher Scientific) following the manufacturer's instructions. Briefly, 100 μL TTR proteins and BSA (0.1 μg/μL) were incubated with 4.7 μL Alexa Fluor 594 succinimidyl ester (12.2 nmole/μL) for 15 min at room temperature, and the conjugated reaction mixture was then purified with resin gel-spin filter. Labeled TTR proteins (0.2 μg) and BSA were added to the cells and detected by fluorescence microscope (Nikon, Tokyo, Japan).

2.15. TTR Overexpression Vector

The region corresponding to the TTR gene open reading frame (ORF) was PCR amplified with TTR ORF primer (Forward: 5'-ATGGCTTCCCTTCGACTCTTCC-3', Reverse: 5'-GATTCTGGGGGTTGCTGACGA-3') and ligated into the pcDNA 3.1/CT-GFP-TOPO vector (Invitrogen, Waltham, MA, USA). The ligated sequence was confirmed by sequencing analysis. The construct (2.5 µg) was transfected using 10 µL lipofectamine (1 mg/mL) and Opti MEM medium (Invitrogen) into C2C12 cells following the manufacturer's directions and positive cells were selected using G418 antibiotics (2 µg/mL, AppliChem GmbH, Darmstadt, Germany).

2.16. Immunocytochemistry

The cells were fixed with 4% formaldehyde (Sigma Aldrich) and permeabilized with 0.2% Triton X 100 (Sigma Aldrich). After blocking with 1% normal goat serum (SeraCare Life Sciences, Milford, MA, USA) for 30 min in a humid environment, cells were incubated with primary antibodies [TTR (1:50), MYOD (1:50), MYOG (1:50), MYL2 (1:50), D2 (1:50), RXRγ (1:50), TRα (1:50), or FNDC5 (1:50)] at 4 °C in a humid environment overnight. Secondary antibody (1: 100; Alexa Fluor 594 goat anti-rabbit or anti-mouse; Thermo Fisher Scientific) was applied for 1 h at room temperature. DAPI was used to stain the cells (Sigma-Aldrich) and imaged using a fluorescence microscope equipped with a digital camera (Nikon, Tokyo, Japan).

2.17. Immunohistochemistry

The sections of paraffin-embedded muscle tissue were deparaffinized and hydrated with xylene (Junsei, Tokyo, Japan) and ethanol (Merck), respectively, and endogenous peroxidase activity was quenched in 0.3% H_2O_2/methanol. The sections were then either stained with hematoxylin and eosin (Thermo Fisher Scientific) for morphological observation or blocked with 1% normal goat serum (SeraCare Life Sciences), incubated with primary antibodies [TTR (1:50), D2 (1:50), or FNDC5 (1:50)] overnight at 4 °C, and then incubated with horse radish peroxidase–conjugated secondary antibody (1:100). Positive signals were visualized by adding horse radish peroxidase-conjugated streptavidin (Vector, CA, USA). Nuclei of stained sections were stained with hematoxylin and then dehydrated, mounted, and observed by a light microscope (Leica, Wetzlar, Germany).

2.18. Microarray Analysis

Microarray analysis was conducted with the Agilent Technologies mouse GE4X 44K (V2) chip to determine the differentially expressed genes in wild-type (TTR$_{wt}$) and TTR$_{kd}$ (TTR knockdown) cells as described previously [30]. Briefly, TTR$_{wt}$ and TTR$_{kd}$ cells were grown in serum (+) differentiation media for two days and RNAs were extracted, synthesized into cDNA with fluorescence using a Low RNA Input Linear Amplification kit (Agilent Technologies, CA, USA) according to the manufacturer's instructions. A total of three hybridizations were performed, and the statistical relevance of gene expression differences was confirmed by SAM (Standard University, Palo Alto, CA, USA). The significance cut-off was a median false discovery rate $\leq$5% for the SAM analysis.

2.19. DAVID Analysis

DAVID was performed as described previously [5]. In brief, enriched biological themes in up- and down-regulated gene lists ($p \leq 0.05$ and 2 fold$\leq$) were categorized by employing the Gene Ontology (GO) terms of cellular component, molecular function, and biological process in DAVID.

2.20. Statistical Analysis

Mean values of normalized expressions were evaluated by Tukey's Studentized range test to categorize expressional differences of genes, considering $p \leq 0.05$ statistically significant. The real-time RT-PCR data was normalized using glyceraldehyde 3-phosphate dehydrogenase (GAPDH) as the internal standard and was analyzed by one-way ANOVA using PROC GLM in SAS 9.0 (SAS Institute, Cary, NC, USA).

3. Results

3.1. TTR Secretion During Myoblast Differentiation

To investigate TTR secretion from cells during C2C12 myoblast differentiation, normal and TTR knockdown cells were cultured in serum-free media for two days, after which the isolated protein level from cultured media was analyzed by Western blotting. The appearance of more TTR protein in cultured media compared to that in cell lysate indicates that TTR is secreted during myoblast differentiation (Figure 1A). Furthermore, TTR mRNA and protein were decreased in TTR_{kd} cells and cultured media, respectively, compared to those in TTR_{wt} cells (Figure 1A). Next, the TTR mRNA level was analyzed in normal cells and exosomes from mouse plasma and media of cultured cells (CM): T_4-treated cells, TTR_{wt}, and TTR_{kd}. TTR mRNA was evident in exosomes isolated from culture media and mouse plasma and was increased by T_4 treatment but decreased by TTR_{kd} (Figure 1B). TTR immunoneutralization using TTR antibody was performed during differentiation. Myotube formation and the expression of the myogenic genes were decreased by TTR neutralization. However, TTR expression was significantly enhanced in neutralized cells (Figure 1C,D). Interestingly, when the T_4 concentration was measured in cells, it was higher in non-neutralized cells than in neutralized cells supplemented with T_4 (Figure 1E). Taken together, these results show that TTR secreted from cells transported T_4 into the cells during myoblast differentiation.

3.2. Enhancement of Myoblast Viability and Differentiation by TTR with T_4

To assess the role of TTR and T_4 on myoblast viability and differentiation, C2C12 cells were grown with T_4 or T_4 + TTR protein for two or three days. Cell viability was increased in T_4 + TTR protein treated cells compared to that in only T_4 treated cells (Figure 2A). The T_4 and T_3 concentrations were measured in CM and cells. A lower T_4 concentration in media with a consequent higher concentration in cells was observed with T_4 + TTR treatment than in those with only T_4 treatment. The results indicate that TTR outside the cell enhances the transport of T_4 to the cell interior in myoblast viability (Figure 2A). Further, cells were cultured in serum-free media with added T_4 or T_4 + TTR protein for three days to induce differentiation. The T_4 + TTR treatment significantly induced myotube formation with elevated mRNA (MYL2) and protein expression of myogenic factors (MYOD and MYL2), RXRγ, and TRα. However, TTR mRNA and protein expression were decreased by TTR + T_4 treatment and their expression in exosomes was also reduced from that of only T_4-treated cells (Figure 2B). T_4 and T_3 concentrations were increased by TTR + T_4 treatment (Figure 2C). TTR in mouse MSCs was assessed to determine its expression during differentiation. For this, MSCs were incubated with differentiation media for zero or two days. Expression of TTR and myogenic genes or proteins were increased on day 2 compared to that on day 0 (Figure 2D). Next, MSCs were cultured in serum-free conditions supplemented with T_4 or T_4 + TTR protein for two days to induce differentiation. Similar to the results with C2C12 cells, MSCs exhibited increased myotube formation with elevated thyroid hormone concentration under T_4 + TTR treatment (Figure 2E). Interestingly, decreased TTR mRNA was observed in the exosomes following T_4 + TTR treatment (Figure 2E). Furthermore, T_3 was present in exosomes isolated from serum-free MSCs culture media supplemented with T_4 (Figure 2F). These data showed that TTR protein with T_4 not only enhanced myoblast proliferation and myogenic differentiation, but also increased MSC differentiation into muscle cells.

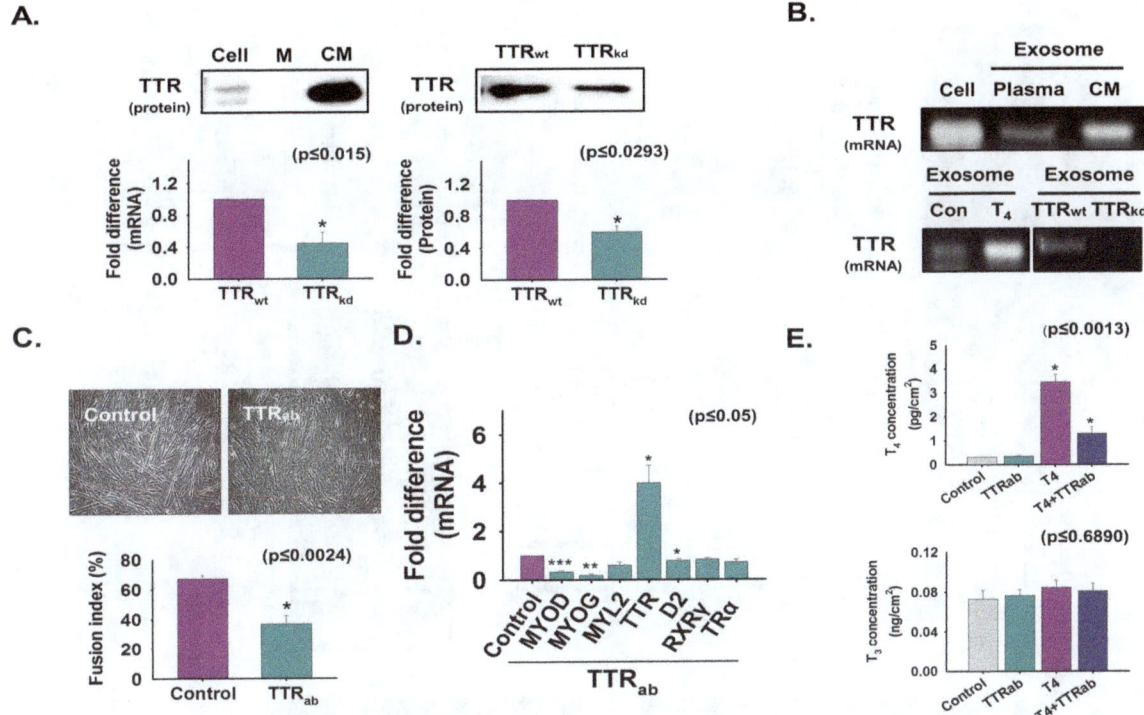

Figure 1. The role of secreted TTR from cells during myogenic differentiation. Normal and TTR knockdown cells were cultured with serum-free media for two days (**A**,**B**). (**A**) Proteins were isolated from cells, DMEM (control) and cultured media (CM). TTR protein level was analyzed by Western blot. TTR mRNA level in cells by real-time RT-PCR, and protein level in cell culture media of TTR_{wt} and TTR_{kd} by Western blot. Band intensity was measured by using ImageJ. (**B**) TTR mRNA levels in normal cell, exosomes isolated from mouse plasma, media of cultured C2C12 cells (CM) with or without T_4 treatment, and TTR_{wt} and TTR_{kd} by RT-PCR. Cells were cultured in 2% FBS or serum-free media supplemented with TTR antibody for two (**C**) or three days (**D**,**E**) for immunoneutralization. (**C**) Myotube formation and fusion index was observed by Giemsa staining. (**D**) Gene expression was observed by real-time RT-PCR. (**E**) T_4 and T_3 concentration in cells was observed by ELISA. TTR_{wt} indicates cells transfected with scrambled vector. Means ± SD ($n = 3$). * $p \leq 0.05$, ** $p \leq 0.001$, *** $p \leq 0.0001$.

3.3. Reduction of T_4 Concentration Inside Cells and Myoblast Differentiation by Bovine Albumin Serum (BSA) Treatment

For comparative assessment of T_4 transport through TTR to the cell interior, C2C12 cells were cultured in serum-free media supplemented with T_4 or T_4 + BSA protein for two days. Myotube formation and MYOG expression were decreased in BSA-treated cells, while TTR and D2 expressions were increased at the translational level (Figure 3A). Interestingly, elevated TTR in both exosomes (mRNA) and CM (protein) was also observed in BSA-treated cells (Figure 3B). High T_4 and T_3 concentrations in T_4 + BSA supplemented media with subsequent low levels in both hormone concentrations in the cell, under the same conditions, indicated that BSA reduced the transport of T_4 to the cell interior (Figure 3C). Furthermore, elevated T_4 concentration was observed in T_4 + BSA + TTR supplemented cells relative to that in T_4 + BSA treated cells (Figure 3D). Interestingly, decreased TTR mRNA was found in exosomes of T_4 + BSA + TTR treated cells (Figure 3E). Additionally, T_3 was present in exosomes, and there was no difference in T_3 concentration in exosomes supplemented with T_4, T_4 + BSA, or T_4 + TTR (Figure 3F). We observed that BSA reduces myotube formation by decreasing T_4 transport.

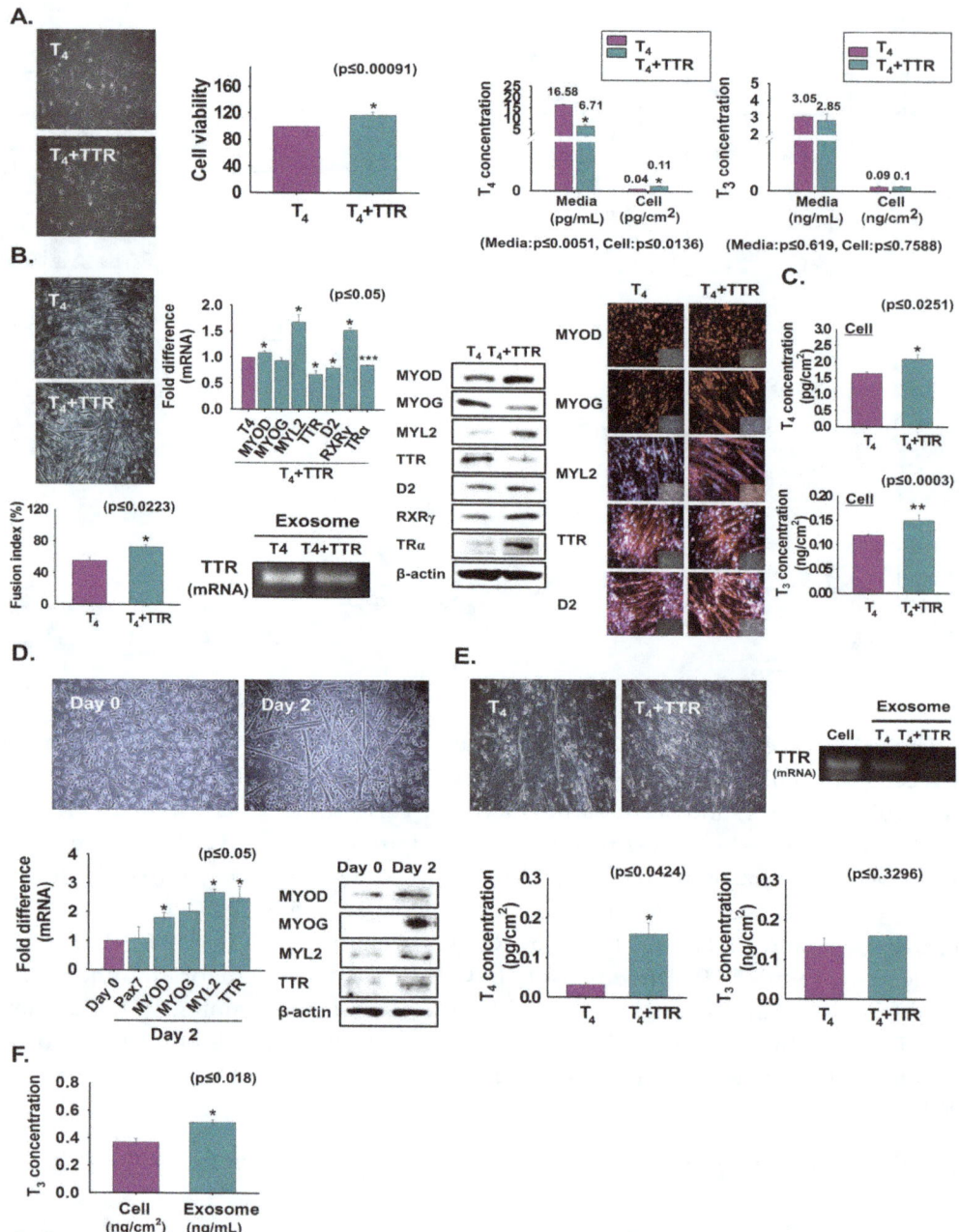

Figure 2. Myoblast viability and differentiation by treatment with TTR proteins. (**A**) C2C12 cells were cultured in 10% FBS media supplemented with T_4 or T_4 + TTR protein for two days. Cell viability was observed by MTT assay. T_4 or T_3 concentration in cultured media and cells were observed by ELISA. Cells were cultured in serum-free media supplemented with T_4 or T_4 + TTR protein for three days (**B**,**C**). (**B**) Myotube formation and fusion index by Giemsa staining, mRNA level in cells by real-time RT-PCR, exosomes by RT-PCR, protein expression by Western blot and immunocytochemistry. (**C**) T_4 or T_3 concentration in cells was observed by ELISA. (**D**) When mouse MSCs reached 100% confluency, media were switched to 2% FBS and cultured for zero and two days. MSC differentiation, TTR mRNA level by real-time RT-PCR and protein expression by Western blot. (**E**) MSCs were cultured in serum-free media supplemented with T_4 or T_4 + TTR protein for two days. T_4 or T_3 concentration in cells was observed by ELISA. (**F**) MSCs were cultured with serum-free media supplemented with T_4 for two days and exosomes were isolated from cultured media. T_3 concentration in cell and exosomes was observed by ELISA. Means ± SD ($n = 3$). * $p \leq 0.05$, ** $p \leq 0.001$, *** $p \leq 0.0001$.

3.4. TTR Internalization Into Myoblast

To elucidate TTR internalization to the cell interior, TTR protein or BSA was fluorescently labeled and C2C12 cells were cultured under serum-free conditions supplemented with labeled TTR protein or BSA for one day. Higher fluorescence of labeled TTR protein was evident in the cells treated with labeled TTR than with BSA or in non-treated cells (Figure 4A). TTR overexpression was achieved by transfection with the TTR ORF plasmid and cultured with 10% FBS for two days. Increased cell viability was observed in TTR-overexpressing cells (Figure 4B). Next, TTR-overexpressing cells were cultured with serum-free media for two days. Increased myotube formation with enhanced TTR mRNA/protein expression was observed in TTR-overexpressing cells (Figure 4C). Additionally, elevated concentrations of THs were observed in TTR-overexpressing cells supplemented with T_4 (Figure 4C).

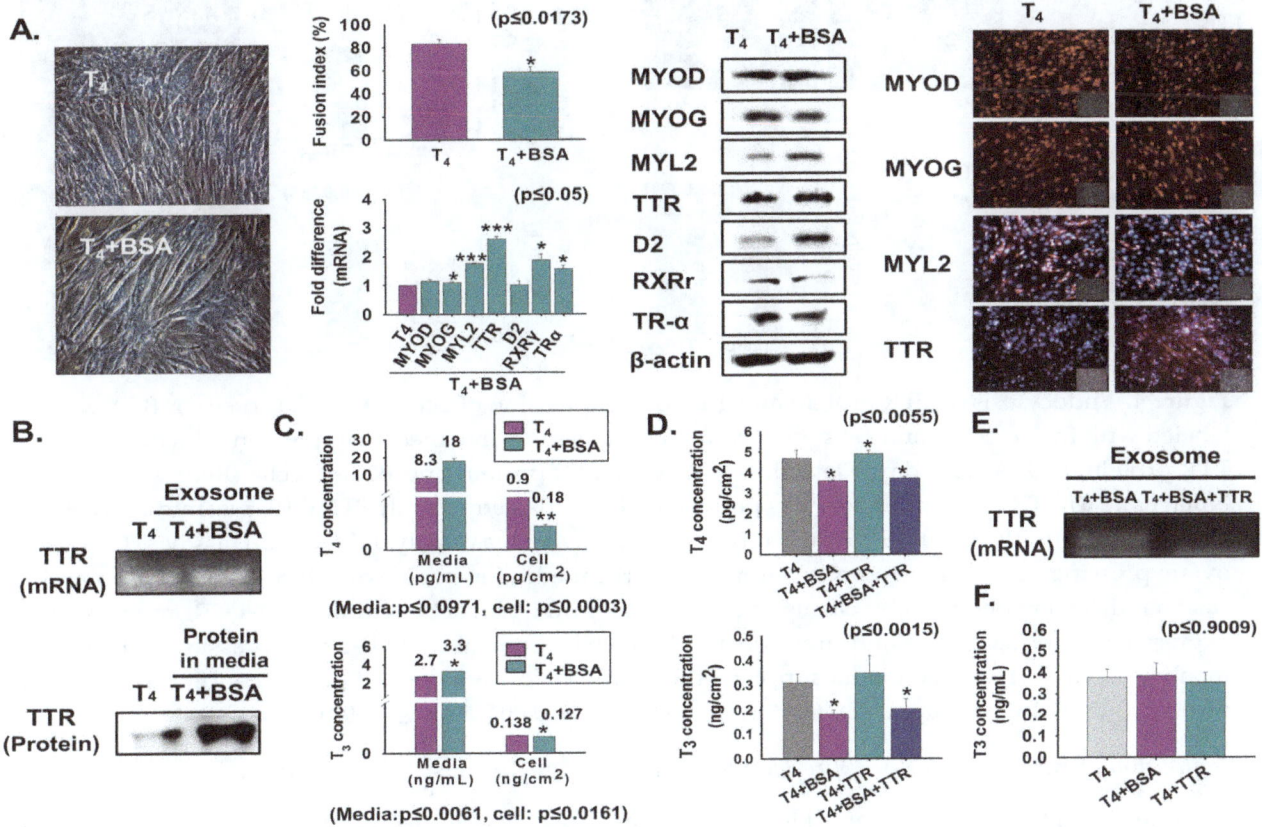

Figure 3. Myoblast differentiation following BSA treatment. Cells were cultured in serum-free media supplemented with T_4 or T_4 + BSA for two days (**A–E**). (**A**) Myotube formation and fusion index were observed by Giemsa staining. mRNA level was observed by real-time RT-PCR and protein expressions by Western blot and immunocytochemistry. (**B**) TTR mRNA in exosomes of cultured media using RT-PCR and protein level in cultured media by Western blot. (**C**) T_4 or T_3 concentration in cultured media or cells was observed by ELISA. (**D,E**) Cells were cultured with serum-free media supplemented with T_4, T_4 + BSA, T_4 + TTR or T_4 + BSA + TTR for two days. T_4 or T_3 concentration in T_4 + BSA or T_4 + BSA + TTR treated cells. TTR mRNA in exosomes of cultured media (in T_4 + BSA or T_4 + BSA + TTR treated cells) using RT-PCR. (**F**) Cells were cultured in serum-free media supplemented with T_4 or T_4 + BSA or T_4 + TTR for two days and exosomes were isolated from each cultured medium. T_3 concentration in exosomes. Means ± SD ($n = 3$). * $p \leq 0.05$, ** $p \leq 0.001$, *** $p \leq 0.0001$.

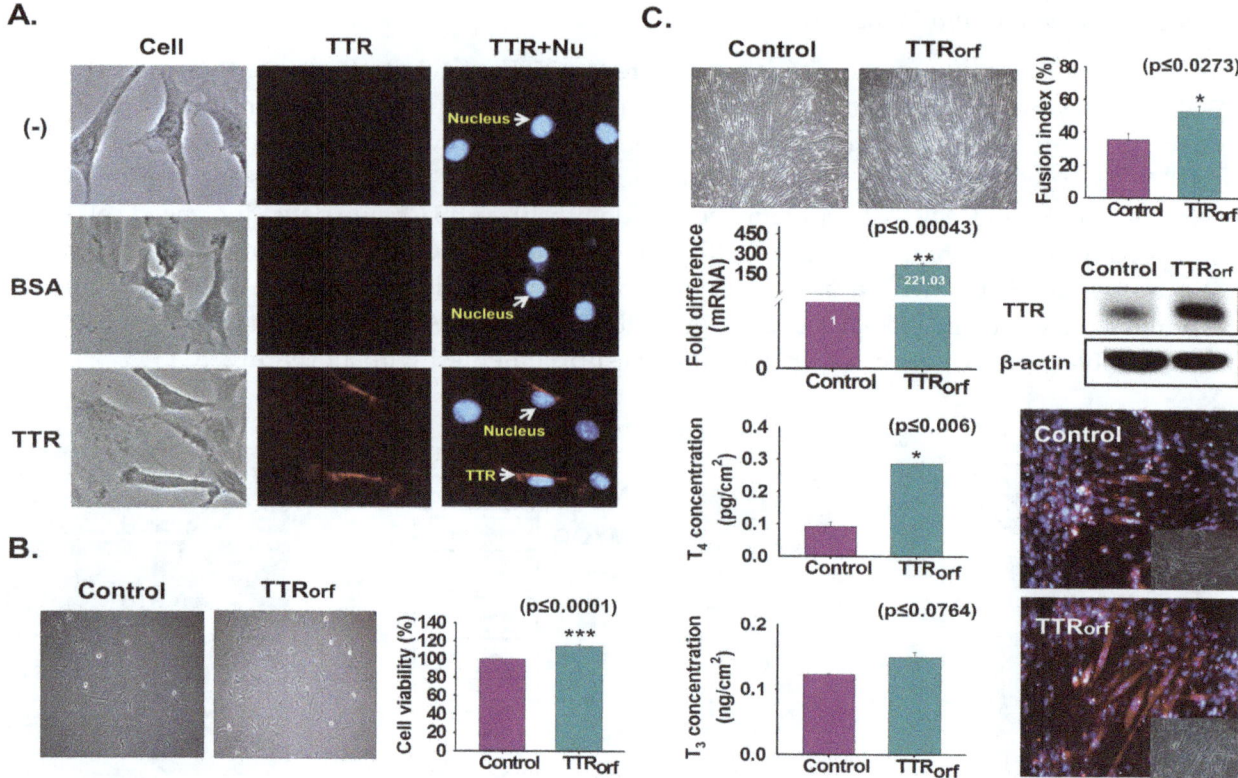

Figure 4. Endocytosis of TTR protein and TTR overexpression effects. (**A**) TTR protein or BSA were labeled with fluorescence and cells were cultured with serum-free media supplemented with labeled TTR protein or BSA for 1 day. Detection of labeled TTR protein and BSA in cells (Red: TTR, Blue: Nucleus). (**B**) TTR overexpression was performed by transfecting with TTR ORF plasmid followed by incubation with 10% FBS for two days. Cell viability was analyzed by MTT assay. (**C**) TTR overexpressing cells were incubated with serum-free media for two days. Myotube formation and fusion index were observed by Giemsa staining, TTR mRNA level by real-time RT-PCR, and protein expression by Western blot and immunocytochemistry. Control or TTR-overexpressing cells were incubated with serum-free media supplemented with T_4 for two days. T_4 or T_3 concentration was measured by ELISA. Means $\pm$ SD ($n = 3$). * $p \leq 0.05$, ** $p \leq 0.001$, *** $p \leq 0.0001$.

3.5. Regulation of RXRγ and TRα Expression by TTR During Myoblast Differentiation

To determine the role of T_4 or TTR on RXRγ and TRα expression, C2C12 cells were grown with or without serum in normal or TTR knockdown cells, and the effects were studied during myoblast differentiation. Increases in mRNA and protein expression of RXRγ and TRα were evident on day 2 compared to the levels on day 0 (Figure 5A). Next, T_4 treatment under serum-free conditions stimulated RXRγ expression at both the transcriptional and translational level. However, TRα protein expression was decreased by T_4 treatment (Figure 5B). Interestingly, TTR knockdown reduced expression of RXRγ and TRα (Figure 5C). Further, RXRγ and TRα knockdown were performed and followed by culturing with 2% FBS for two days. Myotube formation, myogenic genes and D2 expression were decreased by RXRγ or TRα knockdown, whereas TTR and TRα expressions were increased in RXRγ$_{kd}$ cells. Most gene or protein expressions were decreased in TRα knockdown cells (Figure 5D,E). Overall, the above results indicate that expression of RXRγ is controlled by TTR via T_4 transportation into the cell during myoblast differentiation.

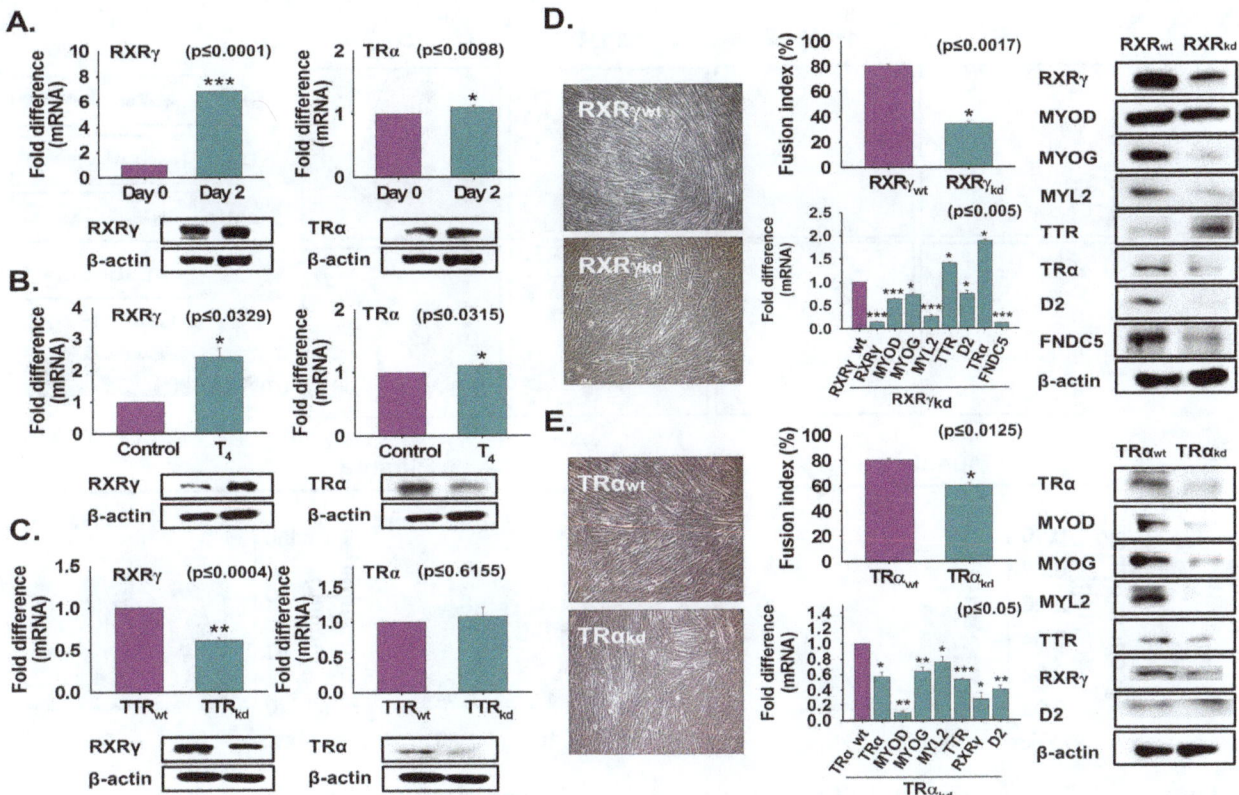

Figure 5. RXRγ and TRα expression during myoblast differentiation. (**A**) Cells were cultured with 2% FBS for two days. RXRγ and TRα expressions using real-time RT-PCR or Western blot. (**B**) Cells were cultured in serum-free media supplemented with T_4 for two days. RXRγ and TRα expression by real-time RT-PCR or Western blot. (**C**) RXRγ and TRα expression in TTR_{kd} and TTR_{wt} cells using real-time RT-PCR or Western blot. (**D**) RXRγ knockdown was performed and followed by culture with 2% FBS for two days. Myotube formation and fusion index were observed by Giemsa staining, mRNA expression by real-time RT-PCR, and protein expression by Western blot in $RXRγ_{kd}$ and $RXRγ_{wt}$ cells. (**E**) TRα knockdown was performed and followed by culture with 2% FBS for two days. Myotube formation and fusion index were observed by Giemsa staining, mRNA expression by real-time RT-PCR, and protein expression by Western blot in $TRα_{kd}$ and $TRα_{wt}$ cells. TTR_{wt}, $RXRγ_{wt}$, or $TRα_{wt}$ indicate cells transfected with the scrambled vector. Means ± SD ($n = 3$). * $p \leq 0.05$, ** $p \leq 0.001$, *** $p \leq 0.0001$.

3.6. Relationship between TTR and D2 According to Muscle Age

To determine the effect of muscle age on TTR and D2 expression, mouse muscle at 16- and 26-weeks were collected. Myofiber size (width) and expression of TTR and D2 were decreased in 26-week muscle compared with 16-week muscle (Figure 6A). Interestingly, a decreased TTR level was observed in exosomes isolated from 26-week plasma (Figure 6A). The T_3 concentration in 16-week muscle was higher than that in 26-week muscle (Figure 6B). Further, a significant increase in the T_4 concentration in the plasma of 26-week mice the was observed, whereas there was no difference in the T_3 concentration in the plasma of either age group (Figure 6B). The above findings suggest that expressions of TTR and D2 correlate with the age-dependent differences of muscle.

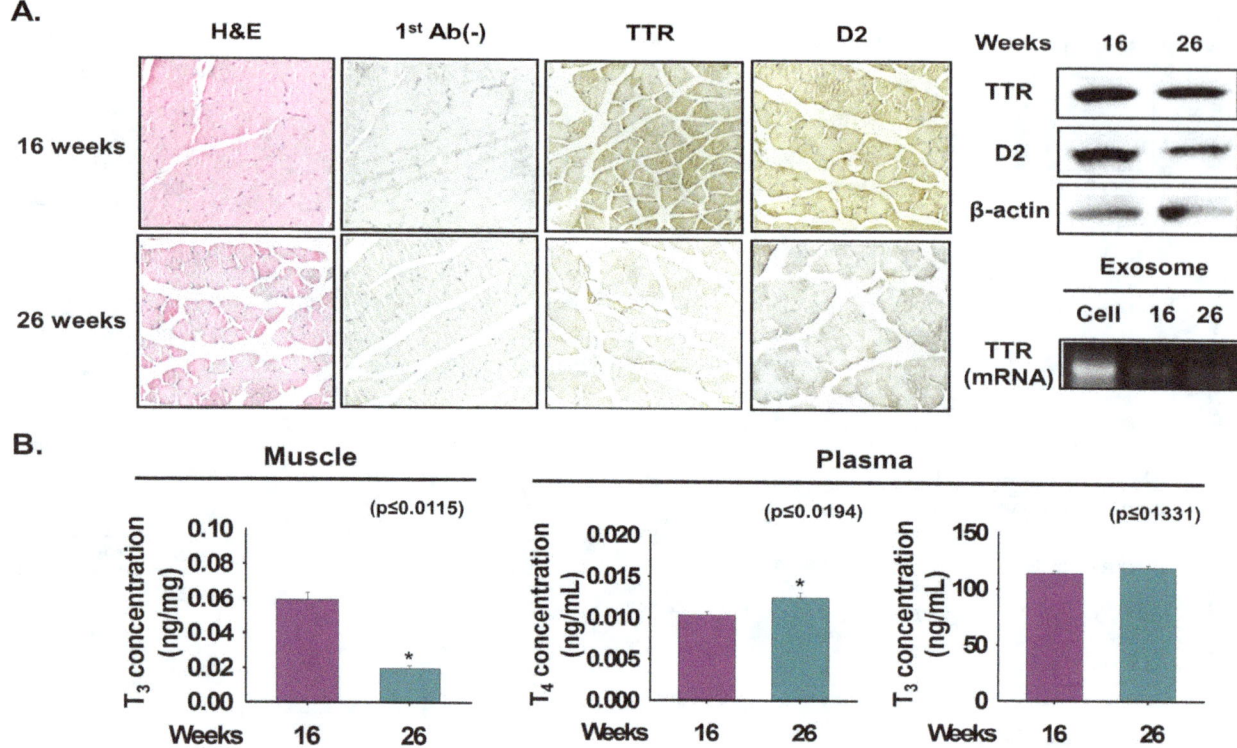

Figure 6. TTR expression and T_3 concentration in age-dependent differences of muscle.. Expression of TTR and D2 proteins were analyzed in 16- and 26-week mouse muscles. (**A**) TTR and D2 proteins expression by Immunohistochemistry and Western blot. Exosomes were isolated from 16- and 26-week plasma. TTR mRNA level in cell and exosomes of 16- or 26-week plasma by RT-PCR. (**B**) T_3 or T_4 concentration in 16- or 26-week muscles or plasma was observed by ELISA. Means ± SD ($n = 3$). * $p \leq 0.05$, ** $p \leq 0.001$, *** $p \leq 0.0001$.

3.7. Microarray Assessment of Gene Expression in TTR$_{kd}$ Cells and Effect of T_4 on Gene Expression

To explore TTR function in myoblast differentiation, TTR$_{kd}$ and TTR$_{wt}$ C2C12 cells were cultured with 2% FBS for two days. TTR/MYOG expression and myotube formation were decreased by TTR$_{kd}$ (Supplementary Figure S1A,B). Microarray analysis was performed with TTR$_{wt}$ and TTR$_{kd}$ cells. After applying two-fold cut-offs for down- and up-regulated genes, analysis of the effects of knocking down TTR on myoblasts revealed that, among the genes involved in sarcomere formation, specific genes are actively up- or down-regulated, and some novel genes that are not involved in sarcomere formation functioned at the onset of myogenesis. Among the identified genes, 29 and 7 genes were down- or up-regulated, respectively, by greater than two-fold in TTR$_{kd}$ cells (Table 1A,B; Supplementary Figure S1C,D). Many genes were previously reported to be involved in MSC maintenance (Heyl, Sox8), myogenesis (Fgf21, Ankrd2, Sox8, Asb2), proliferation (Ankrd2), myokine secretion (Fndc5), neuromuscular junction (Dok7), and Ca^{2+} release of sarcoplasmic reticulum (Asph). Even though some of these genes have identified roles in myogenesis, many novel genes were also affected by TTR$_{kd}$ (R3hdml, Inpp4b, Igf2as, Btbd17, Sema6b and Ddc) (Table 1A; Supplementary Table S4A). However, the upregulated genes were mostly involved in the cell cycle, cell proliferation, and transcription regulation. Interestingly, there was little information indicating that those genes were related to muscle differentiation. Moreover, most of the up-regulated genes were novel genes, but their main functions have been studied in other tissues or organs (Table 1B; Supplementary Table S4B).

Table 1. Microarray analysis of TTR knockdown.

A.

Gene	Set1	Set2	Set3	Set4	Average	p Value	Description
Myh1	0.16	0.31	0.13	0.06	0.16	0.0001	Mus musculus myosin, heavy polypeptide 1, skeletal muscle, adult (Myh1)
Heyl	0.25	0.19	0.15	0.1	0.17	0.0001	Mus musculus hairy/enhancer-of-split related with YRPW motif-like (Heyl)
Myo18b	0.17	0.4	0.13	0.05	0.19	0.0001	Mus musculus myosin XVIIIb (Myo18b)
Myh8	0.2	0.39	0.12	0.08	0.2	0.0001	Mus musculus myosin, heavy polypeptide 8, skeletal muscle, perinatal (Myh8)
Nmrk2	0.16	0.37	0.06	0.22	0.2	0.0001	Mus musculus nicotinamide riboside kinase 2 (Nmrk2)
Fgf21	0.14	0.35	0.06	0.32	0.22	0.0001	Mus musculus fibroblast growth factor 21 (Fgf21)
Ankrd2	0.17	0.36	0.06	0.28	0.22	0.0001	Mus musculusankyrin repeat domain 2 (stretch responsive muscle) (Ankrd2)
Myom3	0.18	0.49	0.11	0.11	0.22	0.0001	Mus musculusmyomesin family, member 3 (Myom3)
Myh3	0.18	0.39	0.14	0.21	0.23	0.0001	Mus musculus myosin, heavy polypeptide 3, skeletal muscle, embryonic (Myh3)
Myh7	0.3	0.33	0.12	0.2	0.24	0.0001	Mus musculus myosin, heavy polypeptide 7, cardiac muscle, beta (Myh7)
Myh3	0.21	0.4	0.15	0.21	0.24	0.0001	Mus musculus myosin, heavy polypeptide 3, skeletal muscle, embryonic (Myh3)
Fndc5	0.44	0.26	0.18	0.1	0.25	0.0001	Mus musculus fibronectin type III domain containing 5 (Fndc5)
R3hdml	0.35	0.4	0.09	0.15	0.25	0.0001	Mus musculus R3H domain containing-like (R3hdml)
Myh7b	0.31	0.39	0.07	0.22	0.25	0.0001	Mus musculus myosin, heavy chain 7B, cardiac muscle, beta (Myh7b)
Rbm24	0.2	0.41	0.15	0.23	0.25	0.0001	Mus musculus RNA binding motif protein 24 (Rbm24)
Sox8	0.45	0.21	0.13	0.22	0.25	0.0001	Mus musculus SRY (sex determining region Y)-box 8 (Sox8)
Dok7	0.21	0.5	0.08	0.29	0.27	0.0002	Mus musculus docking protein 7 (Dok7)
Tnnt1	0.31	0.37	0.12	0.29	0.27	0.0001	Mus musculus troponin T1, skeletal, slow (Tnnt1), transcript variant 1
Ttn	0.17	0.48	0.24	0.2	0.27	0.0001	Mus musculus titin (Ttn), transcript variant N2-B
Asph	0.28	0.46	0.18	0.16	0.27	0.0001	Mus musculus aspartate-beta-hydroxylase (Asph), transcript variant 8
Inpp4b	0.2	0.41	0.33	0.16	0.27	0.0001	Mus musculus inositol polyphosphate-4-phosphatase, type II (Inpp4b)
Igf2os	0.37	0.45	0.15	0.16	0.28	0.0001	Mus musculus insulin-like growth factor 2, opposite strand (Igf2os), antisense RNA
Myh6	0.42	0.23	0.18	0.32	0.28	0.0001	Mus musculus myosin, heavy polypeptide 6, cardiac muscle, alpha (Myh6)
Asb2	0.48	0.39	0.23	0.17	0.32	0.0001	Mus musculusankyrin repeat and SOCS box-containing 2 (Asb2)
Mybpc1	0.45	0.44	0.25	0.13	0.32	0.0001	Mus musculus myosin binding protein C, slow-type (Mybpc1)
Btbd17	0.47	0.45	0.1	0.29	0.33	0.0002	Mus musculus BTB (POZ) domain containing 17 (Btbd17)
Sema6b	0.46	0.39	0.09	0.38	0.33	0.0002	Mus musculussema domain, transmembrane domain (TM), and cytoplasmic domain
Actc1	0.38	0.39	0.33	0.25	0.34	0.0001	Mus musculus actin, alpha, cardiac muscle 1 (Actc1)
Ddc	0.48	0.48	0.22	0.39	0.39	0.0001	Mus musculusdopa decarboxylase (Ddc), transcript variant 1

B.

Gene	Set1	Set2	Set3	Set4	Average	pValue	Description
Gm10536	4.95	7.99	11.97	13.93	9.71	0.0049	Mus musculus predicted gene 10536 (Gm10536), long non-coding RNA
Iws1	3.92	4.7	2.15	10.28	5.26	0.5130	Mus musculus IWS1 homolog (S. cerevisiae) (Iws1)
Dkk2	4.02	3.54	4.95	2.98	3.87	0.0005	Mus musculusdickkopf homolog 2 (Xenopuslaevis) (Dkk2)
Cdc45	3.44	2.22	4.92	3.16	3.43	0.0048	Mus musculus cell division cycle 45 (Cdc45), transcript variant 1
Suv420h1	3.25	2.86	2.71	3.45	3.07	0.0001	Mus musculus suppressor of variegation 4–20 homolog 1 (Drosophila) (Suv420h1)
Cdc42bpa	2.28	2.11	3.11	4.32	2.95	0.0082	Mus musculus CDC42 binding protein kinase alpha (Cdc42bpa)
Zfp318	2.02	2.89	2.23	4.18	2.83	0.0094	Mus musculus zinc finger protein 318 (Zfp318), transcript variant 2

Table 1. *Cont.*

C.			
Term	**Count**	**%**	***p* Value**
Transcription regulation	3	42.9	7.5×10^{-2}
Nucleus	4	57.1	9.8×10^{-2}

D.			
Term	**Count**	**%**	***p* Value**
Muscle protein	8	28.6	1.40×10^{-13}
Thick filament	6	21.4	1.00×10^{-12}
Myosin	7	25	1.40×10^{-11}
Motor protein	7	25	5.90×10^{-9}
Actin-binding	6	21.4	8.50×10^{-6}
ATP-binding	10	35.7	1.20×10^{-5}
Calmodulin-binding	5	17.9	1.80×10^{-5}
Methylation	6	21.4	6.60×10^{-5}
Nucleotide-binding	10	35.7	8.90×10^{-5}
Coiled coil	11	39.3	1.40×10^{-3}
Cytoplasm	10	35.7	4.80×10^{-2}
Isopeptide bond	4	14.3	9.40×10^{-2}

TTR_{wt} or TTR_{kd} were cultured with 2% FBS for two days and microarray analysis was performed on TTR_{wt} or TTR_{kd}. (**A** and **B**) List of down- or up-regulated genes in TTR_{kd} (2-fold$\leq$). (**C** and **D**) Functional analysis by DAVID (2-fold$\leq$). TTR_{wt} indicates cells transfected with scrambled vector. Means $\pm$ SD ($n = 3$).

Down-regulated genes were analyzed at different myogenic times (0, 2, 4 and 6 days). Interestingly, most gene expressions were increased under myogenic conditions than that at the proliferating stage (Day 0). Similar to MYOG (the myogenic marker gene) the expression of 15 genes increased greatly during myogenic differentiation (Supplementary Figure S2). DAVID analysis was performed using the up- and down-regulated genes. More than half of the up-regulated genes were classified as transcription regulators (Table 1C), especially cell-cycle regulators. Although some of the down-regulated genes were identified as being involved in Ca^{2+}-mediated signal transduction and were reported to regulate transcription, most down-regulated genes were classified as components or regulators of the sarcomere motor unit or the ATPase-related group, which are the main structural components of the sarcomere (Table 1D).

Even though genes were selected based on their high statistical significance among all differentially expressed genes, the genes were also cross-examined by performing real-time RT-PCR with TTR_{kd} and comparing the results to those of TTR_{wt} (Figure 7A). To investigate the effect of T_4 on TR expression, cells were grown under serum-free conditions with added T_4 and/or TR-specific antagonist 1-850 and examined both for morphological appearance and for changes in mRNA expression levels of certain genes. Myotube formation and mRNA levels of the myogenic marker genes (MYOD, MYOG and MYL2) were decreased by T_4 + 1-850 treatment (Figure 7B). In contrast, T_4 treatment increased myofibril diameter. The T_4 treatment elevated most of the gene mRNA levels, whereas T_4 + 1-850 treatment had opposite effects. However, T_4 treatment reduced the suppressing effect of 1-850 on mRNA expression of Nmrk2 (40% rescue), Sox8 (40%), Myh1 (20%), and Myh8 (30%) (Figure 7C).

To determine whether the TTR_{kd} effects were produced by TH and its specific receptor, the TR binding site was scanned in genome portions containing the 5' flanking region and the first intron of each gene. For precise analysis, two nuclear receptor scanning software programs, NHR-scan and NUBI-scan, were utilized. All binding site candidates were predicted by using the AGGTCA sequence arranged by the DR0, DR4, IR0, IR4, ER4, and ER6 patterns, as was used in the in silico thyroid hormone response elements (TRE) prediction models. Consequently, most of the genes contained more than one TRE at the 5' flanking region. However, some genes such as Fgf21 did not have a suitable TRE. In addition, Myh1 did not possess a TRE upstream of the first exon (Supplementary Figures S3 and S4). Altogether, these results showed that T_4 transported to the cell interior activated TR to induce gene expression and modulated novel and major transcription regulating genes that markedly increased during myogenic differentiation in a TH-dependent manner.

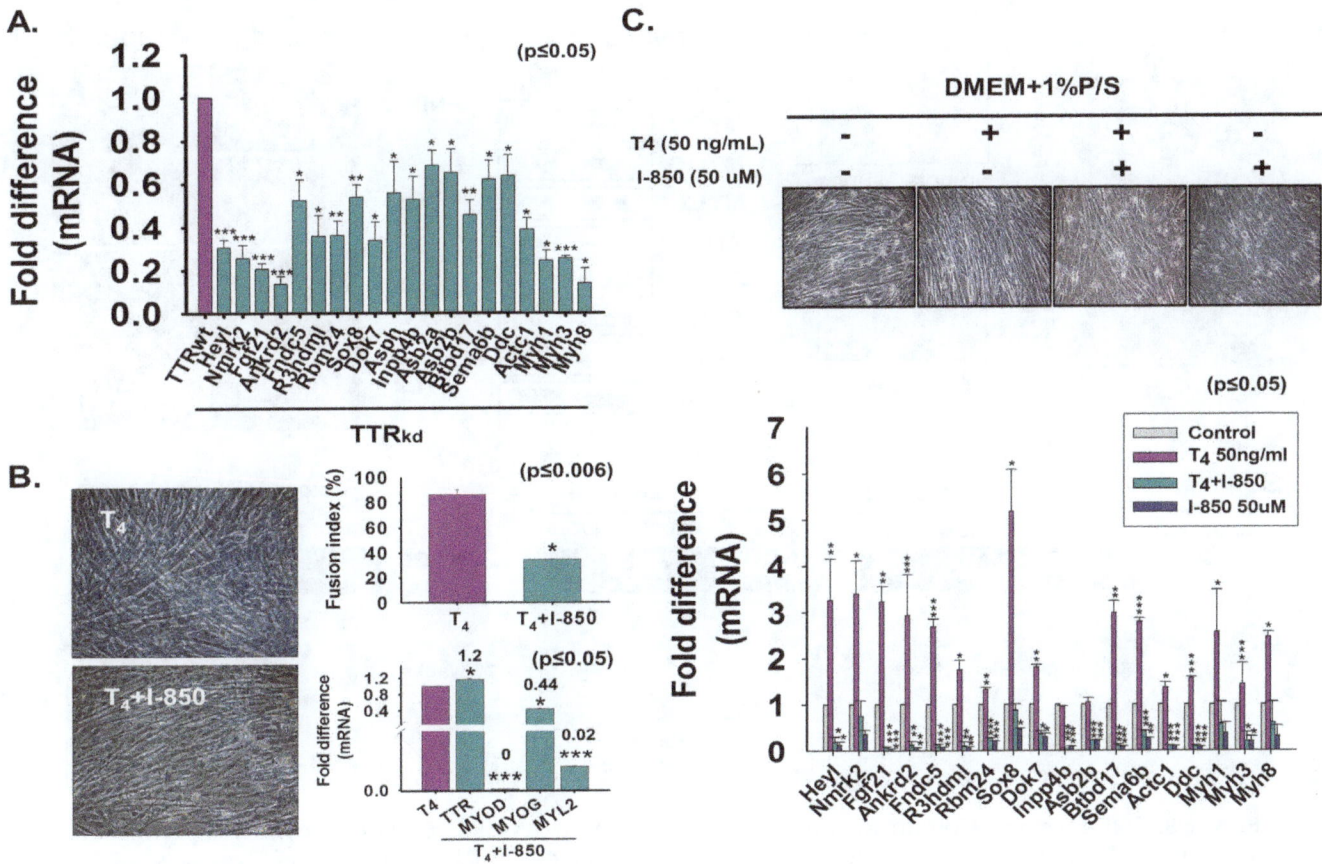

Figure 7. Expression of down-regulated genes in TTR knock-down cells and effect of T_4 treatment on down-regulated genes. (**A**) TTR_{wt} or TTR_{kd} were cultured with 2% FBS for two days. Down-regulated gene expression was assessed by real-time RT-PCR in TTR_{wt} or TTR_{kd}. (**B**) Cells were cultured with serum-free media supplemented with T_4 or T_4 + 1-850 and incubated for two days. Myotube formation and fusion index were observed by Giemsa staining and mRNA expression by real-time RT-PCR. (**C**) Cells were incubated without or with T_4, T_4 + 1-850 or 1-850 for two days. Expression of down-regulated genes without or with T_4, T_4 + 1-850 or 1-850 by real-time RT-PCR. Control indicates non-treated cells. Means ± SD ($n = 3$). * $p \leq 0.05$, ** $p \leq 0.001$, *** $p \leq 0.0001$.

3.8. FNDC5 Expression During Myoblast Differentiation

To confirm the function of the genes that were down-regulated by TTR_{kd}, myokine FNDC5 was selected. FNDC5 knockdown was performed followed by culture with 2% FBS for two days. Myotube formation and myogenic gene expression were decreased in $FNDC5_{kd}$ cells, whereas TTR and TRα expressions were increased at both the transcriptional and translational levels (Figure 8A). Next, cells were grown in serum-free media or supplemented with T_4 for two days, and the FNDC5 mRNA level was analyzed in normal cells and exosomes from plasma and media of cultured cells ($FNDC5_{kd}$ and $FNDC5_{wt}$). FNDC5 mRNA was evident in exosomes from culture media and plasma and decreased in $FNDC5_{kd}$ cells (Figure 8B). Additionally, decreased FNDC5 mRNA was observed in T_4 + TTR treatment in MSCs exosomes (Figure 8B). Expression of FNDC5 was decreased in 26-week muscle compared with that in 16-week muscle (Figure 8C). These results show that FNDC5 positively regulates myoblast differentiation.

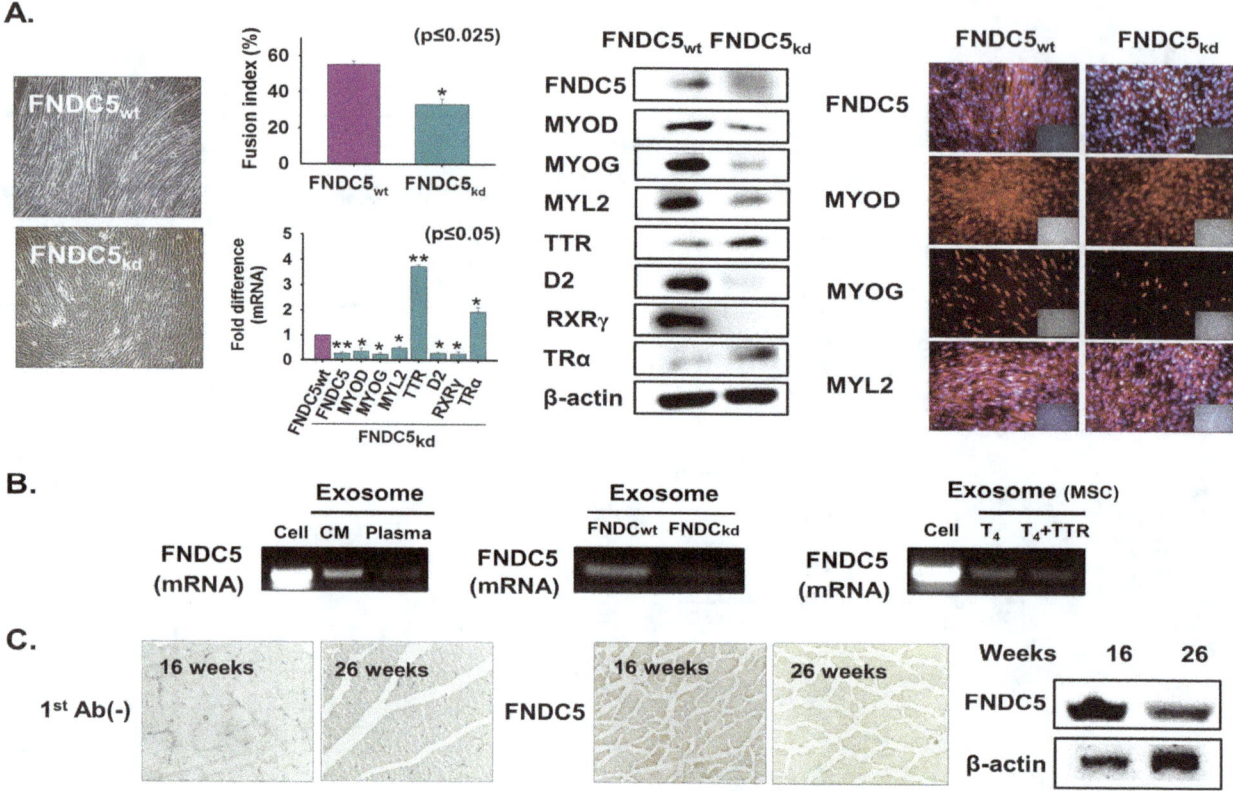

Figure 8. FNDC5 expression during myoblast differentiation. (**A**) FNDC5 knockdown was performed and cells were incubated with 2% FBS for two days. Myotube formation and fusion index were observed by Giemsa staining, mRNA expression using real-time RT-PCR and protein expression were observed by Western blot and immunocytochemistry. (**B**) Cells were cultured with only serum-free media for two days and exosomes were isolated from cultured media. FNDC5 mRNA level in normal cells, exosomes isolated from plasma, and media of cultured cells (FNDC5$_{wt}$ and FNDC5$_{kd}$). MSCs were cultured with only serum-free media or supplemented with T_4 for two days. FNDC5 mRNA level in exosomes from cell, media of cultured cells with T_4 or T_4 + TTR. (**C**) FNDC5 protein expression in 16- or 26-week muscle by immunohistochemistry and Western blot. FNDC5$_{wt}$ indicates cells transfected with scrambled vector. Means ± SD (n = 3). * $p \leq 0.05$, ** $p \leq 0.001$, *** $p \leq 0.0001$.

4. Discussion

Skeletal muscle accounts for nearly half of the body mass and represents the largest protein reservoir in the human body [31]. Although the importance of TH signaling in muscle physiology has been documented for several years, its precise mechanism in skeletal muscle during postnatal myogenesis remains unclear. Initially, we demonstrated the role of TTR in sustaining the cellular T_4 level during myoblast proliferation and differentiation [6,29]. In this study, we give the first direct evidence of TTR secretion and uptake in C2C12 mouse myoblast cells. We also identify TTR mRNA in exosomes and its increased expression following T_4 treatment, which may act as a mediator in this process. In addition, we studied the role of TTR in T_4 transport into C2C12 cells and murine MSCs during the assessment of cell viability and differentiation. The appearance of TTR in cultured serum-free media from myoblasts strongly suggests that TTR synthesized by C2C12 cell is secreted. This suggestion was confirmed by TTR immunoneutralization using TTR antibody, which demonstrated a reduction in myotube formation and mRNA level of some myogenic marker genes (especially, MYOD and MYOG), and T_4 uptake into cells, along with an increase in TTR retained in the cells. Further, it is important to emphasize the presence of T_3 in exosomes, which indicates that T_3 produced in cells is secreted out of the cell through exosomes. These results imply that muscle may not only utilize T_4 but also act as a reservoir of T_3 in order to distribute it to other tissues or to more distant sites.

Cosmo et al. reported that TH uptake by skeletal muscle can occur independently of monocarboxylate transporter 8 (Mct8). However, they found enhanced TH action, T_3 content, and glucose metabolism in Mct8 knockout mice [32]. We speculate that TTR might maintain the TH content in Mct8 knockout mice and, hence, normal muscle metabolism and development. The binding affinity of TTR for T_4 is high, hence, it serves as a primary distributor protein in muscle. We showed that TTR with T_4 treatment significantly increased cell viability and differentiation compared to that of only T_4 treated cells. This was consistent with our previous finding that TTR expression increases myoblast differentiation by increasing T_4 transport into the cell [29]. Similar to what we observed in the C2C12 cell line, the T_4 + TTR protein treated mouse MSCs also showed increased myotube formation with elevated T_4 concentration. Additionally, a progressive increase in TTR expression was observed during differentiation (day 2) in primary MSC cultures. These data confirm that TTR promotes myogenesis by enhancing the transport of T_4.

Kassem et al. showed that the availability of TTR in cerebrospinal fluid (CSF) was associated with enhanced T_4 uptake into the choroid plexus and brain and this uptake was increased in the presence of TTR [33]. Accordingly, in the present study, low T_4 concentration in media with its consequent high concentration in cells supplemented with T_4 + TTR indicated that TTR enhanced the transport of T_4 to the cell interior during myoblast viability. The enhanced cell uptake may be a simple consequence of the increased T_4 level in serum, providing a concentration gradient that promotes TTR secretion and subsequent cell uptake. Furthermore, increased uptake of TH in cells treated with both T_4 and TTR probably involves a T_4 complex with TTR, as well as passive diffusion of T_4, allowing for greater cell uptake than can be accomplished by diffusion only, which is consistent with observations in human ependymoma cells [34]. Although TTR has been reported to be the main component in maintaining high TH levels in CSF and brain [33,35], in this study we observed that TTR also sustained the TH concentration in skeletal muscle and, hence, promoted myogenesis.

TTR is one of three proteins required for T_4 transport: TBG is the major transporter and albumin has the lowest affinity, acting as the third T_4 binding protein in human plasma [25,36]. Consistent with this theory, we found that BSA reduced T_4 transport to the cells, which was also increased with TTR treatment as it has high efficiency for TH. Additionally, BSA treatment decreased myotube formation and myogenic protein expression, while TTR and D2 expressions were increased at the translational level, which might reflect the drop in the T_4 level in the cells. TH regulates several genes that are responsible for muscle development and homeostasis. Among those genes, MYOD, MYOG and contractility-determining proteins are transcriptionally regulated by TH and are important for regeneration and myogenesis [37]. MYOD expression regulated by TH is involved in the fast muscle fiber phenotype, with transcriptional stimulation of the myosin-1, myosin-2 and myosin-4 isoforms [38]. TH metabolizing enzyme D2 can activate TH by outer-ring deiodination and can influence local tissue TH levels [39]. Collectively, our findings suggest that TTR acts to maintain the TH level in myoblast cells.

Evidence of high fluorescence-labeled TTR protein levels in cells reveals that TTR was internalized into the myoblast cells. This supports previous results showing endocytosis of fluorescence-labeled TTR in ependymoma cells [34]. In other reports, ^{125}I-TTR and digoxigenin labeled TTR were internalized by an endocytic process in rat yolk sac and β-cells, respectively [40,41]. Furthermore, increased uptake of T_4 in TTR-overexpressing cells supplemented with T_4 implies that an even distribution of T_4 within the cell is not only dependent on the free fraction of T_4 in serum but also on the T_4 bound to TTR. The presence of T_4 or T_3 significantly enhanced TTR internalization in JEG-3 cells, with TTR entering the cells as a TTR-T_4 complex [27]. In addition, Divino and Schussler [42] reported increased TTR internalization in HepG2 cells with increasing amounts of T_4 and suggested that a T_4-stimulated conformational alteration in TTR somehow enhanced the uptake of TTR.

Reduced T_4 serum concentrations have been reported in old rats [43,44], though their serum T_3 level remains more controversial [43]. We show that TTR and D2 expressions with T_3 concentration have a correlation with muscle age. The reduced D2 activity is suggestive of impaired T_4 conversion in 26-week muscle. Silvestri et al. observed reduced D1 activity in 26-month-old rats relative to that in young (6- and 12-month-old male) rats [44]. Interestingly, decreased TTR expression in 26-week muscle was consistent with the decreased TH transporter Mct8 protein level in liver of 24-month-old rats [44]. Furthermore, higher plasma T_3 or T_4 concentration in 26-week muscle could be associated with the reduced free T_4 concentration in the 16-week muscle, probably due to a higher TBG expression, as described elsewhere [45]. Additionally, decreased T_3 concentration in the 26-week muscle at the cellular level was consistent with the findings of Silvestri et al. [44] in which decreased T_3 concentration was observed in 24-month-old rats. Nevertheless, T_3 generation has been observed in 11-month-old rats relative to that in seven-month-old rats [46], indicating that the mechanisms of T_3 production from T_4 in old muscle remain poorly understood.

TH is the main endocrine regulator that acts by binding to TRs and imposing a signature type of gene expression [11]. TH primarily functions either via nuclear receptor-mediated stimulation that is T_3 dependent or by switching off the gene transcription machinery [13]. In muscle, this signaling pathway is regulated by the THRA1 isoform of TR [47]. The heterodimer complex formed by the TR with RXR- binds to a TRE, leading to activation or suppression of gene transcription [13]. Accordingly, we showed that T_4 treatment induced RXRγ expression. However, myotube formation and myogenic factors were decreased in RXRγ and TRα knockdown cells. Interestingly, RXRγ knockout mice are unable to increase their mass in response to high-fat feeding, suggesting a specific effect of RXRγ in skeletal muscle [48]. In muscle, the proteins whose expression are transcriptionally controlled by T_3 are SERCA1a [12], SERCA2a [49], uncoupling protein 3 (UCP3) [50], GLUT4 [51], cytosolic malic enzyme (ME1) [52], muscle glycerol-3-phosphate dehydrogenase (mGPDH) [53], and myosin-7 [54]. Furthermore, we found that TTR and D2 expression were decreased in TRα_{kd} cells, which explains the retarded transport of TH into the cell. The selective functions of TRs are controlled by local ligand availability [39,55] or by TH transport to the cell interior via Mct8 or other associated transporters [56]. The TH metabolizing enzymes D2 and D3, as well as transporters Mct8 and Mct10, are expressed in both rodent and human skeletal muscle [57,58].

The TTR-affected genes identified by TTR_{kd}-based microarray analysis included important transcription factors or mediators that have the potential to control several other genes. For example, Rbm24 is reported to regulate MYOG expression [59] and mediate skeletal muscle-specific splicing events [60]. In contrast, Sox8, a negative regulator of myogenesis [61], has increased expression during myogenesis of C2C12 cells. In addition, Sox8 and Heyl genes are marker genes of MSCs [61,62]; however, the Heyl gene showed increased expression during myogenic differentiation. Interestingly, those opposing results were also observed for Nmrk2 [63]. Another research group reported that Ddc is not produced by myotubes [64], but in the present study, it was induced by suitable myogenic differentiation. Altogether, some genes that have been reported to be negatively correlated with myogenesis were markedly increased in expression during myogenic differentiation in this study.

Another interesting observation from the time-course expression study is that several novel genes that show increased expression during myogenesis responded to T_4 as they did to TTR. However, Inpp4b and Asb2, genes that contain TREs in proximity to the transcription start site (TSS), did not show any change with T_4 treatment. In the case of Inpp4b, TREs in the proximity of the promoter were only downstream of the TSS, and the first intron was approximately 130 kb. This characteristic indicates a rare aspect of the TTR_{kd}-affected genes. Moreover, Fgf21 and Myh1, which do not seem to contain TREs, showed increased expression levels. The various TRE elements have only been predicted by a one-dimensional arrangement, moreover, a proper, precise, and complete nucleotide matrix for this one-dimensional arrangement is not present in public databases. Due to these limitations, many other researchers [65,66] have reported different nucleotide matrices for TREs and different reactivity of each.

Interaction and cooperation between TR and the mammalian insulator CCCTC-binding factor have already been reported [67,68]. An insulator can mediate multi-dimensional chromosomal changes [69]. In addition, based on the results of the TTR_{kd} microarray analysis, the T_4 affected sarcomere genes Myh1, Myh3 and Myh8 may be suitable candidates for TR-insulator mediated transcriptional regulation. In the case of the Myh1 gene, no TREs were present in its promoter region.

In contrast, the FNDC5 gene, downregulated by TTR_{kd}, also showed a high expression level during myogenic differentiation and after T_4 treatment. The FNDC5 gene encodes the irisin protein, which is considered as a circulating myokine. The most remarkable feature of the FNDC5/irisin protein is that it generates brown fat from white fat [70,71]. Recently, it has been shown that irisin injection stimulated muscle hypertrophy and increased regeneration in injured skeletal muscle [72]. Additionally, enhanced irisin levels have been found during myogenic differentiation and the additional irisin enhances the expression of p-Erk, which has a vital role in the protein synthesis pathway [73]. Thus, knockdown of the FNDC5 gene was undertaken. We showed that interruption of the FNDC5 gene produced a low level of myotube formation. In humans, FNDC5 protein is cleaved to provide detectable irisin levels in circulation. Additionally, increased irisin concentrations occur in response to exercise in humans [74]. Therefore, based on the pro-myogenic role of FNDC5 in the present study, we suggest that FNDC5 may be a potential curative target for the intrusion of muscle dystrophy. Thus, we conclude that one control pathway within TTR myogenesis is mediated by the protein FNDC5.

5. Conclusions

In conclusion, these results suggest that: (1) a portion of the extracellular T_4 enters myoblasts or myocytes via MCT via passive diffusion and is converted to T_3 by the D2 enzyme which, in turn, induces the expression of several genes including TTR; (2) synthesized TTR exocytoses the cell through exosomes; (3) TTR brings T_4 inside the cells as a TTR-T_4 complex through an endocytic mechanism; (4) intracellularly synthesized T_3 can exocytose via exosomes (Figure 9A); and (5) TTR, through the action of T_3 converted from T_4, regulates gene expression of TTR intermediates, such as RXRγ and FNDC5 (irisin), which ultimately induces myogenesis (Figure 9B). In this study, we have shown that muscle cells use a much more active mechanism than previously thought to bring T_4 into cells. Moreover, intracellularly-generated T_3, besides being used in the target muscle cells, also moves out of the cell and affects adjacent cells as well as probably other tissues. Herein, we propose a novel mechanism for the uptake and release of T_4 and T_3 in myoblasts and for TTR to act as a sensor for intracellular T_4 during myogenesis. However, this study has presented a most rudimentary picture of T_4 and T_3 transport into and out of muscle cells, and further studies will undoubtedly reveal more detailed mechanisms.

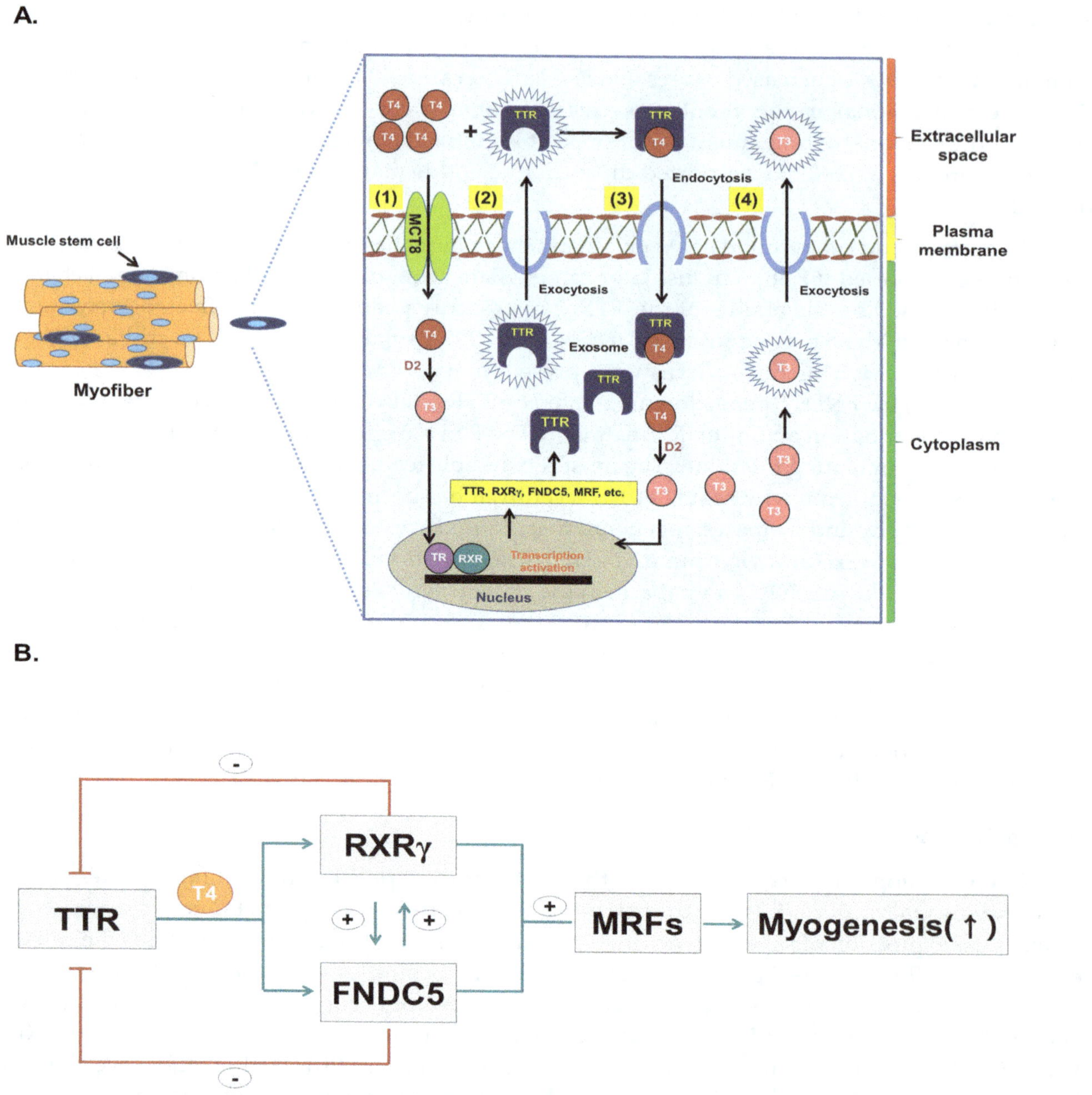

A.

B.

Figure 9. Hypothesis for the role of TTR with T_4 during myoblast differentiation. (**A**) Hypothetical figure depicting role of TTR with T_4 during myoblast differentiation. (1) T_4 enters cells via Mct8 by passive diffusion and is converted to T_3 by D2 enzyme, which in turn triggers the expression of several genes including TTR. (2) Synthesized TTR is exocytosed through exosomes, and (3) subsequently enters the cells as TTR-T_4 complex via an endocytic mechanism. (4) T_3 produced in the cells can exocytose via exosomes. (**B**) TTR positively regulates RXRγ and FNDC5 and triggers myogenic regulatory factors, hence promoting myogenesis. RXRγ and FNDC5 negatively regulate TTR while RXRγ and FNDC5 regulate each other.

Supplementary Materials:
Figure S1: Microarray analysis of TTR_{kd} cells, Figure S2: Time-course study of down-regulated genes during myoblast differentiation, Figure S3: Promoter of down-regulated genes was analyzed to predict TRE binding site, Figure S4: Promoter of down-regulated genes was analyzed to predict TRE binding site, Table S1: shRNA information, Table S2: Primer information, Table S3: Molecular weight of protein, Table S4: Functional analysis of up- or down-regulated genes affected by TTR_{kd}.

Author Contributions: Conceptualization: E.J.L. and I.C.; formal analysis: Y.-W.K. and I.C.; funding acquisition: E.J.L. and I.C.; investigation: E.J.L. and D.C.; methodology: J.H.L., Y.-H.L. and S.-Y.P.; resources: S.J.P. and S.-Y.P.; writing—original draft: E.J.L., S.S. and I.C.; writing—review and editing: E.J.L., S.S., K.A. and M.H.B.

Abbreviations

TTR	Transthyretin
RXR	Retinoid X receptor
MSCs	Muscle satellite cells
MYOG	Myogenin
T_4	Thyroxin
T_3	Triiodothyronine
THs	Thyroid hormones
TR	Thyroid hormone receptors
MYOD	Myoblast determination protein
TBG	Thyroxine binding globulin
FBS	Fetal bovine serum
P/S	Penicillin/Streptomycin
D2	Iodothyronine deiodinase type 2
TRE	Thyroid hormone response elements
Mct8	Monocarboxylate transporter 8
TSS	Transcription start site
CSF	Cerebrospinal fluid
BSA	Bovine serum albumin
FNDC5	Fibronectin type III domain containing 5
CM	Culture media MYL2 (Myosin light chain 2)

References

1. Blau, H.M.; Cosgrove, B.D.; Ho, A.T. The central role of muscle stem cells in regenerative failure with aging. *Nat. Med.* **2015**, *21*, 854–862. [CrossRef] [PubMed]
2. Ahmad, K.; Lee, E.J.; Moon, J.S.; Park, S.Y.; Choi, I. Multifaceted Interweaving between Extracellular Matrix, Insulin Resistance, and Skeletal Muscle. *Cells* **2018**, *8*, 332. [CrossRef] [PubMed]
3. Baig, M.H.; Jan, A.T.; Rabbani, G.; Ahmad, K.; Ashraf, J.M.; Kim, T.; Min, H.S.; Lee, Y.H.; Cho, W.K.; Ma, J.Y.; et al. Methylglyoxal and Advanced Glycation End products: Insight of the regulatory machinery affecting the myogenic program and of its modulation by natural compounds. *Sci. Rep.* **2017**, *7*, 5916. [CrossRef] [PubMed]
4. Zhang, K.; Zhang, Y.; Gu, L.; Lan, M.; Liu, C.; Wang, M.; Su, Y.; Ge, M.; Wang, T.; Yu, Y.; et al. Islr regulates canonical Wnt signaling-mediated skeletal muscle regeneration by stabilizing Dishevelled-2 and preventing autophagy. *Nat. Commun.* **2018**, *9*, 5129. [CrossRef]
5. Lee, E.J.; Jan, A.T.; Baig, M.H.; Ashraf, J.M.; Nahm, S.S.; Kim, Y.W.; Park, S.Y.; Choi, I. Fibromodulin: A master regulator of myostatin controlling progression of satellite cells through a myogenic program. *FASEB J.* **2016**, *30*, 2708–2719. [CrossRef]
6. Lee, E.J.; Bhat, A.R.; Kamli, M.R.; Pokharel, S.; Chun, T.; Lee, Y.H.; Nahm, S.S.; Nam, J.H.; Hong, S.K.; Yang, B.; et al. Transthyretin is a key regulator of myoblast differentiation. *PLoS ONE* **2013**, *8*, e63627. [CrossRef]
7. Mishra, A.; Zhu, X.G.; Ge, K.; Cheng, S.Y. Adipogenesis is differentially impaired by thyroid hormone receptor mutant isoforms. *J. Mol. Endocrinol.* **2010**, *44*, 247–255. [CrossRef]
8. Ambrosio, R.; De Stefano, M.A.; Di Girolamo, D.; Salvatore, D. Thyroid hormone signaling and deiodinase actions in muscle stem/progenitor cells. *Mol. Cell Endocrinol.* **2017**, *459*, 79–83. [CrossRef]

9. Milanesi, A.; Lee, J.W.; Yang, A.; Liu, Y.Y.; Sedrakyan, S.; Cheng, S.Y.; Perin, L.; Brent, G.A. Thyroid Hormone Receptor Alpha is Essential to Maintain the Satellite Cell Niche During Skeletal Muscle Injury and Sarcopenia of Aging. *Thyroid* **2017**, *27*, 1316–1322. [CrossRef]

10. Soukup, T.; Smerdu, V. Effect of altered innervation and thyroid hormones on myosin heavy chain expression and fiber type transitions: A mini-review. *Histochem. Cell Biol.* **2015**, *143*, 123–130. [CrossRef]

11. Salvatore, D.; Simonides, W.S.; Dentice, M.; Zavacki, A.M.; Larsen, P.R. Thyroid hormones and skeletal muscle—new insights and potential implications. *Nat. Rev. Endocrinol.* **2014**, *10*, 206–214. [CrossRef] [PubMed]

12. Simonides, W.S.; Brent, G.A.; Thelen, M.H.; van der Linden, C.G.; Larsen, P.R.; van Hardeveld, C. Characterization of the promoter of the rat sarcoplasmic endoplasmic reticulum Ca2+-ATPase 1 gene and analysis of thyroid hormone responsiveness. *J. Biol. Chem.* **1996**, *271*, 32048–32056. [CrossRef] [PubMed]

13. Brent, G.A. Mechanisms of thyroid hormone action. *J. Clin. Investig.* **2012**, *122*, 3035–3043. [CrossRef] [PubMed]

14. Lazar, M.A. Thyroid hormone receptors: Multiple forms, multiple possibilities. *Endocr. Rev.* **1993**, *14*, 184–193. [PubMed]

15. Weiss, R.E.; Murata, Y.; Cua, K.; Hayashi, Y.; Seo, H.; Refetoff, S. Thyroid hormone action on liver, heart, and energy expenditure in thyroid hormone receptor beta-deficient mice. *Endocrinology* **1998**, *139*, 4945–4952. [CrossRef] [PubMed]

16. Muscat, G.E.; Mynett-Johnson, L.; Dowhan, D.; Downes, M.; Griggs, R. Activation of myoD gene transcription by 3,5,3'-triiodo-L-thyronine: A direct role for the thyroid hormone and retinoid X receptors. *Nucleic Acids Res.* **1994**, *22*, 583–591. [CrossRef]

17. Leid, M.; Kastner, P.; Lyons, R.; Nakshatri, H.; Saunders, M.; Zacharewski, T.; Chen, J.Y.; Staub, A.; Garnier, J.A.; Mader, S.; et al. Purification, cloning, and RXR identity of the HeLa cell factor with which RAR or TR heterodimerizes to bind target sequences efficiently. *Cell* **1992**, *68*, 377–395. [CrossRef]

18. Mangelsdorf, D.J.; Borgmeyer, U.; Heyman, R.A.; Zhou, J.Y.; Ong, E.S.; Oro, A.E.; Kakizuka, A.; Evans, R.M. Characterization of three RXR genes that mediate the action of 9-cis retinoic acid. *Genes Dev.* **1992**, *6*, 329–344. [CrossRef]

19. Simpson, R.J.; Jensen, S.S.; Lim, J.W. Proteomic profiling of exosomes: Current perspectives. *Proteomics* **2008**, *8*, 4083–4099. [CrossRef]

20. Valadi, H.; Ekström, K.; Bossios, A.; Sjöstrand, M.; Lee, J.J.; Lötvall, J.O. Exosome-mediated transfer of mRNAs and microRNAs is a novel mechanism of genetic exchange between cells. *Nat. Cell Biol.* **2007**, *9*, 654–659. [CrossRef]

21. Jan, A.T.; Malik, M.A.; Rahman, S.; Yeo, H.R.; Lee, E.J.; Abdullah, T.S.; Choi, I. Perspective Insights of Exosomes in Neurodegenerative Diseases: A Critical Appraisal. *Front. Aging Neurosci.* **2017**, *9*, 317. [CrossRef] [PubMed]

22. Johnson, S.M.; Connelly, S.; Fearns, C.; Powers, E.T.; Kelly, J.W. The transthyretin amyloidoses: From delineating the molecular mechanism of aggregation linked to pathology to a regulatory-agency-approved drug. *J. Mol. Biol.* **2012**, *421*, 185–203. [CrossRef] [PubMed]

23. Richardson, S.J. Cell and molecular biology of transthyretin and thyroid hormones. *Int. Rev. Cytol.* **2007**, *258*, 137–193. [PubMed]

24. Monk, J.A.; Sims, N.A.; Dziegielewska, K.M.; Weiss, R.E.; Ramsay, R.G.; Richardson, S.J. Delayed development of specific thyroid hormone-regulated events in transthyretin null mice. *Am. J. Physiol. Endocrinol. Metab.* **2013**, *304*, E23–E31. [CrossRef] [PubMed]

25. Alshehri, B.; D'Souza, D.G.; Lee, J.Y.; Petratos, S.; Richardson, S.J. The diversity of mechanisms influenced by transthyretin in neurobiology: Development, disease and endocrine disruption. *J. Neuroendocrinol.* **2015**, *27*, 303–323. [CrossRef] [PubMed]

26. Blaner, W.S.; Bonifacio, M.J.; Feldman, H.D.; Piantedosi, R.; Saraiva, M.J. Studies on the synthesis and secretion of transthyretin by the human hepatoma cell line Hep G2. *FEBS Lett.* **1991**, *287*, 193–196. [CrossRef]

27. Landers, K.A.; McKinnon, B.D.; Li, H.; Subramaniam, V.N.; Mortimer, R.H.; Richard, K. Carrier-mediated thyroid hormone transport into placenta by placental transthyretin. *J. Clin. Endocrinol. Metab.* **2009**, *94*, 2610–2616. [CrossRef] [PubMed]

28. McKinnon, B.; Li, H.; Richard, K.; Mortimer, R. Synthesis of thyroid hormone binding proteins transthyretin and albumin by human trophoblast. *J. Clin. Endocrinol. Metab.* **2005**, *90*, 6714–6720. [CrossRef]

29. Lee, E.J.; Pokharel, S.; Jan, A.T.; Huh, S.; Galope, R.; Lim, J.H.; Lee, D.M.; Choi, S.W.; Nahm, S.S.; Kim, Y.W.; et al. Transthyretin: A Transporter Protein Essential for Proliferation of Myoblast in the Myogenic Program. *Int. J. Mol. Sci.* **2017**, *18*, 115. [CrossRef]

30. Lee, E.J.; Jan, A.T.; Baig, M.H.; Ahmad, K.; Malik, A.; Rabbani, G.; Kim, T.; Lee, I.K.; Lee, Y.H.; Park, S.Y.; et al. Fibromodulin and regulation of the intricate balance between myoblast differentiation to myocytes or adipocyte-like cells. *FASEB J.* **2018**, *32*, 768–781. [CrossRef]

31. Gonzalez-Freire, M.; Semba, R.D.; Ubaida-Mohien, C.; Fabbri, E.; Scalzo, P.; Hojlund, K.; Dufresne, C.; Lyashkov, A.; Ferrucci, L. The Human Skeletal Muscle Proteome Project: A reappraisal of the current literature. *J. Cachexia Sarcopenia Muscle* **2017**, *8*, 5–18. [CrossRef] [PubMed]

32. Di Cosmo, C.; Liao, X.H.; Ye, H.; Ferrara, A.M.; Weiss, R.E.; Refetoff, S.; Dumitrescu, A.M. Mct8-deficient mice have increased energy expenditure and reduced fat mass that is abrogated by normalization of serum T3 levels. *Endocrinology* **2013**, *154*, 4885–4895. [CrossRef] [PubMed]

33. Kassem, N.A.; Deane, R.; Segal, M.B.; Preston, J.E. Role of transthyretin in thyroxine transfer from cerebrospinal fluid to brain and choroid plexus. *Am. J. Physiol. Regul. Integr. Comp. Physiol.* **2006**, *291*, R1310–R1315. [CrossRef] [PubMed]

34. Kuchler-Bopp, S.; Dietrich, J.B.; Zaepfel, M.; Delaunoy, J.P. Receptor-mediated endocytosis of transthyretin by ependymoma cells. *Brain Res.* **2000**, *870*, 185–194. [CrossRef]

35. Chen, R.L.; Kassem, N.A.; Preston, J.E. Dose-dependent transthyretin inhibition of T4 uptake from cerebrospinal fluid in sheep. *Neurosci. Lett.* **2006**, *396*, 7–11. [CrossRef]

36. Palha, J.A. Transthyretin as a thyroid hormone carrier: Function revisited. *Clin. Chem. Lab. Med.* **2002**, *40*, 1292–1300. [CrossRef]

37. Bentzinger, C.F.; Wang, Y.X.; Dumont, N.A.; Rudnicki, M.A. Cellular dynamics in the muscle satellite cell niche. *EMBO Rep.* **2013**, *14*, 1062–1072. [CrossRef]

38. Allen, D.L.; Sartorius, C.A.; Sycuro, L.K.; Leinwand, L.A. Different pathways regulate expression of the skeletal myosin heavy chain genes. *J. Biol. Chem.* **2001**, *276*, 43524–43533. [CrossRef]

39. Bianco, A.C.; Salvatore, D.; Gereben, B.; Berry, M.J.; Larsen, P.R. Biochemistry, cellular and molecular biology, and physiological roles of the iodothyronine selenodeiodinases. *Endocr. Rev.* **2002**, *23*, 38–89. [CrossRef]

40. Dekki, N.; Refai, E.; Holmberg, R.; Kohler, M.; Jornvall, H.; Berggren, P.O.; Juntti-Berggren, L. Transthyretin binds to glucose-regulated proteins and is subjected to endocytosis by the pancreatic beta-cell. *Cell Mol. Life Sci.* **2012**, *69*, 1733–1743. [CrossRef]

41. Sousa, M.M.; Norden, A.G.; Jacobsen, C.; Willnow, T.E.; Christensen, E.I.; Thakker, R.V.; Verroust, P.J.; Moestrup, S.K.; Saraiva, M.J. Evidence for the role of megalin in renal uptake of transthyretin. *J. Biol. Chem.* **2000**, *275*, 38176–38181. [CrossRef] [PubMed]

42. Divino, C.M.; Schussler, G.C. Transthyretin receptors on human astrocytoma cells. *J. Clin. Endocrinol. Metab.* **1990**, *71*, 1265–1268. [CrossRef] [PubMed]

43. Mariotti, S.; Franceschi, C.; Cossarizza, A.; Pinchera, A. The aging thyroid. *Endocr. Rev.* **1995**, *16*, 686–715. [CrossRef] [PubMed]

44. Silvestri, E.; Lombardi, A.; de Lange, P.; Schiavo, L.; Lanni, A.; Goglia, F.; Visser, T.J.; Moreno, M. Age-related changes in renal and hepatic cellular mechanisms associated with variations in rat serum thyroid hormone levels. *Am. J. Physiol. Endocrinol. Metab.* **2008**, *294*, E1160–E1168. [CrossRef]

45. Savu, L.; Vranckx, R.; Rouaze-Romet, M.; Maya, M.; Nunez, E.A.; Treton, J.; Flink, I.L. A senescence up-regulated protein: The rat thyroxine-binding globulin (TBG). *Biochim. Biophys. Acta* **1991**, *1097*, 19–22. [CrossRef]

46. Jang, M.; DiStefano, J.J., 3rd. Some quantitative changes in iodothyronine distribution and metabolism in mild obesity and aging. *Endocrinology* **1985**, *116*, 457–468. [CrossRef]

47. Van Mullem, A.; van Heerebeek, R.; Chrysis, D.; Visser, E.; Medici, M.; Andrikoula, M.; Tsatsoulis, A.; Peeters, R.; Visser, T.J. Clinical phenotype and mutant TRalpha1. *N. Engl. J. Med.* **2012**, *366*, 1451–1453. [CrossRef]

48. Haugen, B.R.; Jensen, D.R.; Sharma, V.; Pulawa, L.K.; Hays, W.R.; Krezel, W.; Chambon, P.; Eckel, R.H. Retinoid X receptor gamma-deficient mice have increased skeletal muscle lipoprotein lipase activity and less weight gain when fed a high-fat diet. *Endocrinology* **2004**, *145*, 3679–3685. [CrossRef]

49. Hartong, R.; Wang, N.; Kurokawa, R.; Lazar, M.A.; Glass, C.K.; Apriletti, J.W.; Dillmann, W.H. Delineation of three different thyroid hormone-response elements in promoter of rat sarcoplasmic reticulum Ca2+ATPase gene. Demonstration that retinoid X receptor binds 5′ to thyroid hormone receptor in response element 1. *J. Biol. Chem.* **1994**, *269*, 13021–13029.

50. Solanes, G.; Pedraza, N.; Calvo, V.; Vidal-Puig, A.; Lowell, B.B.; Villarroya, F. Thyroid hormones directly activate the expression of the human and mouse uncoupling protein-3 genes through a thyroid response element in the proximal promoter region. *Biochem. J.* **2005**, *386*, 505–513. [CrossRef]

51. Zorzano, A.; Palacin, M.; Guma, A. Mechanisms regulating GLUT4 glucose transporter expression and glucose transport in skeletal muscle. *Acta Physiol. Scand.* **2005**, *183*, 43–58. [CrossRef] [PubMed]

52. Desvergne, B.; Petty, K.J.; Nikodem, V.M. Functional characterization and receptor binding studies of the malic enzyme thyroid hormone response element. *J. Biol. Chem.* **1991**, *266*, 1008–1013. [PubMed]

53. Dummler, K.; Muller, S.; Seitz, H.J. Regulation of adenine nucleotide translocase and glycerol 3-phosphate dehydrogenase expression by thyroid hormones in different rat tissues. *Biochem. J.* **1996**, *317*, 913–918. [CrossRef] [PubMed]

54. Morkin, E. Control of cardiac myosin heavy chain gene expression. *Microsc. Res. Tech.* **2000**, *50*, 522–531. [CrossRef]

55. Gereben, B.; Zavacki, A.M.; Ribich, S.; Kim, B.W.; Huang, S.A.; Simonides, W.S.; Zeold, A.; Bianco, A.C. Cellular and molecular basis of deiodinase-regulated thyroid hormone signaling. *Endocr. Rev.* **2008**, *29*, 898–938. [CrossRef] [PubMed]

56. Visser, W.E.; Friesema, E.C.; Visser, T.J. Minireview: Thyroid hormone transporters: The knowns and the unknowns. *Mol. Endocrinol.* **2011**, *25*, 1–14. [CrossRef] [PubMed]

57. Friesema, E.C.; Jansen, J.; Jachtenberg, J.W.; Visser, W.E.; Kester, M.H.; Visser, T.J. Effective cellular uptake and efflux of thyroid hormone by human monocarboxylate transporter 10. *Mol. Endocrinol.* **2008**, *22*, 1357–1369. [CrossRef]

58. Marsili, A.; Ramadan, W.; Harney, J.W.; Mulcahey, M.; Castroneves, L.A.; Goemann, I.M.; Wajner, S.M.; Huang, S.A.; Zavacki, A.M.; Maia, A.L.; et al. Type 2 iodothyronine deiodinase levels are higher in slow-twitch than fast-twitch mouse skeletal muscle and are increased in hypothyroidism. *Endocrinology* **2010**, *151*, 5952–5960. [CrossRef]

59. Jin, D.; Hidaka, K.; Shirai, M.; Morisaki, T. RNA-binding motif protein 24 regulates myogenin expression and promotes myogenic differentiation. *Genes Cells* **2010**, *15*, 1158–1167. [CrossRef]

60. Cardinali, B.; Cappella, M.; Provenzano, C.; Garcia-Manteiga, J.M.; Lazarevic, D.; Cittaro, D.; Martelli, F.; Falcone, G. MicroRNA-222 regulates muscle alternative splicing through Rbm24 during differentiation of skeletal muscle cells. *Cell Death Dis.* **2016**, *7*, e2086. [CrossRef]

61. Schmidt, K.; Glaser, G.; Wernig, A.; Wegner, M.; Rosorius, O. Sox8 is a specific marker for muscle satellite cells and inhibits myogenesis. *J. Biol. Chem.* **2003**, *278*, 29769–29775. [CrossRef] [PubMed]

62. Yamaguchi, M.; Murakami, S.; Yoneda, T.; Nakamura, M.; Zhang, L.; Uezumi, A.; Fukuda, S.; Kokubo, H.; Tsujikawa, K.; Fukada, S. Evidence of Notch-Hesr-Nrf2 Axis in Muscle Stem Cells, but Absence of Nrf2 Has No Effect on Their Quiescent and Undifferentiated State. *PLoS ONE* **2015**, *10*, e0138517. [CrossRef] [PubMed]

63. Li, J.; Mayne, R.; Wu, C. A novel muscle-specific beta 1 integrin binding protein (MIBP) that modulates myogenic differentiation. *J. Cell. Biol.* **1999**, *147*, 1391–1398. [CrossRef] [PubMed]

64. Smith, J.L.; Patil, P.B.; Minteer, S.D.; Lipsitz, J.R.; Fisher, J.S. Possibility of autocrine beta-adrenergic signaling in C2C12 myotubes. *Exp. Biol. Med.* **2005**, *230*, 845–852. [CrossRef] [PubMed]

65. Harbers, M.; Wahlstrom, G.M.; Vennstrom, B. Transactivation by the thyroid hormone receptor is dependent on the spacer sequence in hormone response elements containing directly repeated half-sites. *Nucleic Acids Res.* **1996**, *24*, 2252–2259. [CrossRef] [PubMed]

66. Weth, O.; Weth, C.; Bartkuhn, M.; Leers, J.; Uhle, F.; Renkawitz, R. Modular insulators: Genome wide search for composite CTCF/thyroid hormone receptor binding sites. *PLoS ONE* **2010**, *5*, e10119. [CrossRef]

67. Ali, T.; Renkawitz, R.; Bartkuhn, M. Insulators and domains of gene expression. *Curr. Opin. Genet. Dev.* **2016**, *37*, 17–26. [CrossRef]

68. Lutz, M.; Burke, L.J.; LeFevre, P.; Myers, F.A.; Thorne, A.W.; Crane-Robinson, C.; Bonifer, C.; Filippova, G.N.; Lobanenkov, V.; Renkawitz, R. Thyroid hormone-regulated enhancer blocking: Cooperation of CTCF and thyroid hormone receptor. *EMBO J.* **2003**, *22*, 1579–1587. [CrossRef]

69.　Hou, C.; Zhao, H.; Tanimoto, K.; Dean, A. CTCF-dependent enhancer-blocking by alternative chromatin loop formation. *Proc. Natl. Acad. Sci. USA* **2008**, *105*, 20398–20403. [CrossRef]

70.　Bostrom, P.; Wu, J.; Jedrychowski, M.P.; Korde, A.; Ye, L.; Lo, J.C.; Rasbach, K.A.; Bostrom, E.A.; Choi, J.H.; Long, J.Z.; et al. A PGC1-alpha-dependent myokine that drives brown-fat-like development of white fat and thermogenesis. *Nature* **2012**, *481*, 463–468. [CrossRef]

71.　Roca-Rivada, A.; Castelao, C.; Senin, L.L.; Landrove, M.O.; Baltar, J.; Belen Crujeiras, A.; Seoane, L.M.; Casanueva, F.F.; Pardo, M. FNDC5/irisin is not only a myokine but also an adipokine. *PLoS ONE* **2013**, *8*, e60563. [CrossRef] [PubMed]

72.　Reza, M.M.; Subramaniyam, N.; Sim, C.M.; Ge, X.; Sathiakumar, D.; McFarlane, C.; Sharma, M.; Kambadur, R. Irisin is a pro-myogenic factor that induces skeletal muscle hypertrophy and rescues denervation-induced atrophy. *Nat. Commun.* **2017**, *8*, 1104. [CrossRef] [PubMed]

73.　Huh, J.Y.; Dincer, F.; Mesfum, E.; Mantzoros, C.S. Irisin stimulates muscle growth-related genes and regulates adipocyte differentiation and metabolism in humans. *Int. J. Obes.* **2014**, *38*, 1538–1544. [CrossRef] [PubMed]

74.　Jedrychowski, M.P.; Wrann, C.D.; Paulo, J.A.; Gerber, K.K.; Szpyt, J.; Robinson, M.M.; Nair, K.S.; Gygi, S.P.; Spiegelman, B.M. Detection and Quantitation of Circulating Human Irisin by Tandem Mass Spectrometry. *Cell Metab.* **2015**, *22*, 734–740. [CrossRef] [PubMed]

11

TGF-β Regulates Collagen Type I Expression in Myoblasts and Myotubes via Transient *Ctgf* and *Fgf*-2 Expression

Michèle M. G. Hillege, Ricardo A. Galli Caro, Carla Offringa, Gerard M. J. de Wit, Richard T. Jaspers * and Willem M. H. Hoogaars

Laboratory for Myology, Department of Human Movement Sciences, Faculty of Behavioural and Movement Sciences, Vrije Universiteit Amsterdam, Amsterdam Movement Sciences, 1081 BT Amsterdam, The Netherlands; m.m.g.hillege@vu.nl (M.M.G.H.); r.a.galli@amsterdamumc.nl (R.A.G.C.); c.offringa@vu.nl (C.O.); g.m.j.de.wit@vu.nl (G.M.J.d.W.); w.m.h.hoogaars@umcg.nl (W.M.H.H.)
* Correspondence: r.t.jaspers@vu.nl;

Abstract: Transforming Growth Factor β (TGF-β) is involved in fibrosis as well as the regulation of muscle mass, and contributes to the progressive pathology of muscle wasting disorders. However, little is known regarding the time-dependent signalling of TGF-β in myoblasts and myotubes, as well as how TGF-β affects collagen type I expression and the phenotypes of these cells. Here, we assessed effects of TGF-β on gene expression in C2C12 myoblasts and myotubes after 1, 3, 9, 24 and 48 h treatment. In myoblasts, various myogenic genes were repressed after 9, 24 and 48 h, while in myotubes only a reduction in *Myh3* expression was observed. In both myoblasts and myotubes, TGF-β acutely induced the expression of a subset of genes involved in fibrosis, such as *Ctgf* and *Fgf-2*, which was subsequently followed by increased expression of *Col1a1*. Knockdown of *Ctgf* and *Fgf-2* resulted in a lower *Col1a1* expression level. Furthermore, the effects of TGF-β on myogenic and fibrotic gene expression were more pronounced than those of myostatin, and knockdown of TGF-β type I receptor *Tgfbr1*, but not receptor *Acvr1b*, resulted in a reduction in *Ctgf* and *Col1a1* expression. These results indicate that, during muscle regeneration, TGF-β induces fibrosis via *Tgfbr1* by stimulating the autocrine signalling of *Ctgf* and *Fgf-2*.

Keywords: *Acvr1b*; *Tgfbr1*; myostatin; *Col1a1*; skeletal muscle; fibrosis; myogenesis; atrophy

1. Introduction

Muscle wasting disorders, such as sarcopenia, cachexia and muscle dystrophies, are characterised by muscle fibre injury or atrophy, which results in the gradual replacement of muscle fibres by adipose and fibrotic tissue [1,2]. This leads to progressive muscle weakness and loss of contractile function. Transforming Growth Factor β (TGF-β) is known for its role in the regulation of skeletal muscle size as well as fibrosis and contributes to the progressive pathology of muscle wasting disorders such as Duchenne Muscular Dystrophy (DMD) [3,4].

TGF-β functions by regulating expression of target genes via specific binding of type II and type I receptor kinases and subsequent activation of intracellular receptor-regulated SMAD2 and SMAD3 proteins (R-SMADS) [5]. TGF-β is expressed by multiple cell types, such as macrophages, monocytes, neutrophils, fibroblasts and bone cells [6–9]. While TGF-β is transiently expressed during skeletal muscle regeneration following injury [10], prolonged elevated TGF-β protein levels are associated with pathologies such as DMD [3], limb girdle muscular dystrophy and amyotrophic lateral sclerosis (ALS), as well as sarcopenia [11–13]. TGF-β may affect skeletal muscle size by the inhibition of muscle stem cell (MuSC) differentiation and the induction of the atrophy of muscle fibres. In vitro studies have shown that TGF-β inhibits myoblast differentiation through the repression of myogenic gene expression, whereas differentiated myotubes seem to be insensitive to TGF-β-induced myogenic inhibition [14–16]. Muscle-specific overexpression of TGF-β in mice stimulates the expression of E3 ligase (i.e., atrogin-1) and concomitant muscle atrophy [17,18]. However, whether the induction of atrogin-1 and muscle atrophy is a direct effect of TGF-β expression or an indirect effect via the stimulation of other paracrine factors remains to be assessed.

TGF-β is also known to be involved in fibrosis. Overexpression of TGF-β in mouse skeletal muscle results in excessive collagen deposition [17]. In addition, antibody treatment to neutralise TGF-β in murine X-linked muscular dystrophy (mdx) mice reduces connective tissue deposition compared to that of untreated mdx mice [19]. Moreover, C2C12 myoblasts overexpressing TGF-β transdifferentiate into fibrotic cells after transplantation into skeletal muscle, which indicates that muscle cells may contribute to fibrosis [20].

Another TGF-β family member, muscle specific cytokine myostatin, has been shown to inhibit myoblast differentiation via a similar mechanism as via TGF-β [21]. Furthermore, myostatin is a well-known regulator of muscle mass and has been suggested to be involved in muscle fibrosis [22]. Myostatin signals via distinct type II and type I receptors than TGF-β does, but also through phosphorylation of SMAD2/3 [23,24]. TGF-β signals mainly via the type I receptor TGF-β receptor type-I (TGFR-1) [24]. While in muscle cells myostatin signals mainly via type I receptor Activin receptor type-1B (ACTR-1B), in fibroblasts myostatin signals mainly via TGFR-1 [23,25]. Both proteins have been indicated as possible therapeutic targets for muscle wasting disorders.

While transient TGF-β expression may contribute to muscle regeneration after injury, the chronic elevated expression of TGF-β in skeletal muscle may be detrimental [cf.10]. Although the role of TGF-β in muscle mass regulation and skeletal muscle fibrosis has been studied extensively, the effects on myoblasts and differentiated muscle cells and underlying mechanisms are not well understood. The aim of this study was to assess the time-dependent effects of TGF-β signalling and downstream signalling on the expression of myogenic, atrophic and fibrotic genes in both myoblasts and myotubes. Furthermore, taking into account the functional and mechanistic similarities between TGF-β and myostatin, as well as the fact that both ligands have been implied as possible therapeutic targets for muscle wasting disorders, the effects of TGF-β and myostatin signalling in myoblasts were compared. Our data indicate that TGF-β inhibits myogenic gene expression in both myoblasts and myotubes but does not affect myotube size. Most importantly, our results show that TGF-β stimulates collagen type I, alpha 1 (Col1a1) mRNA expression in both myoblasts and myotubes, which is largely induced via autocrine expression of connective tissue growth factor (Ctgf) and fibroblast growth factor-2 (Fgf-2). Lastly, the effects of TGF-β on myogenic and fibrotic signalling are more pronounced than those of myostatin, and only TGF-β receptor type-I (Tgfbr1) mRNA knockdown, but not Activin receptor type-1B (Acvr1b) mRNA knockdown, decreased Ctgf and Col1a1 expression levels, suggesting that myoblasts are more sensitive to TGF-β than to myostatin.

2. Materials and Methods

2.1. C2C12 Cell Culture

The C2C12 mouse muscle myoblast cell line (ATCC CRL-1772) was obtained from ATCC (Wesel, Germany). Cells were cultured in growth medium (DMEM, 4.5% glucose (Gibco, 11995, Waltham, MA, USA), containing 10% fetal bovine serum (Biowest, S181B, Nuaillé, France), 1% penicillin/streptomycin (Gibco, 15140, Waltham, MA, USA), and 0.5% amphotericin B (Gibco, 15290-026, Waltham, MA, USA)) at 37 °C, 5% CO_2. The cells were used for experiments between passage 4–14. All experiments with C2C12 cells were performed on collagen-coated plates (collagen I rat protein, tail (Gibco, A10483-01, Waltham, MA, USA) diluted in 0.02N acetic acid). C2C12 myoblasts were cultured in differentiation medium (DMEM, 4.5% glucose, 2% horse serum (HyClone, 10407223, Marlborough, MA, USA), 1% penicillin/streptomycin, 0.5% Amphotericin B) for 16 h or allowed to differentiate for 3 days before treatment. Cells were treated with 10 ng/mL TGF-β1 (Peprotech, 100-21C, London, UK) or 300 ng/mL myostatin (Peprotech, 120-00, London, UK) for 0, 1, 3, 9, 24 or 48 h, unless indicated differently. The cells were treated with 10μM Ly364947 (dissolved in dimethyl sulfoxide (DMSO), 1mM). As a control, cells were treated with 0.1% DMSO.

2.2. Isolation of the Extensor Digitorum Longus (EDL) Muscle and Primary Myoblast Culture

EDL muscles were obtained from 6-week to 4-month old mice of a C57BL/6 background. The muscles were incubated in collagenase type I (Sigma-Aldrich, C0130, Saint Louis, MO, USA) at 37 °C, 5% CO_2 for 2 h. The muscles were washed in DMEM, 4.5% glucose (Gibco, 11995, Waltham, MA, USA), containing 1% penicillin/streptomycin (Gibco, 15140, Waltham, MA, USA) and incubated in 5% Bovine serum albumin (BSA)-coated dishes containing DMEM (4.5% glucose, 1% penicillin/streptomycin) for 30 min at 37 °C, 5% CO_2 to inactivate collagenase. Single muscle fibres were separated by gently blowing with a blunt ended sterilized Pasteur pipette. Subsequently, muscle fibres were seeded in a thin layer matrigel (VWR, 734-0269, Radnor, PA, USA)-coated 6-well plate containing growth medium (DMEM, 4.5% glucose (Gibco, 11995, Waltham, MA, USA), 1% penicillin/streptomycin (Gibco, 15140, Waltham, MA, USA), 10% horse serum (HyClone, 10407223, Marlborough, MA, USA), 30% fetal bovine serum (Biowest, S181B, Nuaillé, France), 2.5ng/mL recombinant human fibroblast growth factor (rhFGF) (Promega, G5071, Madison, WI, USA), and 1% chicken embryonic extract (Seralab, CE-650-J, Huissen, The Netherlands)). Primary myoblasts were allowed to proliferate and migrate off the muscle fibres for 3–4 days at 37 °C, 5% CO_2. After gentle removal of the muscle fibres, myoblasts were cultured in matrigel-coated flasks until passage 5. Cells were pre-plated in an uncoated flask for 15 min with each passage to reduce the number of fibroblasts in culture. Cell population was 99% Pax7+. All experiments with primary myoblasts were performed on matrigel-coated plates. Primary myoblasts were cultured in differentiation medium for 6 h or allowed to differentiate for 2 days before treatment with 10 ng/mL TGF-β1 (Peprotech, 100-21C, London, UK) or 300 ng/mL myostatin (Peprotech, 120-00, London, UK).

2.3. Tgfbr1 and Acvr1b siRNA Assay

C2C12 cells were seeded at a density of 7900 cells/cm^2 in a 12-well plate (Greiner Bio-One, 665180, Alphen aan den Rijn, The Netherlands) in antibiotic-free growth medium (DMEM, 1% glucose (Gibco, 31885, Waltham, MA, USA), 10% fetal bovine serum (Biowest, S181B, Nuaillé, France)) at 37 °C, 5% CO_2 and allowed to adhere overnight. SiRNA with a final concentration of 25 nM was prepared according to manufacturer's protocol. Then, 50 nM siControl, 25 nM siAcvr1b + 25 nM siControl, 25 nM siTgfbr1 + 25 nM or 25 nM siAcvr1b + 25 nM siTgfbr1 was added to the medium of the cells. We used 2 µL DharmaFECT1 per well. The cells were treated with siRNA for 24 h in antibiotic-free growth medium. Subsequently, cells were treated with siRNA for 48 h in antibiotic-free differentiation medium (DMEM, 1% glucose (Gibco, 31885, Waltham, MA, USA), 2% horse serum (HyClone, 10407223, Marlborough, MA, USA)). The following reagents for transfection were obtained from Dharmacon (Lafayette, Colorado): ON-TARGET plus Non-targeting Pool (D-001810-10), DharmaFECT1 (T-2001), 5X siRNA Buffer (B-002000-UB-100), mouse ON-TARGET plus Tgfbr1 siRNA (J-040617-05), and mouse ON-TARGET plus Acvr1b siRNA(J-043507-08)

2.4. Ctgf and Fgf-2 siRNA Assay

C2C12 myoblast cells were seeded at a density of 4200 cells/cm^2 and cultured in antibiotic-free growth medium (DMEM, 4.5% glucose (Gibco, 11995, Waltham, MA, USA), 10% fetal bovine serum (Biowest, S181B, Nuaillé, France)) at 37°C, 5% CO_2. The cells were transfected with siRNA targeting Ctgf or Fgf-2 (Ambion® Silencer® Select Pre-Design siRNA, Ctgf siRNA ID: s66077, Fgf-2 siRNA ID: s201344, Carlsbad, CA, USA) or a siRNA-negative control (Silencer® Select Negative Control #1 siRNA, Invitrogen 4390843, Carlsbad, CA, USA). SiRNA was re-suspended to a final concentration of 10 µM and lipofectamine transfection reagent (Lipofectamine® RNAiMAX Reagent, Invitrogen 13778100, Carlsbad, CA, USA) was used to prepare the siRNA–lipid complex according to manufacturer's protocol for a 24-well plate set-up. The cells were cultured for 24 h in antibiotic-free growth medium and transfected with *Ctgf* or *Fgf-2* siRNA–lipid complex for another 24 h. Cells were transfected a second time in antibiotic-free differentiation medium (DMEM, 4.5% glucose, 2% horse serum (HyClone, 10407223, Marlborough, MA, USA). After 16 h, the cells were treated with TGF-β1 (10ng/mL) for 0 h, 3 h and 48 h.

2.5. RNA Isolation and Reverse Transcription

Cells were lysed in TRI reagent (Invitrogen, 11312940, Carlsbad, CA, USA). After this, 10% bromochloropropane (Sigma-Aldrich, B9673, Saint Louis, MO, USA) was added. Lysates were inverted and incubated at room temperature for 5 min and centrifuged (4 °C, 12,000 g, 10 min). The RNA containing supernatant was transferred to a new centrifuge tube and washed with 100% ethanol 2:1. RNA was further isolated using the RiboPure RNA purification kit (Thermo Fisher Scientific, AM1924, Waltham, MA, USA). Then, 500 ng RNA and 4 µL SuperScript VILO Mastermix (Invitrogen, 12023679, Carlsbad, CA, USA) were diluted to 20 µL in RNAse free water and reverse transcription was performed in a 2720 thermal cycler (Applied Biosystems, Foster City, CA, USA), using the following program: 10 min 25 °C, 60 min 42 °C, 5 min 85 °C. The cDNA was diluted 10x in RNAse free water.

2.6. Quantitative Real Time PCR

We added 7.5 µL Fast SYBR Green master mix (Fischer Scientific, 10556555, Pittsburgh, PA, USA), 2.5 µL primer mix and 5 µL cDNA in duplo in a 48-well plate. The program ran on the StepOne real time PCR (Applied Biosystems, Foster City, CA, USA) was 20 s at 95 °C holding stage, 40 times 3 s 95 °C step 1 and 30 s 60 °C step 2 cycle stage, 15 s 95 °C, 1 min 60 °C and 15 s 95 °C. *Gapdh* was used as a housekeeping gene to correct for cDNA input. The efficiency of all used primers (Table 1) was tested.

Table 1. Primers for qPCR.

Primer	Sequence
mGapdh-forward	TCCATGACAACTTTGGCATTG
mGapdh-reverse	TCACGCCACAGCTTTCCA
Myod1-forward	AGCACTACAGTGGCGACTCA
Myod1-reverse	GCTCCACTATGCTGGACAGG
Myog-forward	CCCAACCCAGGAGATCATTT
Myog-reverse	GTCTGGGAAGGCAACAGACA
Myh3-forward	CGCAGAATCGCAAGTCAATA
Myh3-reverse	CAGGAGGTCTTGCTCACTCC
Ctgf-forward	CCACCCGAGTTACCAATGAC
Ctgf-reverse	GCTTGGCGATTTTAGGTGTC
Fgf-2-forward	AAGCGGCTCTACTGCAAGAA
Fgf-2-reverse	GTAACACACTTAGAAGCCAGCAG
Col1a1-forward	ATGTTCAGCTTTGTGGACCT
Col1a1-reverse	CAGCTGACTTCAGGGATGT
Id1-forward	ACCCTGAACGGCGAGATCA
Id1-reverse	TCGTCGGCTGGAACACAT
Nox4-forward	CTTTTCATTGGGCGTCCTC
Nox4-reverse	GGGTCCACAGCAGAAAACTC

2.7. Western Blotting

Cells were lysed in RIPA buffer (Sigma-Aldrich, R0278, Saint Louis, MO, USA) containing 1 tablet of protease inhibitor (Sigma-Aldrich, 11836153001, Saint Louis, MO, USA) and 1 tablet of phosStop (Sigma-Aldrich, 04906837001, Saint Louis, MO, USA) per 10 mL. The total protein concentration in the lysates was determined using a Pierce BCA Protein Assay kit (Thermo Scientific, 23225, Waltham, MA, USA). The absorbance was measured using a microplate spectrophotometer (Epoch Biotek, Winooski, VT, USA) and the protein concentration was calculated using Gen5 software (BioTek, Winooski, VT,

USA). An 8% polyacrylamide gel was made. Then, 15 μL sample mix, containing 9 μg total protein and 5 μL sample buffer (5.7 mL water, 1.6 mL glycerol, 1.1 mL 10% SDS, 1.3 mL 0.5 M Tris (pH6.8), 25 mg dithiotreitol (DTT), 300 μL bromophenol blue) was heated to 90 °C for 5 min, cooled on ice and loaded onto the gel. The gel was run in electrophoresis buffer (25 mM Tris base, 190 mM glycine, 0.1% SDS) at 70 V until the samples reached the separating gel and then run at 150 V until the samples reached the bottom of the gel. Next, the proteins were transferred onto a polyvinylidene fluoride (PVDF) membrane (GE Healthcare, 15269894, Chicago, IL, USA) for 1 h at 80V on ice in cold blot buffer (25 mM Tris base, 190 mM glycine, 20% ethanol). The membrane was rinsed in water and washed 2x in Tris-buffered saline and Tween-20 (TBS-T) (20 mM Tris/HCl, 137 mM NaCl, 0.1% Tween-20). The membrane was incubated for 1 h in 2% enhanced chemiluminescence (ECL) prime blocking agent (GE Healthcare, RPN418, Chicago, IL, USA) in TBS-T at 4 °C while shaking. Subsequently, the membrane was incubated overnight in 2% blocking agent in TBS-T with primary antibody (Table 2) at 4 °C while shaking. The membrane was washed 3×5 min in TBS-T and incubated in 2% blocking agent in TBS-T with secondary antibody (Table 2) for 1 h at room temperature. ECL solution A and B (GE Healthcare, RPN2235, Chicago, IL, USA) were mixed 1:1 at room temperature and the membrane was incubated for 5 min. Images were taken by the ImageQuant LAS500 (GE healthcare, life sciences, Chicago, IL, USA) and relative intensity of protein bands was quantified using ImageJ [26]. Pan actin was used as a loading control.

Table 2. Antibodies for Western Blotting and immunofluorescence.

AB	Dilution	Experiment	Company
Phospho-SMAD2 (Ser465/467) Rabbit mAb	1:1000	WB	cell signaling/3108, Leiden, The Netherlands
SMAD2 Rabbit mAb	1:1000, 1:200	WB, IF	cell signaling/5339
Phospho-SMAD3 (S423/425) Rabbit mAb	1:1000	WB	cell signaling/9520
SMAD3 Rabbit mAb	1:1000	WB	cell signaling/9523
Phospho-Akt (Ser473) Rabbit mAb	1:2000	WB	cell signaling/4060
Akt (pan) Rabbit mAb	1:1000	WB	cell signaling/4691
Phospho-ERK1/2 Rabbit mAb	1:2000	WB	cell signaling/4370
ERK1/2 Rabbit mAb	1:4000	WB	cell signaling/4695
Pan actin Rabbit mAb	1:1000	WB	cell signaling/8456
Myosin, sarcomere (MHC)	2.5 μg/mL	IF	DSHB/MF20-s, Iowa City, IA, USA
Anti-Rabbit IgG-POD (LumiLightPLUS Western Blotting Kit)	1:2000	WB	Roche/12015218001, Basel, Switzerland
Goat anti-Rabbit IgG (H + L), Alexa Fluor® 555 conjugate	1:500	IF	ThermoFisher Scientific/A21428, Waltham, MA, USA
Goat anti-Mouse IgG (H + L), Alexa Fluor® 488 conjugate	1:250	IF	ThermoFisher Scientific/A11001

2.8. Immunofluorescence

Cells were washed 2x with cold phosphate-buffered saline (PBS) (Gibco, 14190250, Waltham, MA, USA) and fixated for 10 min in 4% paraformaldehyde (PFA) (Fisher Scientific, Pittsburgh, PA, USA) at room temperature. Cells were washed 3x in PBS and permeabilised in 0.1% Triton X-100 in PBS for 10 min. After this, the cells were washed 3x in PBS with 0.05% Tween20 (PBS-T) and incubated for 1 h in 5% normal goat serum (ThermoFisher Scientific, 50062Z, Waltham, MA, USA) in PBS at room temperature. The cells were incubated overnight with primary antibody (Table 2) in 5% normal goat serum in PBS at 4 °C. Then, the cells were washed 3×5 min in PBS-T and incubated with secondary antibody (Table 2) in PBS-T for 1 h at room temperature. Cells were washed again 3×5 min in PBS-T and incubated in PBS with 4′,6-diamidino-2-phenylindole (DAPI) (100 ng/mL). After this, the cells were rinsed with PBS and stored in PBS at 4 °C. Images were taken with a fluorescent microscope (Zeiss Axiovert 200M, Hyland Scientific, Stanwood, WA, USA) using the program Slidebook 5.0 (Intelligent Imaging Innovations, Göttingen, Germany). The images were analysed using ImageJ [26].

2.9. Statistical Analysis

Graphs were made in Prism version 8 (GraphPad software, San Diego, CA, USA). All data were presented as mean + standard error of the mean (SEM). The data were normalised by the values of a control group or of control cells at 0 h. In graphs of time-dependent relative mRNA expression, values of control cells at 0 h were not presented. Statistical analysis was performed in SPSS version 25 (IBM,

Amsterdam, The Netherlands). Significance in the difference between two groups was determined by independent t-test. Statistical significance for multiple comparisons was determined by one-way analysis of variance (ANOVA) or two-way ANOVA with post-hoc Bonferroni corrections. Significance was set at * $p < 0.05$.

3. Results

3.1. TGF-β Inhibits Expression of Myogenic Genes in both C2C12 Myoblasts and Myotubes

TGF-β reduced both the fusion index (number of myotubes with two or more nuclei per total number of nuclei) and differentiation index (number of nuclei within the myotubes per total number of nuclei) of C2C12 cells (Figure 1a–d). After 1 h of TGF-β treatment, in both myoblasts and myotubes SMAD2 and SMAD3 were phosphorylated (Figure 1e–i), indicating that both myoblasts and myotubes are sensitive to TGF-β. SMAD phosphorylation was inhibited by TGF-β receptor type I inhibitor Ly364947.

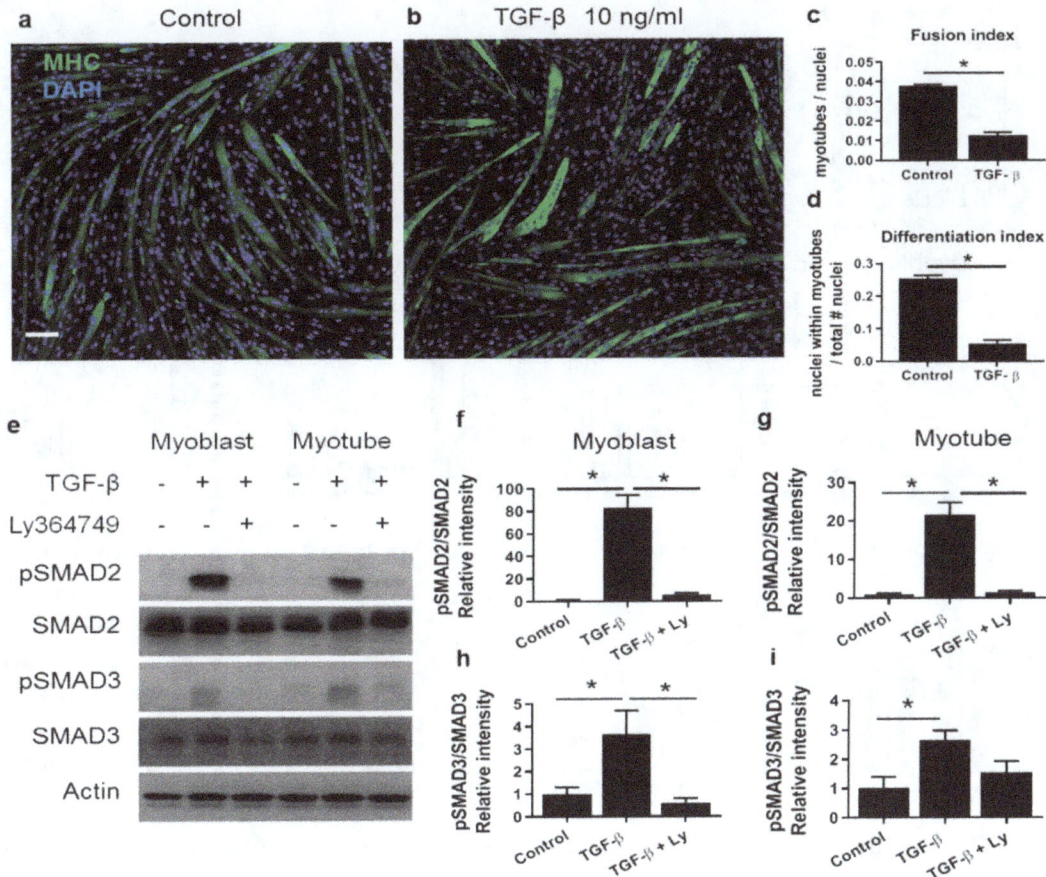

Figure 1. Transforming Growth Factor β (TGF-β) inhibits C2C12 differentiation. (**a,b**) C2C12 cells were induced to differentiate in control medium (**a**) or medium supplemented with TGF-β (**b**). Myotubes stained for myosin heavy chain (MHC) (green). Nuclei were stained using DAPI (blue). Scale indicates 100 μm. (**c,d**) Fusion index, defined as number of myotubes ≥ 2 nuclei/total number of nuclei and differentiation index defined as number of nuclei within MHC+ myotubes/total number of nuclei were reduced after TGF-β. (**e,f,g,h,i**) In both myoblasts and myotubes, phosphorylation levels of SMAD2 (**f,g**) and SMAD3 (**h,i**) were increased upon 1 h of TGF-β treatment. Pan actin served as loading control. Phosphorylation levels are displayed as relative intensity of pSMAD/total SMAD. Data were normalized to values of control condition. Error bars indicate standard error of the mean; * indicates significant difference at $p < 0.05$; $n = 4$ experiments per condition.

Subsequently, to assess acute and delayed effects in both myoblasts and myotubes, the time-dependent effects of TGF-β on myogenic gene expression were examined after 1, 3, 9, 24 and 48 h of treatment. After 9, 24 and 48 h of TGF-β treatment, *Myod* mRNA expression levels in myoblasts were reduced compared to those in untreated cells, although, after 48 h, *Myod* mRNA expression levels were increased compared to those at earlier time points (Figure 2a). After 24 and 48 h, myogenin (*Myog*) and embryonic myosin heavy chain (*Myh3*) mRNA expression levels in myoblasts were reduced compared to those in untreated cells, although expression levels did gradually increase compared to earlier time points (Figure 2b,d). These results show that TGF-β does not acutely reduce the expression levels of *Myod*, *Myog* and *Myh3* in myoblasts, but rather reduces or attenuates differentiation-related increases in mRNA expression levels of *Myod*, *Myog* and *Myh3* at later time points. In myotubes, *Myog* mRNA expression levels were not significantly affected by TGF-β (Figure 2c). However, after 24 and 48 h of TGF-β treatment, *Myh3* expression levels were reduced compared to those in untreated myotubes (Figure 2e). Thus, TGF-β represses *Myh3* mRNA expression, even in differentiated myotubes.

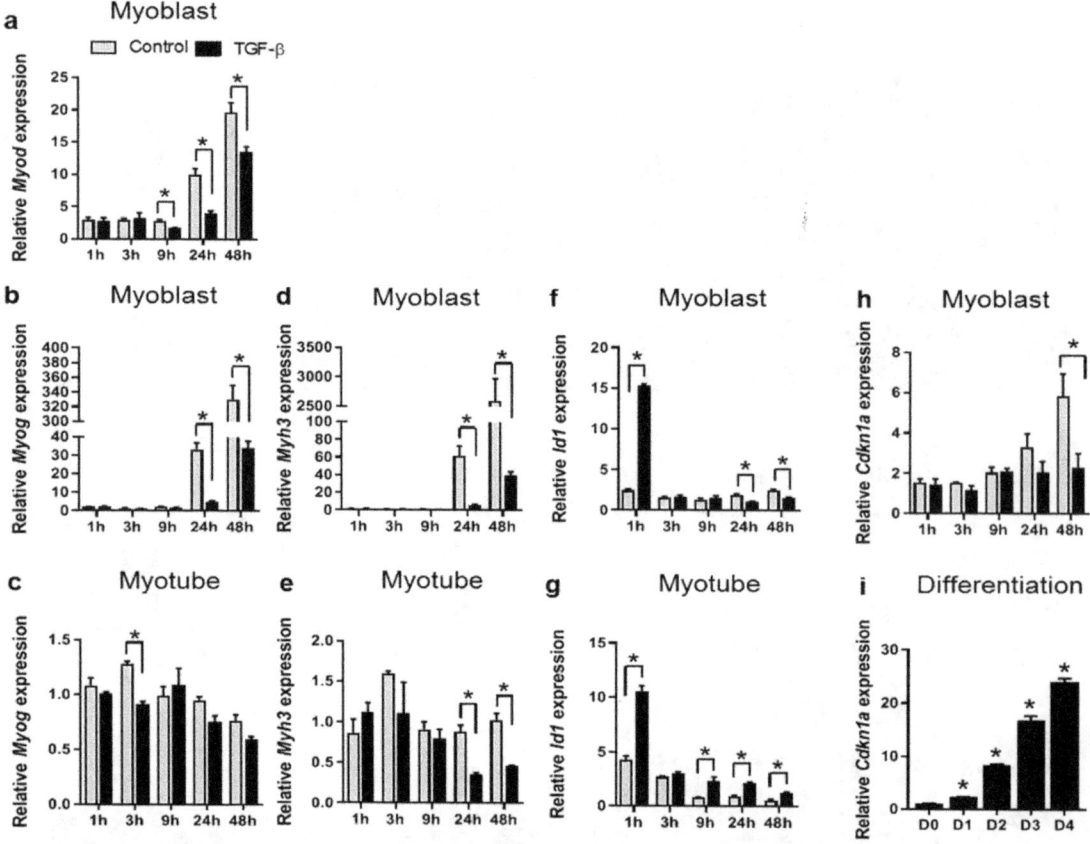

Figure 2. TGF-β reduces myogenic gene expression. (**a,b,d,f**) In myoblasts, expression levels of *Myod* (**a**) were reduced by TGF-β after 9 h compared to those of untreated cells, while expression levels of *Myog* (**b**) and *Myh3* (**d**) were reduced after 24 h. *Id1* expression levels (**f**) were induced after 1 h and repressed after 24 and 48 h. (**c,e,g**) In myotubes, the expression levels of *Myog* (**c**) were unaffected by TGF-β, while expression levels of *Myh3* (**e**) were reduced compared to those of untreated cells after 24 and 48 h. Expression levels of *Id1* (**g**) were induced after 1 h and remained slightly elevated at later time points. (**h**) In untreated myoblasts, the expression levels of *Cdkn1a* significantly increased, while this increase was inhibited in TGF-β treated cells. (**i**) *Cdkn1a* mRNA expression increased during myoblast differentiation, where D0 is the start of differentiation and D1, 2, 3 and 4 are days 1 to 4 of differentiation. *Gapdh* served as housekeeping gene. Data were normalized to values of control cells at 0 h; * indicates significant difference at $p < 0.05$; $n = 3$ experiments per condition.

Regarding the mechanisms underlying effects on differentiation, inhibitor of differentiation 1 (*Id1*) overexpression has been suggested to inhibit differentiation [27]. Since TGF-β induces *Id1* expression in various cell types via SMAD1/5 [28], we quantified *Id1* expression levels. In both C2C12 myoblast and myotubes, TGF-β transiently upregulated *Id1* expression after 1 h (Figure 2f,g), which corresponded with observed SMAD1/5 phosphorylation (Figure S1). In myoblasts, after 24 and 48 h of TGF-β treatment *Id1* mRNA expression levels were slightly reduced compared to those in untreated cells, whereas in myotubes *Id1* mRNA expression levels remained elevated. Based on these results, together with the known function of *Id1*, it is conceivable that *Id1* is involved in TGF-β mediated inhibition of differentiation.

In addition, effects of TGF-β on cell cycle inhibitor cyclin-dependent kinase inhibitor 1A (*Cdk1na*) mRNA expression was examined, because myostatin has been suggested to inhibit myoblast differentiation through inhibition of cyclin-dependent kinase inhibitor 1A [21]. In untreated C2C12 myoblasts, after 48 h *Cdk1na* mRNA expression levels were increased, while this increase was inhibited by TGF-β treatment (Figure 2h). However, *Cdk1na* expression increased during myoblast differentiation (Figure 2i) and no significant effects were observed at earlier time points. This indicates that effects on *Cdkn1a* mRNA expression were likely related to inhibited differentiation, rather than a direct effect of TGF-β on *Cdkn1a* mRNA expression. This suggests that TGF-β does not inhibit differentiation via the regulation of *Cdkn1a* expression.

3.2. TGF-β Does Not Affect Myotube Size In Vitro

TGF-β does not only negatively regulate muscle mass via the inhibition of myoblast differentiation, but TGF-β overexpression in adult mouse muscle has also been shown to result in increased expression of E3 ligase atrogin-1, as well as a reduction in muscle fibre cross sectional area [18]. Furthermore, myostatin is well known to stimulate the expression of E3 ligases, both in adult muscle as well as in myotubes in vitro [29]. E3 ligases are involved in protein degradation via Akt/FOXO signalling and play a role in muscle atrophy [30]. These studies indicate that TGF-β may induce protein degradation and subsequent muscle fibre atrophy via a similar mechanism as myostatin does. In addition, TGF-β-induced protein degradation in differentiating myoblasts may attenuate further myoblast differentiation. Since it remains to be assessed whether TGF-β induces muscle atrophy directly via upregulation of E3 ligase expression, time-dependent effects of TGF-β treatment on expression of muscle specific E3 ligases were determined. In myoblasts, after 3, 9, 24 and 48 h of TGF-β treatment mRNA expression levels of muscle RING-finger 1 (*Murf-1*) were reduced, while after 24 h *Atrogin-1* mRNA expression was transiently repressed (Figure 3a,b). In myotubes, the expression levels of *Atrogin-1* were not affected by TGF-β, whereas after 24 and 48 h mRNA expression levels of *Murf-1* were reduced compared to those in untreated myotubes (Figure 3c,d). These results suggest that TGF-β may protect myotubes against E3 ligase-induced protein degradation. However, our results also show that the endogenous expression of *Murf-1* and *Atrogin-1* increased during differentiation, which suggests that the observed effects of TGF-β on *Murf-1* and *Atrogin-1* expression levels were likely related to its inhibitory effect on differentiation (Figure 3e,f). In both myoblasts and myotubes, TGF-β transiently increased the expression levels of the ligase *Musa1* (Figure 3g,h). In myoblasts, *Musa1* expression levels were significantly increased after 9 h. In myotubes, expression levels were increased after 3 and 9 h.

Subsequently, myotube thickness was measured in C2C12 myoblasts that were differentiated in the presence or absence of TGF-β for three days (cells shown in Figure 1a). There was no significant difference in diameter between myotubes treated with TGF-β and controls (Figure 3n). Furthermore, while SMAD2 and SMAD3 were phosphorylated after 1 h of TGF-β treatment, no significant effects on Akt or ERK1/2 phosphorylation were observed (Figure 3j–m). Together, these results indicate that in vitro TGF-β alone does not affect myotube size.

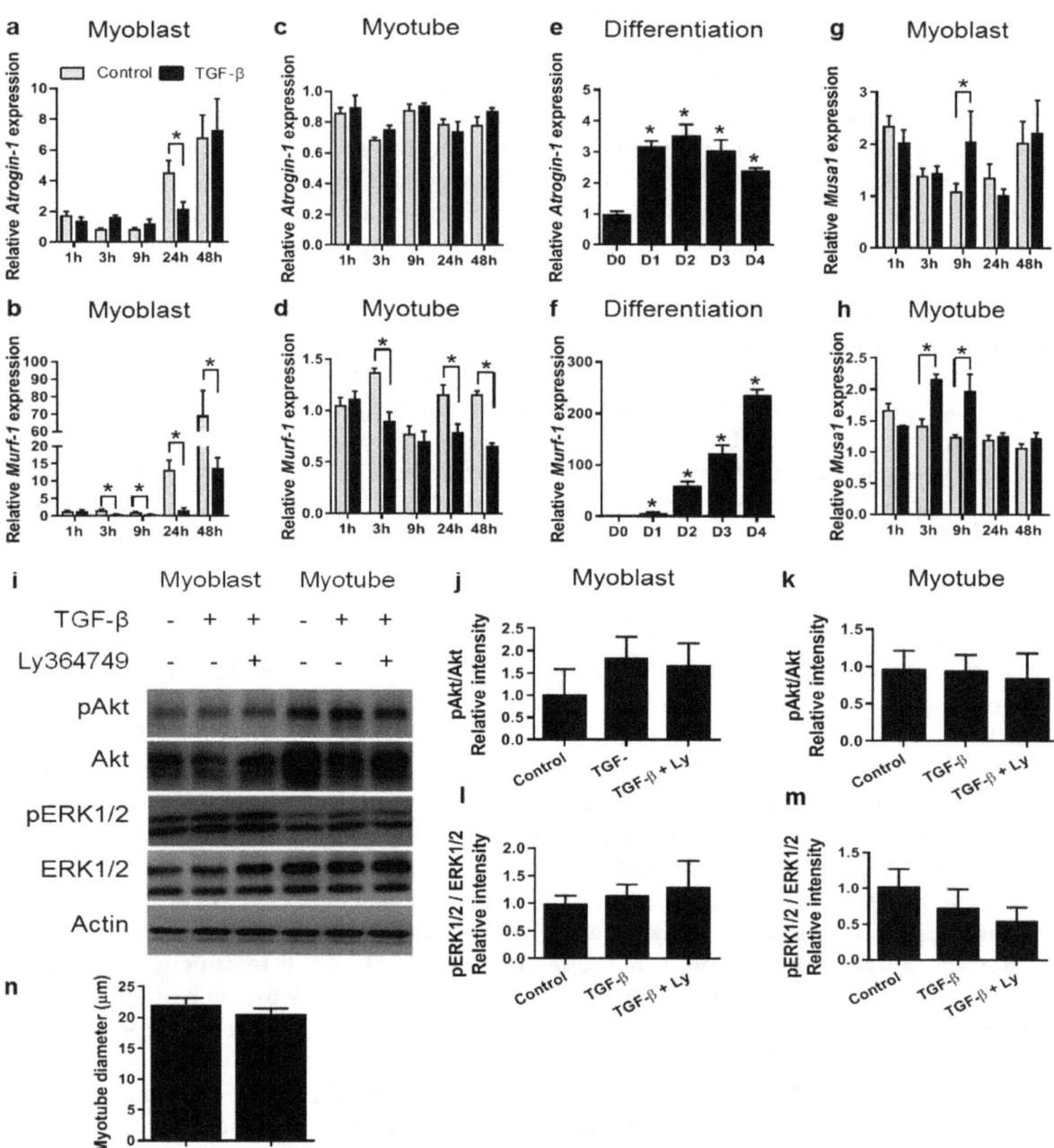

Figure 3. TGF-β does not affect myotube size. (**a,b**) In myoblasts, relative expression levels of *Atrogin-1* (**a**) and *Murf-1* (**b**) were inhibited by TGF-β. (**c,d**) In myotubes, *Atrogin-1* (**c**) expression was unaffected by TGF-β, while *Murf-1* (**d**) expression levels were inhibited after 3, 24 and 48 h. (**e,f**) mRNA expression of *Atrogin-1* (**e**) and *Murf-1* (**f**) increased during differentiation, where D0 is the start of differentiation and D1, 2, 3 and 4 are days 1 to 4 of differentiation. (**g,h**) In both myoblasts (**g**) and myotubes (**h**), TGF-β transiently increased *Musa1* expression levels. *Gapdh* served as housekeeping gene. Data were normalized to values of control cells at 0 h; * indicates significant difference at $p < 0.05$; $n = 3$ experiments per condition (**a–h**). (**i,j**) Western blot quantification of Akt phosphorylation in myoblasts, (**k**) Akt phosphorylation in myotubes, (**l**) ERK1/2 phosphorylation in myoblasts, (**m**) ERK1/2 phosphorylation in myotubes. Pan actin served as loading control. Phosphorylation levels are displayed as relative intensity of phospho/total protein. Data were normalized to values of the control condition. Error bars indicate standard error of the mean; $n = 4$ experiments per condition. **n** After 3 days of TGF-β treatment, the myotube diameters displayed in Figure 1a were not significantly different from those of control condition. $n = 80$ per experimental condition.

3.3. TGF-β Affects Fibrotic Gene Expression in a Time-Dependent Manner in Both Myoblasts and Myotubes

Time-dependent effects of TGF-β on fibrotic gene expression in C2C12 myoblasts and myotubes were studied. In both myoblasts and myotubes, TGF-β acutely and transiently induced the expression of *Ctgf* and *Fgf-2* (Figure 4a–d). Expression levels peaked between 3 and 9 h of treatment and remained significantly increased for at least 48 h compared to levels in untreated cells. In myoblasts, after 3 h TGF-β treatment, *Col1a1* expression levels were 1.9-fold higher compared to those in untreated cells. This effect gradually increased, and after 48 h, *Col1a1* expression levels were 5.6-fold higher in comparison to levels in untreated cells (Figure 4e). In myotubes, *Col1a1* mRNA expression levels were 10-fold higher compared to those in myoblasts (Figure 4i). After 9 and 48 h of TGF-β treatment, *Col1a1* expression levels were 1.5-fold higher compared to those in untreated cells (Figure 4f). NAPDH oxidase 4 (*Nox4*) is a TGF-β target gene that is required for TGF-β-induced expression of components of extracellular matrix (ECM) [31]. Our results show that in both myoblasts and myotubes, *Nox4* mRNA expression levels were significantly higher compared to those in untreated cells, after 9 or 3 h of TGF-β treatment, respectively. The effect of TGF-β treatment gradually increased and after 48 h, in myoblasts, *Nox4* expression levels were 7.9-fold higher and, in myotubes, 3.1-fold higher compared to those of untreated cells (Figure 4g,h). These results suggest that TGF-β stimulates fibrosis by increasing collagen type I expression in both myoblasts and myotubes.

3.4. TGF-β Induces Col1a1 Expression via Ctgf and Fgf-2 in Myoblasts

To investigate whether TGF-β induces *Col1a1* expression in C2C12 myoblasts directly or via the autocrine expression of *Ctgf* or *Fgf-2*, the effects of TGF-β treatment on *Col1a1* expression were studied in the presence of siRNA targeting *Ctgf* or *Fgf-2*. At all time points, treatment with siRNA reduced *Ctgf* or *Fgf-2* mRNA expression levels compared to levels of control siRNA treatment by >90% and >80%, respectively (Figure 4j,m). At 48 h of TGF-β treatment the induction of *Col1a1* mRNA expression was substantially lower (approximately 50%) in the presence of siRNA targeting either *Ctgf* or *Fgf-2* compared to controls (Figure 4k,n), suggesting that *Col1a1* mRNA expression is at least in part regulated by TGF-β dependent *Ctgf* and *Fgf-2* expression. In addition, after 3 h of TGF-β treatment, *Ctgf* knockdown did not affect *Fgf-2* mRNA expression, although after 48 h *Fgf-2* mRNA expression was significantly lower (approximately 70%) in the presence of siRNA targeting *Ctgf*, compared to controls (Figure 4l). *Ctgf* mRNA expression was significantly lower (>55%) in the presence of siRNA against *Fgf-2* compared to controls at all time points (Figure 4o).

3.5. TGF-β Has a Larger Effect on Muscle Differentiation and Fibrosis than Myostatin

Due to the functional and mechanistic similarities between TGF-β and myostatin, the effects of myostatin and TGF-β on C2C12 and primary myoblasts were studied. C2C12 and primary myoblasts, as well as myotubes, were treated with different doses of myostatin or TGF-β. Although a higher concentration of myostatin was needed compared to that of TGF-β in C2C12 and primary myoblasts, as well as myotubes, both proteins induced the translocation of SMAD2 to the nucleus. Figure 5a shows that in primary myotubes and undifferentiated myoblasts, 1 h of 10 ng/mL TGF-β or 300 ng/mL myostatin treatment resulted in the nuclear translocation of SMAD2. Little effect was observed for 0.01 ng/mL TGF-β or 10 ng/mL myostatin. Both of these ligands have a molecular weight of 25 kDa. In primary myoblasts, the comparison of effects of 3 and 48 h myostatin or TGF-β treatment on myogenic and fibrotic gene expression levels showed that after 48 h TGF-β reduced *Myh3* expression by approximately twofold compared to controls, while myostatin did not affect *Myh3* expression (Figure 5b,c). Furthermore, although in primary myoblasts after 3 h of treatment both myostatin and TGF-β significantly enhanced *Ctgf* mRNA expression levels, TGF-β increased *Ctgf* expression levels by 2.2-fold, while myostatin increased *Ctgf* expression levels only by 1.6-fold (Figure 5d,e). These results indicate that TGF-β has a stronger effect on fibrotic and myogenic gene expression levels than myostatin.

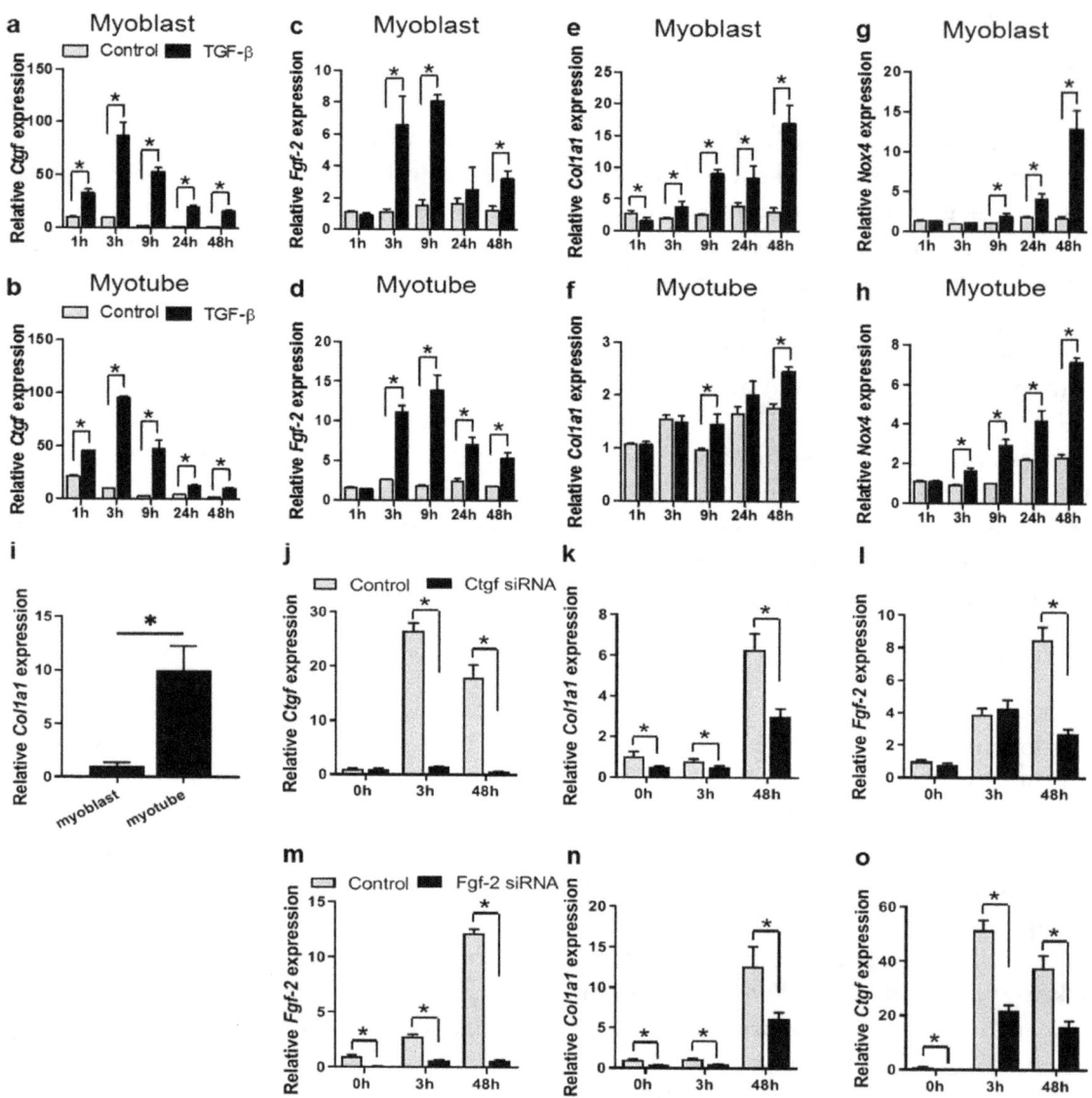

Figure 4. TGF-β affects fibrotic gene expression levels in myoblasts and myotubes in a time-dependent matter. (**a–h**) mRNA expression levels of (**a**) *Ctgf* in myoblasts, (**b**) *Ctgf* in myotubes, (**c**) *Fgf-2* in myoblasts, (**d**) *Fgf-2* in myotubes, (**e**) *Col1a1* in myoblasts, (**f**) *Col1a1* in myotubes, (**g**) *Nox4* in myoblasts, (**h**) *Nox4* in myotubes. (**a–d**) In myoblasts and myotubes, expression levels of *Ctgf* and *Fgf-2* were acutely induced by TGF-β. (**e–h**) *Col1a1* and *Nox4* expression levels were gradually induced by TGF-β. *Gapdh* served as housekeeping gene; data were normalized to values of control cells at 0 h; * indicates significant difference at $p < 0.05$; $n = 3$ experiments per condition (**a–h**). (**i**) *Col1a1* mRNA expression levels in myotubes were approximately 10-fold higher compared to those in myoblasts. *Gapdh* served as housekeeping gene; data were normalized to expression values in myoblasts. * p indicates significant difference at <0.05; $n = 6$ experiments per condition. (**j**) At all time points after siRNA treatment, *Ctgf* expression was knocked down by >90%. (**k**) *Col1a1* expression was reduced in the presence of siRNA targeting *Ctgf*. (**l**) After 3 h of TGF-β treatment, *Fgf-2* expression increased independent of *Ctgf*. After 48 h of TGF-β treatment, in the presence of siRNA targeting *Ctgf*, *Fgf-2* expression was significantly reduced. **m** At all time points after siRNA treatment, *Fgf-2* expression was knocked down by >81%. Both *Col1a1* (**n**) and *Ctgf* (**o**) expression levels were significantly reduced in the presence of siRNA targeting *Fgf-2* compared to those of control siRNA condition. *Gapdh* served as housekeeping gene; data were normalized to values of control cells at 0 h; * indicates significant difference at $p < 0.05$; $n = 6$ experiments per condition (**j–o**).

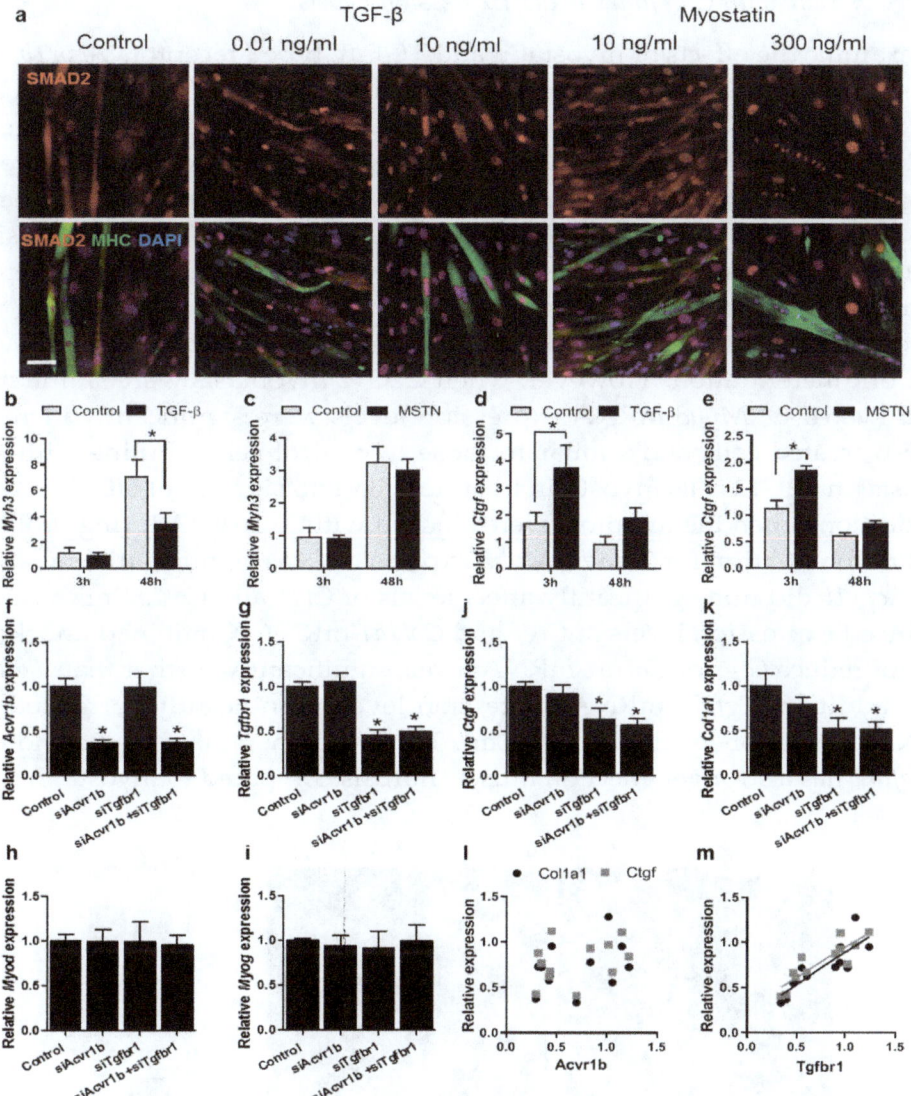

Figure 5. TGF-β has a larger effect on myoblasts compared to myostatin. (**a**) Primary cells were induced to differentiate for 2 days and subsequently treated with TGF-β (0.01 or 10 ng/mL) or myostatin (10 or 300 ng/mL). Myotubes were stained for MHC (green) and nuclei were stained using DAPI (blue). SMAD2 is visible in red. The scale indicates 100 μm. After TGF-β or myostatin treatment, SMAD2 was translocated to the nucleus in both myotubes and undifferentiated myoblasts compared to controls. (**b,c**) In primary mouse myoblasts, expression levels of *Myh3* mRNA were reduced after 48 h TGF-β treatment compared to those in untreated cells (**b**), while no differences were observed for myostatin (MSTN) (**c**). (**d,e**) Expression levels of *Ctgf* were increased after 3 h TGF-β (**d**) or myostatin treatment (**e**) compared to those in untreated cells, although TGF-β had a larger effect. (**f,g**) Treatment with specific siRNAs reduced levels of *Acvr1b* (**f**) or *Tgfbr1* (**g**). (**h,i**) Knockdown of *Acvr1b* or *Tgfbr1* did not affect *Myod* (**h**) or *Myog* (**i**) expression levels. (**j,k**) *Tgfbr1* knockdown slightly reduced *Ctgf* (**j**) and *Col1a1* (**k**) expression levels, while *Acvr1b* knockdown had little effect. The combined knockdown of *Tgfbr1* and *Acvr1b* did significantly reduce *Ctgf* and *Col1a1* expression levels. *Gapdh* served as housekeeping gene; error bars indicate standard error of the mean; * indicates significant difference at $p < 0{,}05$; $n = 3$ experiments per condition; data were normalized to values of control cells at 0 h. (**l,m**) There is a significant correlation between *Tgfbr1* expression level and *Ctgf* and *Col1a1* expression levels (**l**), while no such correlations were found between *Acvr1b* expression levels and *Ctgf* or *Col1a1* expression levels (**m**).

3.6. Tgfbr1 Levels Correlate with Ctgf and Col1a1 Expression Levels

To further examine the effects of myostatin and TGF-β, type I receptors *Acvr1b* and *Tgfbr1* were individually or simultaneously blocked in myoblasts using specific siRNAs. C2C12 myoblasts were treated with siRNA against *Acvr1b* or *Tgfbr1* for 24 h in growth medium and were additionally treated with siRNA for 48 h in differentiation medium. *Acvr1b* and *Tgfbr1* siRNA reduced receptor mRNA levels by >60% and >50%, respectively, without affecting expression of the other receptor (Figure 5f,g). No significant effects of siRNA treatment on *Myod* or *Myog* expression levels were observed (Figure 5h,i). In line with these results, receptor blocking during differentiation using chemical blocker Ly364947 did not affect fusion or differentiation index nor myotube thickness after 3 days of differentiation (Figure 6a–e). In addition, Ly364947 treatment did not affect *Myh3* expression levels after 48 h of differentiation. However, when C2C12 myoblasts were simultaneously treated with TGF-β and Ly364749, *Myh3* mRNA expression levels were significantly increased compared to those in TGF-β treated cells and similar to those in control cells. In line with observations in primary myoblasts, in C2C12 cells myostatin treatment had no significant effect on *Myh3* expression (Figure 6f). In addition, when the receptors were blocked with Ly364947 during proliferation for 24 h and subsequent differentiation for 2 days, *Myh3* expression was significantly increased (Figure 6g). Knockdown of *Acvr1b* did not significantly affect levels of *Ctgf* and *Col1a1* mRNA, whereas *Tgfbr1* knockdown reduced expression levels of *Ctgf* and *Col1a1* mRNA. Combined knockdown of *Acvr1b* and *Tgfbr1* did not reduce *Ctgf* or *Col1a1* mRNA levels significantly further than *Tgfbr1* knockdown (Figure 5j,k). In addition, *Tgfbr1* mRNA expression levels significantly correlated with both *Ctgf* and *Col1a1* mRNA expression levels (Figure 5l,m). Taken together, these results indicate that TGF-β signalling via *Tgfbr1* has a stronger effect on muscle fibrosis compared to myostatin.

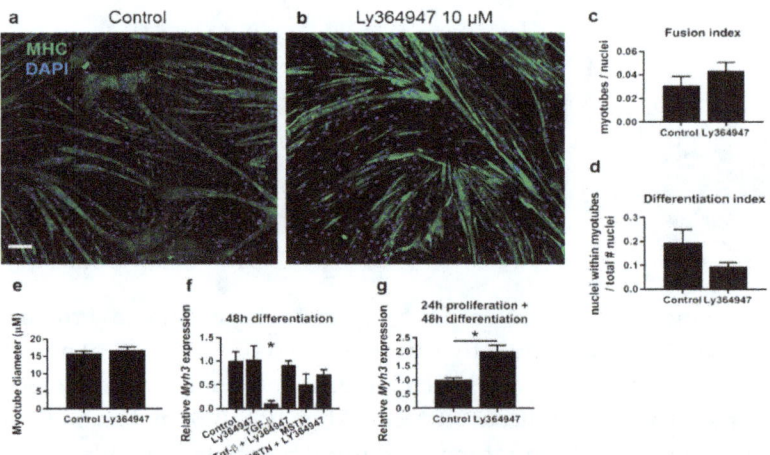

Figure 6. Effects of type I receptor blocking on myoblast differentiation is time-dependent. (**a,b**) C2C12 cells were induced to differentiate in control medium (**a**) or in medium supplemented with the TGF-β receptor inhibitor Ly364947 (**b**). Myotubes were stained for MHC (green) and nuclei were stained using DAPI (blue). Scale indicates 100 μm. (**c**) Fusion index, defined as number of myotubes ≥ 2 nuclei/total number of nuclei and (**d**) differentiation index defined as number of nuclei within MHC+ myotubes/total number of nuclei were not significantly affected by Ly364947 treatment. Error bars indicate standard error of the mean; * indicates significant difference at $p < 0.05$; $n = 4$ experiments per condition. (**e**) Myotube thickness was not affected by Ly36447 treatment, compared to control condition. (**f**) 48 h of Ly364947 treatment did not affect *Myh3* expression levels in differentiating C2C12 myoblasts. *Myh3* expression levels were significantly increased in cells simultaneously treated with TGF-β and Ly364947 compared to those of cells treated with TGF-β and similar to those of untreated cells. Myostatin did not significantly affect *Myh3* expression levels. (**g**) *Myh3* expression levels were significantly increased when C2C12 myoblasts were treated with Ly364947 during proliferation for 24 h and subsequent culture in differentiation medium for 48 h.

4. Discussion

The aim of this study was to assess the time-dependent effects of TGF-β signalling on gene expression in myoblasts and myotubes and compare the effects of TGF-β and myostatin signalling in myoblasts. Here we show that in vitro TGF-β treatment inhibits the expression of a subset of myogenic genes in both myoblasts and myotubes, but does not affect myotube thickness. Most importantly, our results show that TGF-β regulates the expression of fibrotic genes in both myoblasts and myotubes in a time-dependent manner. TGF-β regulates *Col1a1* mRNA expression at least in part via *Ctgf* and *Fgf-2* and, in addition, *Ctgf* and *Fgf-2* are also required to induce the expression of each other. Moreover, our results show a more prominent role for TGF-β in SMAD signalling, as well as myogenic and fibrotic gene expression in comparison to myostatin.

4.1. TGF-β Affects Myogenic Gene Expression in Both Myoblasts and Myotubes

TGF-β is known for its inhibitory effect on myoblast differentiation in vitro through inhibition of MyoD [14,32]. As expected, TGF-β inhibited myoblast differentiation and myogenic gene expression. Also, in myotubes, a reduction in *Myh3* expression was observed after 24 and 48 h of TGF-β treatment. Embryonic myosin heavy chain (eMHC), which is encoded by *Myh3*, is normally only expressed during embryonic/fetal and neonatal development, but is transiently re-expressed during muscle regeneration. The loss of eMHC in adult muscle in vivo has been shown to change MHC isoform expression, while in vitro *Myh3* knockdown may result in reduced fusion index and a reduced number of reserve cells, which suggests that loss of *Myh3* results in the early differentiation of MuSCs, depleting the MuSC pool [33]. Together, these results suggest that long-term TGF-β expression in muscle fibres after injury or in chronic disease may impede proper regeneration through repression of *Myh3* expression.

Additionally, TGF-β has been known from previous studies to interfere with MyoD function via two different mechanisms. First, TGF-β-induced SMAD3 can directly interact with MyoD. Second, TGF-β/SMAD3 interferes with the interaction between MyoD and myocyte enhancer factor 2 (MEF2), which is required for the expression of many myogenic genes [14,32]. Here, we show that TGF-β induces *Id1* expression acutely and transiently in both myoblasts and myotubes. *Id1* is known to inhibit myoblast differentiation by interfering with the formation of MyoD/E complexes, which are required for MyoD function [27]. Our data suggest that the upregulation of *Id1* mRNA may be another mechanism through which TGF-β interferes with MyoD function.

4.2. TGF-β Does Not Affect Myotube Size In Vitro

TGF-β overexpression within mouse muscle has been shown to result in the stimulation of atrogin-1 expression and atrophy in vivo [17,18]. To investigate whether this increase in atrogin-1 expression was a direct or indirect effect of TGF-β, time-dependent effects of TGF-β on E3 ligase mRNA expression were studied. In contrast to what has been shown in vivo, C2C12 myotubes did not show evidence for any effect of TGF-β on muscle atrophy. TGF-β treatment resulted in a reduction in *Atrogin-1* and *Murf-1* mRNA expression, rather than an increase. Moreover, an increase in both *Atrogin-1* and *Murf-1* expression was observed during differentiation, which suggests that the observed TGF-β-induced effects on E3 ligase mRNA expression were likely related to inhibition of differentiation. In both myoblasts and myotubes, expression levels of the ligase *Musa1* were transiently increased. Furthermore, TGF-β did not affect Akt or ERK1/2 phosphorylation nor myotube size. Together, these data indicate that in C2C12 myotubes, TGF-β does not directly contribute to atrophy. However, in vivo long term overexpression of TGF-β may lead to a reduction in muscle fibre size [17,18]. Based on our data, this observed in vivo TGF-β overexpression-induced atrophy is possibly mediated via *Musa1* rather than by elevated *Murf-1* or *Atrogin-1* expression levels. Furthermore, we show that TGF-β stimulates *Nox4* and *Id1* mRNA expression. These genes have been implied to play a role in muscle atrophy [34,35]. TGF-β has been shown to induce caspase 3 expression and DNA fragmentation in C2C12 cells [36]. As such, myonuclear apoptosis and loss of muscle stem cells induced by TGF-β may contribute to muscle atrophy as well. The role of TGF-β in the regulation of muscle fibre size requires further investigation.

4.3. TGF-β Contributes to Fibrosis by Stimulation of Fibrotic Gene Expression in Myoblasts and Myotubes

Our data show that both myoblasts and myotubes express various pro-fibrotic genes and TGF-β stimulates the expression of these genes in a time-dependent manner. This suggests that, in addition to its effect on fibroblasts, TGF-β likely also contributes to muscle fibrosis through effects on myoblasts and muscle fibres. The stimulatory effects of TGF-β on *Col1a1* mRNA expression in myotubes were relatively small compared to those in myoblasts. Nevertheless, myotubes may contribute substantially to collagen type I production. Basal expression levels of *Col1a1* in myotubes were approximately 10-fold higher than in myoblasts. Moreover, MuSCs comprise approximately 2%–5% of the myonuclei within mature muscle [37] and the number of fibroblasts is roughly 10-fold lower than the number of myonuclei [38,39]. Therefore, it is conceivable that within mature skeletal muscle, differentiating myoblasts and muscle fibres contribute substantially to the production of collagen type I.

Collagen type I is found in the endo-, peri- and epimysium surrounding muscle fibre [40,41]. Collagen fibres reinforce the ECM surrounding muscle fibres, which is essential in providing a niche for MuSCs, giving structure to the muscle and is even crucial for proper muscle function [42–44]. It is conceivable that during myogenesis and muscle regeneration, muscle fibres will secrete collagen type I to contribute to the deposition of connective tissue that provides a scaffold for the regenerating parts of the muscle fibre. However, chronic high expression of TGF-β in skeletal muscle may contribute to muscle fibrosis via the continuous elevated expression of collagen. In muscular dystrophies and aged muscle, TGF-β expression in damaged areas of the muscle may cause excessive collagen deposition. This may result in locally enhanced stiffness along the muscle fibre, which may cause strain distributions along the length of the muscle fibre. As a consequence, muscle fibres are likely to become susceptible to further injuries. In addition, excessive collagen deposition will result in enhanced stiffness of the muscle stem cell niche and likely alter MuSC mechanosensitivity, which may reduce myoblast differentiation and thus impair muscle regeneration capacity [44–47].

Besides pro-fibrotic growth factors and ECM genes, TGF-β also induced the expression of *Nox4*. *Nox4* expression is induced by TGF-β within various cell types such as endothelial cells or lung mesenchymal cells [31,48]. *Nox4* is part of an enzyme family which catalyses the reduction of oxygen into reactive oxygen species (ROS). In lung fibrosis, *Nox4*-dependent H_2O_2 generation is required for TGF-β mediated myofibroblast differentiation and ECM production [31]. Furthermore, *Nox4* is a known source for oxidative stress in many tissues and in chronic kidney disease both *Nox4* and oxidative damage markers are increased in muscle [49]. Therefore, we suggest that prolonged TGF-β expression in muscle wasting disorders may contribute to oxidative damage via *Nox4* upregulation.

4.4. TGF-β Induces Col1a1 Expression via Autocrine Ctgf and Fgf-2 Signalling

In lung fibrosis, TGF-β is known to induce collagen 1 expression via CTGF [50–52]. This, in combination with the observed expression patterns for *Ctgf*, *Fgf-2* and *Col1a1* in our myoblasts and myotubes, raised the question regarding whether in muscle cells TGF-β directly induced *Col1a1* expression or indirectly via enhancement of expression of these growth factors. *Ctgf* and *Fgf-2* were significantly knocked down using siRNA. After 48 h of TGF-β treatment, *Col1a1* mRNa expression levels were significantly reduced when *Ctgf* or *Fgf-2* was knocked down. This suggests that *Col1a1* expression is at least in part dependent on both *Ctgf* and *Fgf-2* expression in an autocrine manner. In corneal endothelial cells and human vertebral bone marrow stem cells, FGF-2 has been implied to stimulate collagen production [53,54], while in muscle FGF-2 is best known to stimulate MuSC activation and proliferation [55,56]. In this study, we show for the first time that in C2C12 muscle cells *Fgf-2* is required for TGF-β induced *Col1a1* mRNA expression.

Our results show that after 3 h of TGF-β treatment, *Ctgf* knockdown did not significantly affect *Fgf-2* expression; however, *Fgf-2* expression was significantly reduced after 48 h of TGF-β treatment in the presence of siRNA against *Ctgf*. These data suggest that TGF-β acutely induces *Fgf-2* expression independently of changes in *Ctgf* expression, though chronic expression of *Fgf-2* depends on *Ctgf* expression levels. *Ctgf* expression was shown to depend on *Fgf-2* levels both acutely and chronically. To the best of our knowledge, this interaction has not been reported before. See Figure 7 for a schematic of the proposed mechanism for TGF-β induced regulation of *Ctgf*, *Fgf-2* and *Col1a1*. We suggest that TGF-β stimulates *Col1a1* expression largely via the autocrine and paracrine signalling of *Ctgf* and *Fgf-2* and that *Ctgf* and *Fgf-2* may regulate the expression of each other via a positive feedback loop.

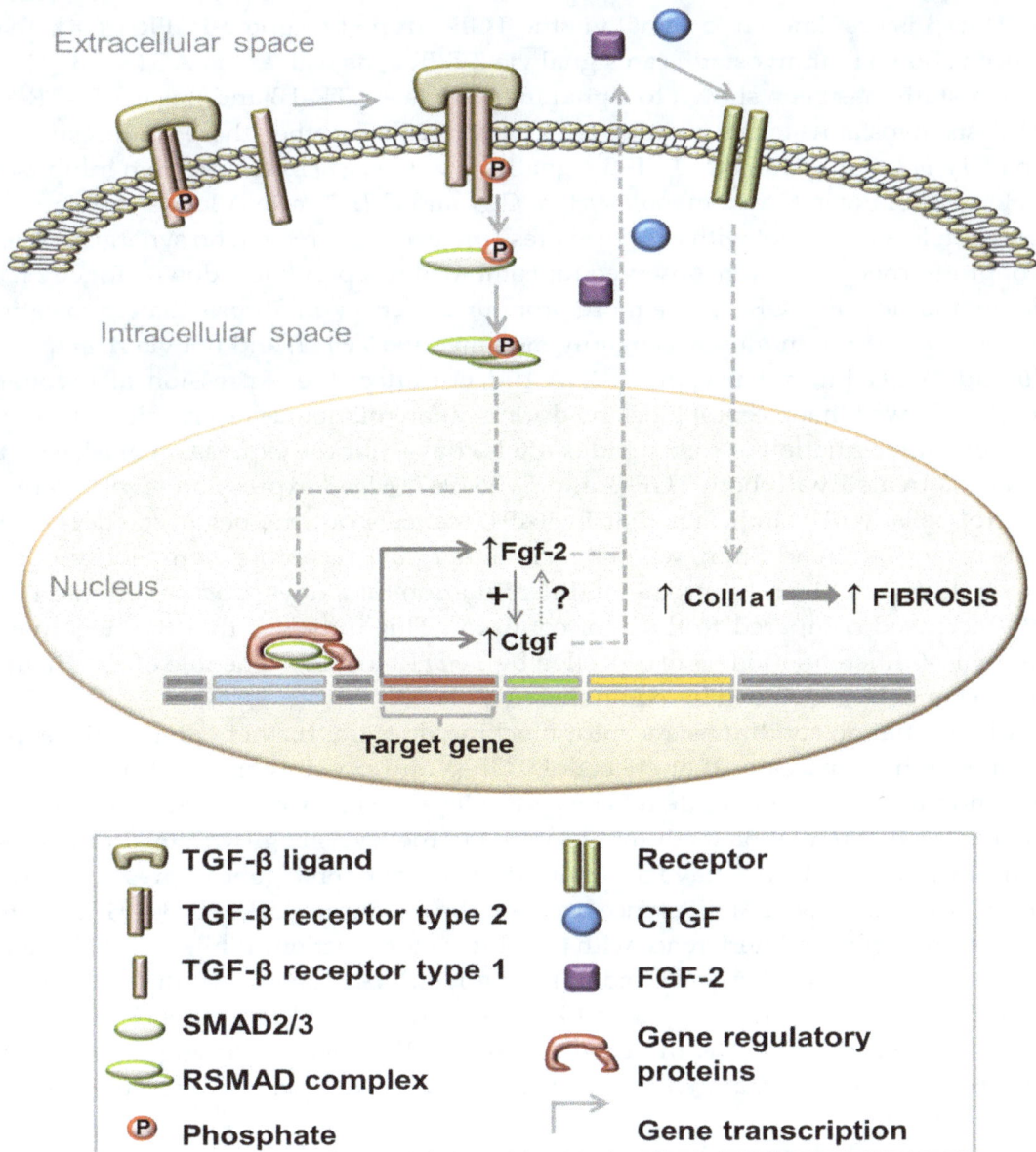

Figure 7. Schematic illustration of a proposed mechanism of how TGF-β regulates *Col1a1* mRNA expression. TGF-β binds to its receptors and activates downstream SMAD2/3 signalling. Subsequently, R-SMAD complexes translocate into the nucleus to regulate mRNA expression of growth factors such as *Ctgf* and *Fgf-2*. CTGF and FGF-2 proteins are secreted by the muscle cell and subsequently induce *Col1a1* expression via autocrine or paracrine signalling. Furthermore, expression levels of *Fgf-2* and *Ctgf* are dependent on each other.

4.5. TGF-β Has a More Pronounced Effect than Myostatin on Myoblast Differentiation and Fibrotic Gene Expression

Because of overlap in functional implications and mechanistic similarities between TGF-β and myostatin signalling in myoblasts, we compared the effects of both growth factors on myogenic and fibrotic gene expression. In order to induce downstream activation of SMAD2 signalling, a higher concentration of myostatin was required compared to TGF-β. Furthermore, in myoblasts, TGF-β had a larger effect on *Myh3* and *Ctgf* expression compared to myostatin. To further compare effects of TGF-β and myostatin signalling on myoblasts, these ligands were inhibited by using siRNA against their type I receptors. TGF-β is best known to signal via the TGF-β type I receptor TGFR-1 [24]. In epithelial cells, it has been shown that myostatin can signal via TGFR-1, as well as via ACTR-1B [23]. In mouse myoblasts, myostatin has been shown to signal mainly via ACTR-1B and not via TGFR-1, while in mouse fibroblasts myostatin signals mainly via ACTR-1B [25]. Together, these studies suggest that the knockdown of *Tgfbr1* mainly inhibits TGF-β signalling, while *Acvr1b* knockdown inhibits myostatin signalling. Here, we show in C2C12 myoblasts that *Ctgf* and *Col1a1* mRNA levels correlate with *Tgfbr1* mRNA expression levels, but not with *Acvr1b* expression levels. Moreover, no synergistic effects on the expression of pro-fibrotic genes were observed for combined receptor knockdown. Together, these data indicate that in muscle cells TGF-β has a more pronounced effect on fibrosis than myostatin and that pro-fibrotic gene expression in muscle is mainly mediated via *Tgfbr1*, and not via *Acvr1b*.

Acvr1b and *Tgfbr1* inhibition using siRNA did not affect the expression of myogenic genes. Furthermore, we showed that receptor blocking during differentiation using chemical blocker Ly364947 did not affect the differentiation or fusion index after 3 days, nor the expression of *Myh3* after 2 days. However, in cells treated with both TGF-β and Ly364947, *Myh3* expression levels were similar to those of control cells, which indicates that Ly364947 cancels out the negative effect of TGF-β on *Myh3* expression levels. In addition, when *Acvr1b* and *Tgfbr1* receptors were blocked by Ly364947 during proliferation for 24 h and subsequent differentiation for 2 days, *Myh3* expression levels were significantly increased compared to those of controls. This indicates that the negative effects of TGF-β on myoblast differentiation were cancelled by *Tgfbr1* blocking. The role of *Acvr1b* in myoblast differentiation cannot be concluded based on these results.

Under differentiation conditions, receptor blocking does not further enhance the expression of myogenic genes, which indicates that effects of TGF-β and possibly myostatin on differentiation are dose-dependent and time-dependent. The serum levels (i.e., growth factors such as TGF-β) are relatively low in the differentiation medium compared to the levels in growth medium. This suggests that low concentrations of TGF-β have a minor effect on myogenic gene expression and myoblast differentiation. Note that there is a difference between the chemical blocker Ly364947 and the siRNAs targeting *Acvr1b* and *Tgfbr1* in interference with type I receptor function. While Ly364947 blocks TGF-β signalling within one hour, as demonstrated in Figure 1, siRNAs interfere with the translation of the target mRNA, which may result in a delayed knockdown of type I receptors (Figure 5). This may explain why the presence of siRNA in growth medium did not affect myogenic gene expression. Based on our results, it seems that myoblast differentiation is less sensitive to myostatin signalling than to TGF-β signalling.

4.6. Implications in Therapeutic Treatments

Altogether, our results demonstrate that TGF-β signalling has an inhibitory effect on myoblast differentiation and contributes substantially to fibrosis. Therefore, the TGF-β pathway proves to be an interesting potential therapeutic target for treatment of muscular dystrophies. The inhibition of the TGF-β pathway may relieve and attenuate progressive muscle pathology characterized by severe fibrosis and loss of muscle mass. However, taking into account that TGF-β affects various cellular processes throughout the body, generic inhibition of the protein may have serious consequences. Our data show that TGF-β inhibits differentiation and induces fibrosis directly via its receptor in myoblasts and differentiated myotubes. This indicates that the inhibition of TGF-β exclusively within muscle tissue may be an effective approach to improve muscle regeneration in muscular dystrophy. Furthermore, our data demonstrate that TGF-β has a larger effect on differentiation and fibrosis than myostatin. Moreover, *Tgfbr1*, but not *Acvr1b* inhibition, significantly reduced *Ctgf* and *Col1a1* mRNA expression levels, while simultaneous receptor knockdown did not reduce expression levels even further. This suggests that solely blocking *Tgfbr1* and concomitant inhibition of TGF-β signalling may be sufficient to reduce fibrosis in muscular dystrophy. However, when in pathological conditions, both the inhibition of fibrosis and improved regeneration are required, thus simultaneous blocking of the *Tgfbr1* and *Acvr1b* receptor may be desirable. It has been shown that both myostatin and activins signal via *Acvr1b* and that these ligands synergistically inhibit regulation of muscle size [57,58]. Thus, simultaneous targeting of *Tgfbr1* and *Acvr1b* in vivo may still have a synergistic effect on overall muscle function improvement.

5. Conclusions

In conclusion, our data show that TGF-β inhibits myogenic gene expression in both myoblasts and myotubes, but does not affect myotube size in vitro. Most importantly, our results show that TGF-β stimulates *Col1a1* mRNA expression largely via autocrine expression of *Ctgf* and *Fgf-2*. Moreover, the effects of TGF-β on myogenic and fibrotic signalling are more pronounced than those of myostatin. Knockdown of *Tgfbr1* was sufficient to decrease *Ctgf* and *Col1a1* expression levels, while knockdown of *Acvr1b* had little effect. These results indicate that during muscle regeneration, TGF-β induces fibrosis via *Tgfbr1* by stimulating autocrine signalling of *Ctgf* and *Fgf-2*.

Author Contributions: Conceptualization, M.M.G.H., R.T.J. and W.M.H.H.; methodology, M.M.G.H. and W.M.H.H.; formal analysis, M.M.G.H.; investigation, M.M.G.H., R.A.G.C., C.O. and G.M.J.d.W.; resources, R.T.J. and W.M.H.H.; writing—original draft preparation, M.M.G.H.; writing—review and editing, M.M.G.H., R.A.G.C., R.T.J. and W.M.H.H.; visualization, M.M.G.H. and R.A.G.C.; supervision, R.T.J. and W.M.H.H.; project administration, W.M.H.H.; funding acquisition, W.M.H.H. and R.T.J. All authors have read and agreed to the published version of the manuscript.

Acknowledgments: We thank students M. Bulut and K. Doetjes for their contribution to this research.

References

1.   Ryall, J.G.; Schertzer, J.D.; Lynch, G.S. Cellular and molecular mechanisms underlying age-related skeletal muscle wasting and weakness. *Biogerontology* **2008**, *9*, 213–228. [CrossRef] [PubMed]

2.   Lima, J.; Simoes, E.; de Castro, G.; Morais, M.; de Matos-Neto, E.M.; Alves, M.J.; Pinto, N.I.; Figueredo, R.G.; Zorn, T.M.T.; Felipe-Silva, A.S.; et al. Tumour-derived transforming growth factor-beta signalling contributes to fibrosis in patients with cancer cachexia. *J. Cachexia Sarcopenia Muscle* **2019**, *10*, 1045–1059. [CrossRef]

3.   Bernasconi, P.; Torchiana, E.; Confalonieri, P.; Brugnoni, R.; Barresi, R.; Mora, M.; Cornelio, F.; Morandi, L.; Mantegazza, R. Expression of transforming growth factor-beta 1 in dystrophic patient muscles correlates with fibrosis. Pathogenetic role of a fibrogenic cytokine. *J. Clin. Investig.* **1995**, *96*, 1137–1144. [CrossRef]

4.   Chen, Y.W.; Nagaraju, K.; Bakay, M.; McIntyre, O.; Rawat, R.; Shi, R.; Hoffman, E.P. Early onset of inflammation and later involvement of tgfbeta in duchenne muscular dystrophy. *Neurology* **2005**, *65*, 826–834. [CrossRef]

5.   Shi, Y.; Massague, J. Mechanisms of tgf-beta signaling from cell membrane to the nucleus. *Cell* **2003**, *113*, 685–700. [CrossRef]

6.   Robertson, T.A.; Maley, M.A.; Grounds, M.D.; Papadimitriou, J.M. The role of macrophages in skeletal muscle regeneration with particular reference to chemotaxis. *Exp. Cell Res.* **1993**, *207*, 321–331. [CrossRef]

7.   Grotendorst, G.R.; Smale, G.; Pencev, D. Production of transforming growth factor beta by human peripheral blood monocytes and neutrophils. *J. Cell. Physiol.* **1989**, *140*, 396–402. [CrossRef]

8.   Lawrence, D.A.; Pircher, R.; Kryceve-Martinerie, C.; Jullien, P. Normal embryo fibroblasts release transforming growth factors in a latent form. *J. Cell. Physiol.* **1984**, *121*, 184–188. [CrossRef]

9.   Shur, I.; Lokiec, F.; Bleiberg, I.; Benayahu, D. Differential gene expression of cultured human osteoblasts. *J. Cell. Biochem.* **2001**, *83*, 547–553. [CrossRef]

10.   Zimowska, M.; Duchesnay, A.; Dragun, P.; Oberbek, A.; Moraczewski, J.; Martelly, I. Immunoneutralization of tgfbeta1 improves skeletal muscle regeneration: Effects on myoblast differentiation and glycosaminoglycan content. *Int. J. Cell Biol.* **2009**, *2009*, 659372. [CrossRef]

11. Pasteuning-Vuhman, S.; Putker, K.; Tanganyika-de Winter, C.L.; Boertje-van der Meulen, J.W.; van Vliet, L.; Overzier, M.; Plomp, J.J.; Aartsma-Rus, A.; van Putten, M. Natural disease history of mouse models for limb girdle muscular dystrophy types 2d and 2f. *PLoS ONE* **2017**, *12*, e0182704. [CrossRef]

12. Gonzalez, D.; Contreras, O.; Rebolledo, D.L.; Espinoza, J.P.; van Zundert, B.; Brandan, E. ALS skeletal muscle shows enhanced tgf-beta signaling, fibrosis and induction of fibro/adipogenic progenitor markers. *PLoS ONE* **2017**, *12*, e0177649. [CrossRef]

13. Carlson, M.E.; Hsu, M.; Conboy, I.M. Imbalance between pSmad3 and Notch induces CDK inhibitors in old muscle stem cells. *Nature* **2008**, *454*, 528–532. [CrossRef]

14. Liu, D.; Black, B.L.; Derynck, R. Tgf-beta inhibits muscle differentiation through functional repression of myogenic transcription factors by smad3. *Genes Dev.* **2001**, *15*, 2950–2966. [CrossRef]

15. Olson, E.N.; Sternberg, E.; Hu, J.S.; Spizz, G.; Wilcox, C. Regulation of myogenic differentiation by type beta transforming growth factor. *J. Cell Biol.* **1986**, *103*, 1799–1805. [CrossRef]

16. Massague, J.; Cheifetz, S.; Endo, T.; Nadal-Ginard, B. Type beta transforming growth factor is an inhibitor of myogenic differentiation. *Proc. Natl. Acad. Sci. USA* **1986**, *83*, 8206–8210. [CrossRef]

17. Narola, J.; Pandey, S.N.; Glick, A.; Chen, Y.W. Conditional expression of tgf-beta1 in skeletal muscles causes endomysial fibrosis and myofibers atrophy. *PLoS ONE* **2013**, *8*, e79356. [CrossRef]

18. Mendias, C.L.; Gumucio, J.P.; Davis, M.E.; Bromley, C.W.; Davis, C.S.; Brooks, S.V. Transforming growth factor-beta induces skeletal muscle atrophy and fibrosis through the induction of atrogin-1 and scleraxis. *Muscle Nerve* **2012**, *45*, 55–59. [CrossRef]

19. Andreetta, F.; Bernasconi, P.; Baggi, F.; Ferro, P.; Oliva, L.; Arnoldi, E.; Cornelio, F.; Mantegazza, R.; Confalonieri, P. Immunomodulation of tgf-beta 1 in mdx mouse inhibits connective tissue proliferation in diaphragm but increases inflammatory response: Implications for antifibrotic therapy. *J. Neuroimmunol.* **2006**, *175*, 77–86. [CrossRef]

20. Li, Y.; Foster, W.; Deasy, B.M.; Chan, Y.; Prisk, V.; Tang, Y.; Cummins, J.; Huard, J. Transforming growth factor-beta1 induces the differentiation of myogenic cells into fibrotic cells in injured skeletal muscle: A key event in muscle fibrogenesis. *Am. J. Pathol.* **2004**, *164*, 1007–1019. [CrossRef]

21. Langley, B.; Thomas, M.; Bishop, A.; Sharma, M.; Gilmour, S.; Kambadur, R. Myostatin inhibits myoblast differentiation by down-regulating myod expression. *J. Biol. Chem.* **2002**, *277*, 49831–49840. [CrossRef]

22. Li, Z.B.; Kollias, H.D.; Wagner, K.R. Myostatin directly regulates skeletal muscle fibrosis. *J. Biol. Chem.* **2008**, *283*, 19371–19378. [CrossRef]

23. Rebbapragada, A.; Benchabane, H.; Wrana, J.L.; Celeste, A.J.; Attisano, L. Myostatin signals through a transforming growth factor beta-like signaling pathway to block adipogenesis. *Mol. Cell. Biol.* **2003**, *23*, 7230–7242. [CrossRef]

24. ten Dijke, P.; Yamashita, H.; Ichijo, H.; Franzen, P.; Laiho, M.; Miyazono, K.; Heldin, C.H. Characterization of type I receptors for transforming growth factor-beta and activin. *Science* **1994**, *264*, 101–104. [CrossRef]

25. Kemaladewi, D.U.; de Gorter, D.J.; Aartsma-Rus, A.; van Ommen, G.J.; ten Dijke, P.; t Hoen, P.A.; Hoogaars, W.M. Cell-type specific regulation of myostatin signaling. *FASEB J.* **2012**, *26*, 1462–1472. [CrossRef]

26. Schneider, C.A.; Rasband, W.S.; Eliceiri, K.W. NIH image to imagej: 25 years of image analysis. *Nat. Methods* **2012**, *9*, 671–675. [CrossRef]

27. Jen, Y.; Weintraub, H.; Benezra, R. Overexpression of Id protein inhibits the muscle differentiation program: In vivo association of Id with E2A proteins. *Genes Dev.* **1992**, *6*, 1466–1479. [CrossRef]

28. Ramachandran, A.; Vizan, P.; Das, D.; Chakravarty, P.; Vogt, J.; Rogers, K.W.; Muller, P.; Hinck, A.P.; Sapkota, G.P.; Hill, C.S. Tgf-beta uses a novel mode of receptor activation to phosphorylate smad1/5 and induce epithelial-to-mesenchymal transition. *Elife* **2018**, *7*, e31756. [CrossRef]

29. McFarlane, C.; Plummer, E.; Thomas, M.; Hennebry, A.; Ashby, M.; Ling, N.; Smith, H.; Sharma, M.; Kambadur, R. Myostatin induces cachexia by activating the ubiquitin proteolytic system through an NF-kappaB-independent, FoxO1-dependent mechanism. *J. Cell. Physiol.* **2006**, *209*, 501–514. [CrossRef]

30. Glass, D.J. Skeletal muscle hypertrophy and atrophy signaling pathways. *Int. J. Biochem. Cell Biol.* **2005**, *37*, 1974–1984. [CrossRef]

31. Hecker, L.; Vittal, R.; Jones, T.; Jagirdar, R.; Luckhardt, T.R.; Horowitz, J.C.; Pennathur, S.; Martinez, F.J.; Thannickal, V.J. NAPDH oxidase-4 mediates myofibroblast activation and fibrogenic responses to lung injury. *Nat. Med.* **2009**, *15*, 1077–1081. [CrossRef] [PubMed]

32. Liu, D.; Kang, J.S.; Derynck, R. TGF-beta-activated Smad3 represses MEF2-dependent transcription in myogenic differentiation. *EMBO J.* **2004**, *23*, 1557–1566. [CrossRef] [PubMed]

33. Sharma, A.; Agarwal, M.; Kumar, A.; Kumar, P.; Saini, M.; Kardon, G.; Mathew, S.J. Myosin heavy chain-embryonic is a crucial regulator of skeletal muscle development and differentiation. *bioRxiv* **2018**.

34. Kadoguchi, T.; Shimada, K.; Koide, H.; Miyazaki, T.; Shiozawa, T.; Takahashi, S.; Aikawa, T.; Ouchi, S.; Kitamura, K.; Sugita, Y.; et al. Possible role of NAPDH oxidase 4 in angiotensin II-induced muscle wasting in mice. *Front. Physiol.* **2018**, *9*, 340. [CrossRef]

35. Gundersen, K.; Merlie, J.P. Id-1 as a possible transcriptional mediator of muscle disuse atrophy. *Proc. Natl. Acad. Sci. USA* **1994**, *91*, 3647–3651. [CrossRef]

36. Cencetti, F.; Bernacchioni, C.; Tonelli, F.; Roberts, E.; Donati, C.; Bruni, P. Tgfbeta1 evokes myoblast apoptotic response via a novel signaling pathway involving S1P4 transactivation upstream of Rho-kinase-2 activation. *FASEB J.* **2013**, *27*, 4532–4546. [CrossRef]

37. Zammit, P.S.; Heslop, L.; Hudon, V.; Rosenblatt, J.D.; Tajbakhsh, S.; Buckingham, M.E.; Beauchamp, J.R.; Partridge, T.A. Kinetics of myoblast proliferation show that resident satellite cells are competent to fully regenerate skeletal muscle fibers. *Exp. Cell Res.* **2002**, *281*, 39–49. [CrossRef]

38. Mackey, A.L.; Magnan, M.; Chazaud, B.; Kjaer, M. Human skeletal muscle fibroblasts stimulate in vitro myogenesis and in vivo muscle regeneration. *J. Physiol.* **2017**, *595*, 5115–5127. [CrossRef]

39. Frese, S.; Ruebner, M.; Suhr, F.; Konou, T.M.; Tappe, K.A.; Toigo, M.; Jung, H.H.; Henke, C.; Steigleder, R.; Strissel, P.L.; et al. Long-term endurance exercise in humans stimulates cell fusion of myoblasts along with fusogenic endogenous retroviral genes in vivo. *PLoS ONE* **2015**, *10*, e0132099. [CrossRef]

40. Listrat, A.; Picard, B.; Geay, Y. Age-related changes and location of type I, III, IV, V and VI collagens during development of four foetal skeletal muscles of double-muscled and normal bovine animals. *Tissue Cell* **1999**, *31*, 17–27. [CrossRef]

41. Light, N.; Champion, A.E. Characterization of muscle epimysium, perimysium and endomysium collagens. *Biochem. J.* **1984**, *219*, 1017–1026. [CrossRef] [PubMed]

42. Purslow, P.P. The structure and functional significance of variations in the connective tissue within muscle. *Comp. Biochem. Physiol. A Mol. Integr. Physiol.* **2002**, *133*, 947–966. [CrossRef]

43. Huijing, P.A.; Jaspers, R.T. Adaptation of muscle size and myofascial force transmission: A review and some new experimental results. *Scand J. Med. Sci. Sports* **2005**, *15*, 349–380. [CrossRef] [PubMed]

44. Thomas, K.; Engler, A.J.; Meyer, G.A. Extracellular matrix regulation in the muscle satellite cell niche. *Connect. Tissue Res.* **2015**, *56*, 1–8. [CrossRef] [PubMed]

45. Gillies, A.R.; Lieber, R.L. Structure and function of the skeletal muscle extracellular matrix. *Muscle Nerve* **2011**, *44*, 318–331. [CrossRef]

46. Boers, H.E.; Haroon, M.; Le Grand, F.; Bakker, A.D.; Klein-Nulend, J.; Jaspers, R.T. Mechanosensitivity of aged muscle stem cells. *J. Orthop. Res.* **2018**, *36*, 632–641.

47. Romanazzo, S.; Forte, G.; Ebara, M.; Uto, K.; Pagliari, S.; Aoyagi, T.; Traversa, E.; Taniguchi, A. Substrate stiffness affects skeletal myoblast differentiation in vitro. *Sci. Technol. Adv. Mater.* **2012**, *13*, 064211. [CrossRef]

48. Yan, F.; Wang, Y.; Wu, X.; Peshavariya, H.M.; Dusting, G.J.; Zhang, M.; Jiang, F. Nox4 and redox signaling mediate tgf-beta-induced endothelial cell apoptosis and phenotypic switch. *Cell Death Dis.* **2014**, *5*, e1010. [CrossRef]

49. Avin, K.G.; Chen, N.X.; Organ, J.M.; Zarse, C.; O'Neill, K.; Conway, R.G.; Konrad, R.J.; Bacallao, R.L.; Allen, M.R.; Moe, S.M. Skeletal muscle regeneration and oxidative stress are altered in chronic kidney disease. *PLoS ONE* **2016**, *11*, e0159411. [CrossRef]

50. Lin, C.H.; Yu, M.C.; Tung, W.H.; Chen, T.T.; Yu, C.C.; Weng, C.M.; Tsai, Y.J.; Bai, K.J.; Hong, C.Y.; Chien, M.H.; et al. Connective tissue growth factor induces collagen I expression in human lung fibroblasts through the Rac1/MLK3/JNK/AP-1 pathway. *Biochim. Biophys. Acta* **2013**, *1833*, 2823–2833. [CrossRef]

51. Yang, Z.; Sun, Z.; Liu, H.; Ren, Y.; Shao, D.; Zhang, W.; Lin, J.; Wolfram, J.; Wang, F.; Nie, S. Connective tissue growth factor stimulates the proliferation, migration and differentiation of lung fibroblasts during paraquat-induced pulmonary fibrosis. *Mol. Med. Rep.* **2015**, *12*, 1091–1097. [CrossRef]

52. Ponticos, M.; Holmes, A.M.; Shi-wen, X.; Leoni, P.; Khan, K.; Rajkumar, V.S.; Hoyles, R.K.; Bou-Gharios, G.; Black, C.M.; Denton, C.P.; et al. Pivotal role of connective tissue growth factor in lung fibrosis: MAPK-dependent transcriptional activation of type I collagen. *Arthritis Rheum.* **2009**, *60*, 2142–2155. [CrossRef]

53. Ko, M.K.; Kay, E.P. Regulatory role of FGF-2 on type I collagen expression during endothelial mesenchymal transformation. *Invest. Ophthalmol. Vis. Sci.* **2005**, *46*, 4495–4503. [CrossRef]

54. Park, D.S.; Park, J.C.; Lee, J.S.; Kim, T.W.; Kim, K.J.; Jung, B.J.; Shim, E.K.; Choi, E.Y.; Park, S.Y.; Cho, K.S.; et al. Effect of FGF-2 on collagen tissue regeneration by human vertebral bone marrow stem cells. *Stem Cells Dev.* **2015**, *24*, 228–243. [CrossRef]

55. Yablonka-Reuveni, Z.; Rivera, A.J. Proliferative dynamics and the role of FGF2 during myogenesis of rat satellite cells on isolated fibers. *Basic Appl. Myol.* **1997**, *7*, 189–202.

56. Liu, Y.; Schneider, M.F. FGF2 activates TRPC and Ca(2+) signaling leading to satellite cell activation. *Front. Physiol.* **2014**, *5*, 38. [CrossRef]

57. Chen, J.L.; Walton, K.L.; Hagg, A.; Colgan, T.D.; Johnson, K.; Qian, H.; Gregorevic, P.; Harrison, C.A. Specific targeting of tgf-beta family ligands demonstrates distinct roles in the regulation of muscle mass in health and disease. *Proc. Natl. Acad. Sci. USA* **2017**, *114*, E5266–E5275.

58. Watt, K.I.; Jaspers, R.T.; Atherton, P.; Smith, K.; Rennie, M.J.; Ratkevicius, A.; Wackerhage, H. Sb431542 treatment promotes the hypertrophy of skeletal muscle fibers but decreases specific force. *Muscle Nerve* **2010**, *41*, 624–629. [CrossRef]

12

Mechanisms Regulating Muscle Regeneration: Insights into the Interrelated and Time-Dependent Phases of Tissue Healing

Laura Forcina, Marianna Cosentino and Antonio Musarò *

Laboratory affiliated to Istituto Pasteur Italia—Fondazione Cenci Bolognetti, DAHFMO-Unit of Histology and Medical Embryology, Sapienza University of Rome, Via Antonio Scarpa, 14, 00161 Rome, Italy; laura.forcina@uniroma1.it (L.F.); marianna.cosentino@uniroma1.it (M.C.)
* Correspondence: antonio.musaro@uniroma1.it;

Abstract: Despite a massive body of knowledge which has been produced related to the mechanisms guiding muscle regeneration, great interest still moves the scientific community toward the study of different aspects of skeletal muscle homeostasis, plasticity, and regeneration. Indeed, the lack of effective therapies for several physiopathologic conditions suggests that a comprehensive knowledge of the different aspects of cellular behavior and molecular pathways, regulating each regenerative stage, has to be still devised. Hence, it is important to perform even more focused studies, taking the advantage of robust markers, reliable techniques, and reproducible protocols. Here, we provide an overview about the general aspects of muscle regeneration and discuss the different approaches to study the interrelated and time-dependent phases of muscle healing.

Keywords: muscle regeneration; inflammatory response; satellite cells; cell precursors; experimental methods; stem cell markers; muscle homeostasis

1. Introduction

Muscle regeneration represents an important homeostatic process of adult skeletal muscle, which retains, after development, the ability to regenerate in response to different injured stimuli, restoring damaged myofibers [1–3]. This property of the adult muscle tissue has drawn great scientific attention over time, since the impairment of skeletal muscle regenerative potential characterizes a suite of physiopathologic conditions severely affecting human health. A significant contribution to regenerative studies is derived from the development of experimental protocols to induce controlled muscle damage and from the validation of cellular, molecular, and histological analysis to reveal, monitor, and characterize each step of tissue repair. Several models of muscle injury have been developed in rodents; however, the complex dynamic of events following different types of muscle injury has still to be clarified. Confounding interpretations can derive from the indiscriminate use of experimental damaging techniques, since an increasing body of evidence suggests that skeletal muscle can differentially respond to injuries which affect, at various degree, the distinct cellular and structural components.

In this review, we integrated the principles of the physiologic muscle regeneration with a technical approach, reporting key experimental methods and markers employed to study cellular and molecular interactors dominating each stage of muscle healing.

2. From Tissue Destruction to Recovery: Highlighting the Stages of Muscle Regeneration

The dynamic response of skeletal muscle to damaging events can be roughly divided into two main stages: tissue destruction and the stage of reconstruction. However, a suite of cellular and molecular events has been identified in these stages, leading to a more refined classification of the regenerative process. Indeed, muscle regeneration occurs in five interrelated and time-dependent phases, namely degeneration-necrosis, inflammation, regeneration, maturation/remodelling, and functional recovery, reflecting the hierarchy of the overall process dominating the tissue (Figure 1). Although the kinetics and amplitude of each phase can vary among organisms and may depend on the characteristic and intensity of the damaging agent, the overall dynamic of the phases of muscle healing is similar in different mammals (e.g., mouse, rat, and human) and can be monitored at morphologic, molecular, and functional levels.

2.1. Muscle Degeneration

Muscle necrosis occurs when the integrity of myofibers is severely compromised, and the irreversible damage generally involves alteration of plasmalemma permeability, associated with the uncontrolled ionic flux, organelle disfunction, and the loss of a proper architecture. Although necrotic fibers can be histologically identified as pale and enlarged, reflecting internal abnormalities, other methods can be used to rigorously evaluate and quantify the degree of muscle damage upon injury.

Evans Blue Dye (EBD) has been described as a necrosis-avid agent in mammal muscles since it showed the ability to penetrate only the damaged, necrotic myofibers [4–10]. EBD, also called T-1824 or Direct Blue 53, is a synthetic bis-azo dye characterized by a high-water solubility, a strong affinity for serum albumin, and a slow excretion. When injected intravenously or intraperitoneally in living animals, EBD can bind serum albumin, remaining stable and confined in the blood, and can be distributed throughout the entire body. However, at the site of the lesion, the dye can permeate altered cell membranes, accumulating in the cytoplasm of damaged cells [6]. A satisfactory labelling of permeable myofibers can be obtained in mice with a single intraperitoneal injection of a 1% EBD solution, injected at 1% volume relative to body mass and administered between 16 and 24 h prior to tissue sampling [10,11]. Moreover, EBD presents a double advantage for its visualization. It can be both easily identified macroscopically, by the striking blue color within tissue, or revealed through fluorescent microscopy in tissue sections or even in a whole muscle [12,13]. Indeed, EBD can emit a bright red fluorescence (620 nm excitation/680 nm emission) and the amount of biological dye penetrating in a damaged tissue can be quantified as a total intensity of fluorescence in a tissue sample by using confocal microscopy [11,14]. Since it is well known that serum proteins can cross into damaged fibers, sharing the same basic principle of the EBD, the presence of necrotic fibers in skeletal muscle sections can be histologically highlighted by immunofluorescence analysis for the intracellular accumulation of albumin or immunoglobulin G (IgG). For instance, in the mouse, IgG uptake has been recognized as a marker for necrosis in muscle tissue (Figure 1) [5,15].

Markers of tissue damage can be also detected in serum, since skeletal muscle proteins such as creatine kinase (CK), lactate dehydrogenase (LDH), and troponin, when systemically distributed, are well-recognized indexes of muscle tissue alterations, the intensity of which can vary under different physiopathologic conditions (Table 1) [16]. The most commonly used serum marker of myocellular damage is serum CK, a globular protein catalyzing the exchange of high-energy phosphate bonds between phosphocreatine and ADP produced during contraction [16,17]. Based on the critical role of CK in the maintenance of the energy homeostasis of muscle tissue, a specific isoform of the enzyme CK3 (CK-MM) is highly abundant in myofibers and it is released in the extracellular space when the sarcolemma loses the physiologic integrity.

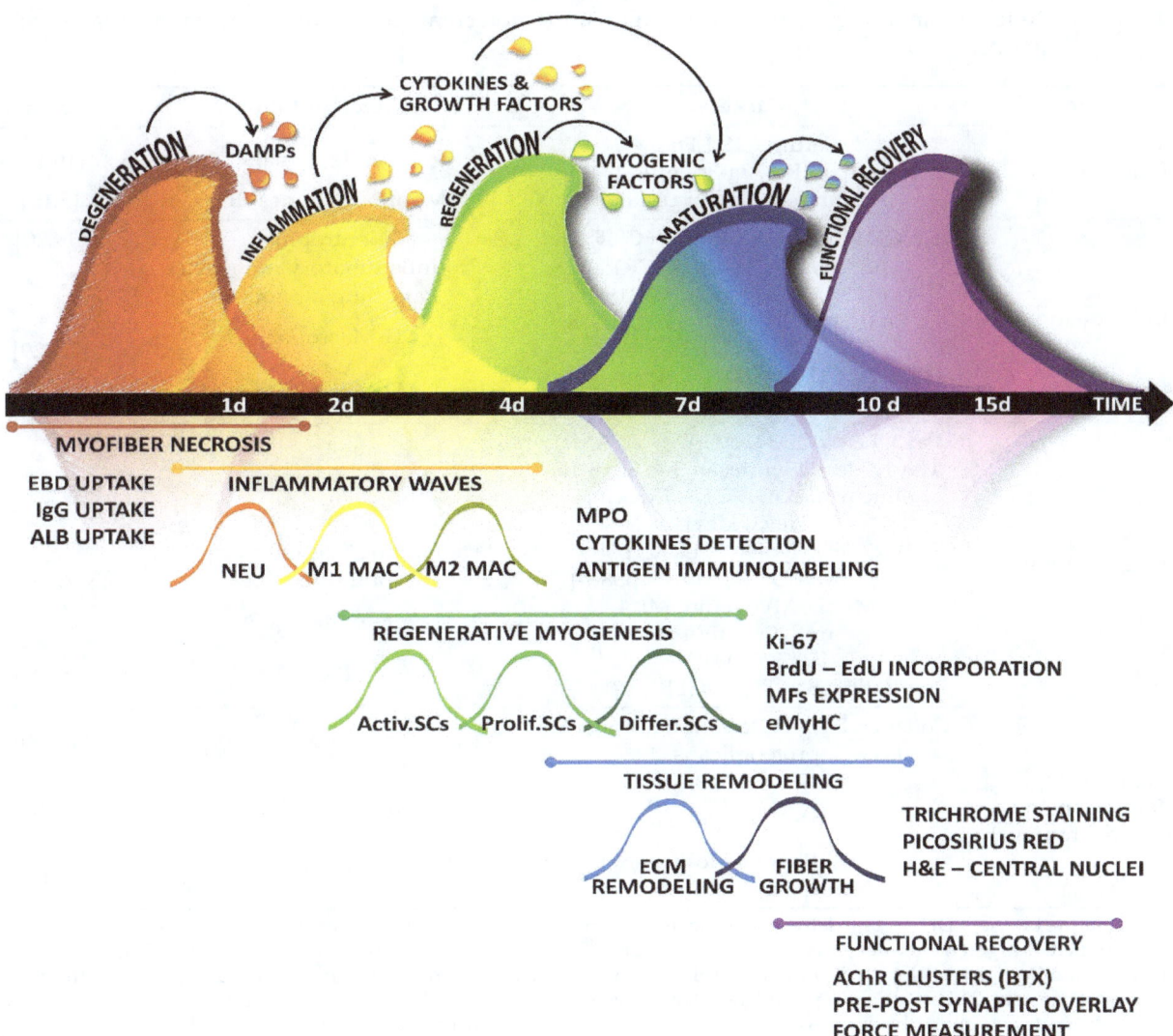

Figure 1. A simplified "wave on wave" model of skeletal muscle healing: The regenerative program activated by muscle tissue in response to damage can be outlined in five interrelated and time-dependent waves, namely degeneration, inflammation, regeneration, maturation-remodelling, and functional recovery, which can be highlighted by using different methodologies. Tissue injury leads to myofiber degeneration/necrosis. Damage stimuli activate the so-called sterile inflammation, characterized by the infiltration of different immune cells dominating in succession the lesion. Inflammation triggers also the regenerative stage, in which satellite cells, along with the support of other stem cells and precursors, undergo activation, expansion, and differentiation. The maturation of myofibers is accompanied by the fine remodelling of tissue architecture, with matrix rearrangement and angiogenesis. The last step of the healing process is characterized by the reconstitution of neuromuscular connections, necessary to regain tissue functionality. DAMPs: Damage-associated molecular patterns; EBD: Evans Blue Dye; IgG: Immunoglobulin G; ALB: Albumin; NEU: neutrophils; MAC: macrophages; MPO: myeloperoxidase; SCs: satellite cells; Activ.SCs: activated SCs; Prolif.SCs: proliferating SCs; Diff.SCs: differentiating SCs; BrdU: 5-bromo-2'-deoxyuridine; EdU: 5-ethynyl-2'-deoxyuridine; MFs: myogenic factors; eMyHC: embryonal myosin heavy chain; H&E: Haematoxylin and Eosin; AchR: Acetylcholine receptor; BTX: Bungarotoxin.

Table 1. Relevant markers of pivotal cellular and molecular actors in the different stages of muscle healing.

Stage	Markers	Recognition	References
Degeneration	Serum CK, LDH, troponin, miR-378a-3p, miR-434-3p	Muscle damage	[16,18]
	Albumin, IgG fiber uptake	Myofiber permeability	[5,15]
Inflammation	CD11b$^{pos.}$/Ly6G$^{pos.}$/Ly6C$^{neg.}$	Neutrophils	[19,20]
	Ly6C^{high}/CCR2$^{pos.}$/CX3CR1^{low}	Pro-inflammatory monocytes	[21–26]
	Ly6C^{low}/CCR2$^{neg.}$/CX3CR1^{high}	Patrolling monocytes	
	CD11b, Ly6C, F4/80, CD68, CD38, Gpr18, Fpr2	M1 Macrophages	[27–29]
	CD206, CD11c, CD163, Arginase1, Egr2, c-Myc	M2 Macrophages	
Regeneration	Pax3, Pax7, CD34, NCAM, VCAM-1, Cav1, Mcad, Syndecan 3-4, Sox8-15, Integrin α7-β1, CTR, Emerin, Hey1, Heyl	Quiescent SCs	[1,12,30–39]
	Pax7^{high}/MyoD^{low}, DGC, p38γ	Proliferating/Self renewing SCs	[1,12,40–43]
	Pax7^{low}/MyoD^{high}, Myf-5, p38α-β	Committed SCs	
	MyoD, Myogenin, Mrf4, miR206, miR486	Differentiating SCs	
	CD45$^{neg.}$/CD31$^{neg.}$/ α7 int$^{neg.}$/Sca$^{pos.}$/PDGFR $\alpha^{pos.}$	FAPs	[1,11,44,45]
Remodeling, Maturation and Functional retrieval	Collagen I–III–IV, laminin, fibronectin, proteoglicans	ECM	[46–50]
	eMyHC	Regenerating Myofibers	[12]
	AchRs/Synaptohysin/ Neurofilament markers	NMJs	[51]

CK: creatine kinase; LDH: lactate dehydrogenase; IgG: immunoglobulin G; CD: cluster of differentiation; Ly6C, Ly6G: lymphocyte antigen 6 complex, locus C, locus G; CCR2: C-C chemokine receptor type 2; CX3CR1: C-X3-C Motif Chemokine Receptor 1; Gpr18: G-protein coupled receptor 18; Fpr2: formyl peptide receptor 2; Egr2: early growth response protein 2; Pax3, Pax7: paired box transcription factor 3, 7; NCAM: neural cell adhesion molecule; VCAM: Vascular Cell Adhesion protein; Cav1: caveolin 1; Mcad: M-cadherin; Sox 8, 15: SRY-Box transcription Factor 8, 15; CTR: calcitonin receptor; SCs: Satellite cells; Hey1, Heyl: hairy/enhancer-of-split related with YRPW motif proteins; MyoD: myoblast determination protein; DGC: dystrophin-associated glycoprotein complex; Myf-5: myogenic factor 5; Mrf4: myogenic regulatory factor 4; Int: integrin; Sca: stem cell antigen; PDGFRα: platelet derived growth factor receptor alpha; FAPs: fibroadipogenic progenitors; eMyHC: embryonal myosin heavy chain; AchRs: acetylcholine receptors; NMJs: neuromuscular junctions.

Among biochemical markers of muscle damage, the serum levels of muscle-specific or muscle-enriched microRNAs (miRNAs) has been proposed [18]. Indeed, a number of miRNAs, including miR-1, miR-133, and miR-206 (myomiRs), have been involved in the regulation of critical myocellular processes such as satellite cell activity, skeletal muscle growth, adaptation, and regeneration [42,43,52,53]. Furthermore, in a recent profiling study, performed on notexin-injured rats, Siracusa and colleagues identified circulating miR-378a-3p and miR-434-3p as reliable biomarkers of acute muscle damage [18] (Table 1).

2.2. Inflammatory Waves

Tissue necrosis is known to stimulate a host inflammatory response named sterile inflammation because no exogenous infectious agents participate in the immune process. Necrotic cell death is mainly characterized by the swelling of organelles, increased cell volume, and the disruption of the plasma membrane, which leads to the release of the intracellular content. When intracellular components are dispersed throughout the extracellular space, they can act as signals, which have been termed as damage-associated molecular patterns (DAMPs), triggering inflammatory reactions [54,55]. Although it has been recognized as a contributor to pathologic changes, inflammation represents an important physiologic process playing a critical role in muscle homeostasis and regeneration. Indeed, the sequential recruitment of specific myeloid cell populations at the site of the lesion is considered the second of five interrelated phases of muscle regeneration (Figure 1) [12,56–60]. The first sensor of the innate immunity to be activated early after injury is the complement system, which allows the immediate immune response against damaged tissue and leads to the infiltration of inflammatory cells at the site of the lesion [21,61]. Neutrophils, along with mast cells, represent the first inflammatory myeloid cells that invade the site of muscle injury [21]. In particular, resident mast cell degranulate in response to muscle injury and release pro-inflammatory factors such as TNF-α (tumor necrosis factor alpha), IFN-γ (Interferon-γ), and IL-1β (interleukin-1β) [21], which stimulate the recruitment of peripheral neutrophils to the lesion site [12,62–66]. Furthermore, it has been recently demonstrated that ADAM8, a member of a disintegrin and metalloprotease (ADAM) family, contributes to the invasiveness of neutrophils into injured muscle fibers by reducing their adhesiveness to blood vessels after the infiltration into interstitial tissues [19]. The pro-inflammatory action of neutrophils is necessary to allow the removal of myofiber debris and to stimulate the homing of other pivotal inflammatory cells, facilitating the progress of muscle regeneration. The phagocytic activity of neutrophils involves the release of high concentrations of free radicals and proteases as well as the secretion of pro-inflammatory cytokines such as IL-1, IL-8, IL-6, and the soluble interleukin-6 receptor alpha (sIL6R). In particular, sIL6R can stimulate, within 24 h after damage, the homing of other inflammatory cell populations, namely monocytes and macrophages [21,59,67,68].

Macrophages becomes the predominant inflammatory cell type 2 days after injury, while neutrophils decline [21,59,67]. Although macrophages are generally recognized as highly specialized cells with phagocytic activity, responsible for tissue debris removal, this inflammatory population cannot be unequivocally labelled because of its heterogeneity, which still lack a comprehensive classification. A differential phagocytic activity has been described in resident macrophages, with ED1[pos.] cells highly participating in tissue response to acute damage and ED2[pos.]/ED3[pos.] cells showing no phagocytic activity and abundantly present in uninjured muscles [69]. Furthermore, macrophages found at the lesion can also derive from blood monocytes. Circulating monocytes derive from bone marrow and can be classed into at least two populations, based on the variable expression levels of specific markers, namely lymphocyte antigen 6 complex locus C (Ly6C) and chemokine receptors (CCR2 and CX3CR1) (Table 1) [21–23].

It has been proposed that Ly6C[high] monocytes can be recruited to the lesion thanks to the elevated expression of C-C chemokine receptor type 2 (CCR2) that then differentiate into pro-inflammatory macrophages M1 [24,26]. In contrast, patrolling Ly6C[low] monocytes are characterized by a low expression of CCR2 and can enter the damaged tissue in a CX3CR1-dependent manner, participating in tissue repair during the third wave of regenerative inflammation, as M2 pro-regenerative macrophages [25]. Other studies support the hypothesis that only inflammatory monocytes are recruited in injured skeletal muscle and then switch to anti-inflammatory subtype to support myogenesis [67,70]. Thus, the origin, the distinction, and even the existence of M1 and M2 populations are still controversial. However, it has been widely accepted that a first outbreak of macrophages works initially to remove the muscle debris and to secrete pro-inflammatory cytokines, while a subsequent appearance of non-phagocytic macrophages contributes to the shift of the inflammatory response toward resolutive events.

Thus, the enhanced expression of inflammatory mediators, mainly TNF-α, IL-6, and IL-1β, can clearly indicate an ongoing inflammatory response; however, these factors can be secreted by a wealth of cellular agents in a damaged muscle, being unspecific markers of cellular interactors in the pro-inflammatory stage of muscle regeneration. On the other hand, the detection and identification of different inflammatory population at the site of the lesion and thus the temporary collocation of the regenerative event can be obtained through the expression of specific markers.

Histological analysis is frequently performed to reveal the presence of inflammatory cells in regenerative studies. Immunofluorescence analysis for lymphocyte antigen 6 complex locus G

(Ly6G) and F4/80 expression in damaged murine muscle sections has been extensively used to detect neutrophils and macrophages, respectively. Additionally, other histological methods, such as the cytochemical myeloperoxidase (MPO) staining, can be used to detect the extent of infiltrating myeloid cells in damaged muscles. Indeed, MPO is a lysosomal enzyme contained in cytoplasmic primary granules of myeloid cells and can be detected through the oxidation of benzidine or the reaction of p-phenylenediamine and catechol in the presence of hydrogen peroxide (H_2O_2). This staining has been widely used to reveal the presence of neutrophils. However, although MPO mainly characterize azurophil neutrophilic granules, the assay can detect mammal monocytes without guaranteeing a fine discrimination of single cell types [71]. Of note, primary granules are absent in lymphocytes; thus, the MPO biochemical assay can be used as a marker for discerning myeloid from lymphoid cells.

Cytofluorimetric analysis can be useful to evaluate the quality of inflammation and to obtain an accurate quantification of inflammatory cell populations. Neutrophils have been identified as CD11b$^{pos.}$/Ly6G$^{pos.}$/Ly6C$^{neg.}$, whereas CD11b positive cells expressing Ly6C but not Ly6G have been identified as monocytes [19,29].

Of note, novel technologies are contributing to expanding the current knowledge about inflammatory cell function and fate. Intravital microscopy, high specific markers, along with the generation of novel transgenic animals allowed the visualization of fast-moving cells, providing promising tools to unravelling inflammatory-associated processes [20,72,73]. In a recent study, Wang and colleagues [74] marked Ly6G$^{pos.}$ cells with a photoactivatable green fluorescent protein (Ly6G-PA-GFP). Using this advanced technique, they combined intravital imaging and photoactivation methods to demonstrate that murine neutrophils do not die at the site of the lesion as previously thought [74,75]. Conversely, it has been shown that neutrophils, fulfilling their inflammatory tasks, are able to perform reverse migration from the local lesion, moving back to circulation and eventually home back to the bone marrow [20,74].

Macrophages (Mac) are a heterogeneous population of cells and their distinction often require the setup of a panel of markers, for which the combination specifically identifies a Mac subset. A marker panel for the detection of macrophages in skeletal muscle can be comprised of Siglec-F, CD11b, Ly6C, F4/80, and CD206 (Table 1) [28,29]. Other markers are required to detect M1 or M2 macrophages. For instance, it has been reported that M1 phenotype expresses CD68 whereas M2 macrophages express CD163. Furthermore, Jablonski and colleagues identified genes common or exclusive to either subset [27]. They report also a validated M1-exclusive pattern of expression for CD38, G-protein coupled receptor 18 (Gpr18), and Formyl peptide receptor 2 (Fpr2), whereas Early growth response protein 2 (Egr2) and c-Myc were recognized as M2 exclusive. Interestingly, they observed that Egr2, rather than the canonical M2 macrophage marker Arginase-1, labelled preferentially M2 macrophages (~70%), indicating that the unambiguous identification of macrophages still deserves further research. Of note, Insulin-like growth factor 1 (IGF-1) is a potent enhancer of tissue regeneration hastening the resolution of the inflammatory phase. It has been demonstrated that local macrophage-derived IGF-1 represents a key factor in inflammation resolution and macrophage polarization during muscle regeneration [76].

2.3. Regeneration

2.3.1. The Role of Satellite Cells

The reconstruction of injured muscle relies on the muscle stem cells, known as satellite cells (SCs), which reside between the basal lamina and sarcolemma of myofibers and are mitotically quiescent until required for growth or repair [77].

Although satellite cells can be easily recognized in healthy skeletal muscle tissue, in light of their sublaminar position, a wealth of markers has been identified to characterize the biology of these myogenic progenitors and to study their behavior during regenerative events. Quiescent satellite cells are characterized by the expression of Paired box transcription factors (Pax3 and Pax7), Neural cell adhesion molecule (NCAM), M-cadherin (Mcad), Forkhead box protein K (FoxK), tyrosine-protein kinase Met (c-Met), Vascular Cell Adhesion protein 1 (VCAM-1), CD34, Syndecan 3 and 4, Sox 8, Sox 15, Integrins (α7 and β1), Caveolin-1, Calcitonin receptor (CTR), Lamin A/C, Emerin, and hairy/enhancer-of-split related with YRPW motif proteins Hey1 and Heyl (Table 1) [1,12,30–39,41]. However, the transition of SCs from the quiescent state toward activation, commitment, and differentiation involves the genetic and epigenetic adaptation to novel biologic functions, entailing dynamic changes in the protein expression profile. Indeed, activated SCs retain the expression of Pax7, Mcad, VCAM1, Caveolin 1, and Integrin α7 along with the induction of proliferative and myogenic markers such as desmin, Myogenic factor 5 (Myf-5), and Myoblast determination protein (MyoD) [78–80].

Proliferating satellite cells can be also effectively identified by using non cell-specific markers of proliferation such as the Ki-67 and Proliferating cell nuclear antigen (PCNA). Ki-67 protein has been detected during all active phases of the cell cycle, namely G(1), S, G(2), and mitosis, but not in resting cells (G(0)), making its expression an excellent marker for determining the cycling fraction of a cell population [81]. Other cell proliferation assays involved the use of the thymidine analog 5-bromo-2'-deoxyuridine (BrdU) or 5-ethynyl-2'-deoxyuridine (EdU) and are based on the de novo synthesis of DNA occurring during cell duplication, which will be labelled by the incorporated nucleosides [82].

It is worth to report that the proliferation of satellite cells has a dual role: the generation of committed cells participating in regenerative processes and the replenishment of the stem cell pool after the exploitation. To achieve this activity, SCs are able to both symmetrically and asymmetrically divide. The symmetric division gives rise to an identical progeny with stem cell properties. Otherwise, through the asymmetric process, a single SC can generate a self-renewing daughter cell, retaining the expression of Pax7 and repressing MyoD (Pax7^{high}/MyoD^{low}) and a committed cell which downmodulates Pax7 and expresses MyoD (Pax7^{low}/MyoD^{high}). When the fine balance between self-renewal and commitment is altered, muscle homeostasis is impaired, leading to failure of the regenerative process and/or to the exhaustion of the stem cell pool. These conditions have been observed in Pax7$^{CreER/+}$:p38$\gamma^{fl/fl}$ mice and in dystrophin-deficient mice, respectively lacking p38γ and dystrophin expression [40]. This is because both dystrophin, as a pivotal member of the dystrophin-associated glycoprotein complex (DGC), and the γ isoform of the p38 MAP kinases are determinants which regulate SC asymmetric division, through the polarized restriction of factors involved in the cell fate decision. Indeed, it has been described that, during the asymmetric division, the apical daughter cell, retaining the expression of the DGC and presenting the phosphorylated p38γ isoform, sequestrates in the cytoplasm molecular mediators of the progression of the myogenic program, undergoing self-renewing. In contrast, other members of the p38 family, such as the α and β isoforms, participate to the commitment and differentiation of satellite cells [40].

The specificity of surface antigens can be used to quantify and isolate satellite cells by Fluorescence Activated Cell Sorting (FACS analysis). This method that has been described as robust and reliable for the isolation of SCs has been widely used, and different panels of antigen detection have been reported [11,32]. Among them, two panels for mouse skeletal muscle analysis, designed to exclude hematopoietic and stromal cells (CD45, CD11b, Ter119, CD31, and Sca-1) and to recognize surface markers present on satellite cells (β1-integrin/CXCR4, α7-integrin/CD34, and VCAM1) have been recently reported and validated [32]. Since it has been well established that satellite cells represent about 2–5% of the total nuclei in skeletal muscle tissue, an accurate evaluation of the muscle stem cell pool can provide indications about the physiopathologic state of the muscle. An abnormal number of SCs can be considered an index of ongoing regenerative events.

Besides the specific analysis of satellite cell activity and fate, overall signs of muscle regeneration can be histologically highlighted by the presence of central nuclei and cytoplasm basophilia. Both characteristics are easily evaluable through Hematoxylin and Eosin (H&E) staining, a standard staining for microscope examination of tissues (Figure 2) [74]. Hematoxylin presents a deep blue-purple color and stains nucleic acids, whereas eosin is pink and stains proteins. Although unspecific, this common staining can allow the visualization of both central nuclei and basophilic small fibers, readily identifying regenerating myofibers [83].

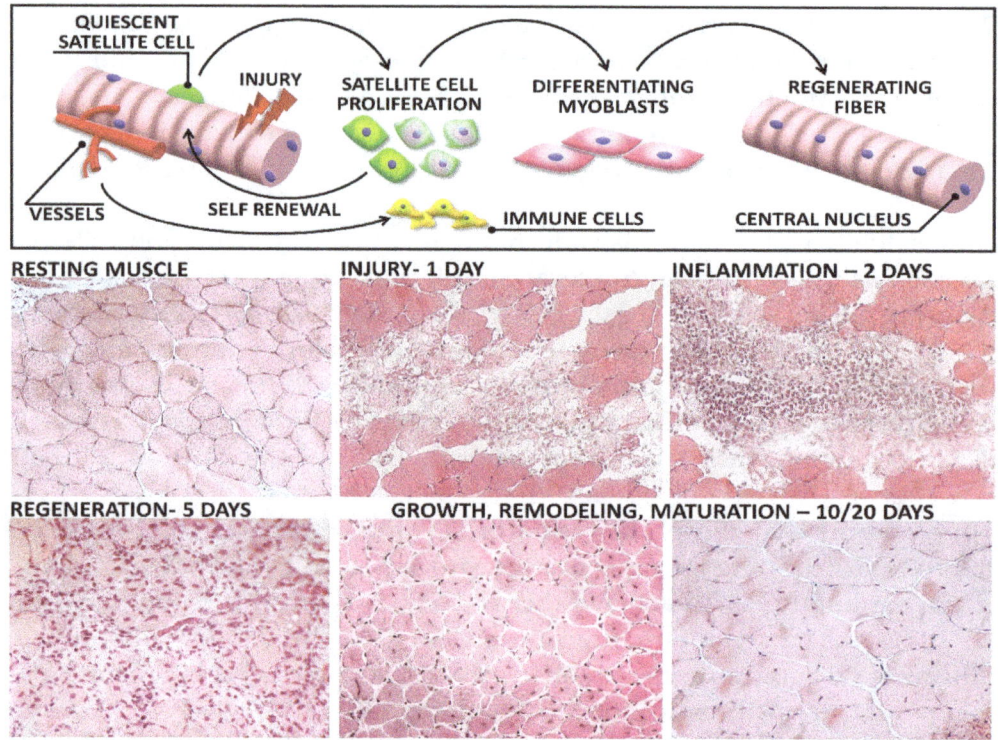

Figure 2. Skeletal muscle regeneration upon acute injury: The upper panel shows a schematic representation of relevant biological responses activated in muscle tissue following damage. Lower panel reports haematoxylin and eosin images of muscle sections, representative of each step of muscle degeneration and regeneration after cardiotoxin (CTX) injection. Early, after the injection (1 day), necrotic myofibers are evident in damaged muscle. During the second day after damage, the lesion is dominated by inflammatory infiltrated cells. Activated satellite cells undergo active proliferation, and newly regenerating fibers appears within the first week. Ten days after injection, the overall tissue architecture is restored and most of myofibers display centrally located nuclei. Regenerated myofibers then undergo progressive growth and maturation, highlighted by the increasing cross-sectional area and the nuclear relocation towards the periphery.

The downmodulation of proliferative genes ratifies the exit of satellite cells from the cell cycle. Committed and differentiating cells, based on the expression levels of Pax7 and MyoD, have been recognized as $Pax7^{low}/MyoD^{high}$ and are characterized by the activation of late markers of the myogenic program, such as myogenin and the myogenic regulatory factor 4 (Mrf4).

The committed population of myoblasts can either fuse with existing myofibers, repair damaged muscle fibers, or alternatively fuse to each other to form new myofibers. This is a complex mechanism not yet fully elucidated which involves tightly regulated events of cell migration, recognition, and adhesion, resulting in an efficacious fusion process [84,85]. In addition to the recognized role of transforming growth factor beta (TGFβ) and IL-4 in myoblast fusion, a crucial role in muscle differentiation is also played by actin cytoskeleton and by components of the contractile apparatus [84–88]. Of note, regenerating myofibers can be also identified by the immunohistochemical detection of the embryonal myosin heavy chain (eMyHC) (Table 1). Indeed, it is well known that the embryonal isoform of the cytoskeletal protein, expressed during muscle development, can be transiently re-expressed in adult muscle upon injury. Newly formed myofibers express eMyHC within 2–3 days after damage and the embryonic protein can be detected for 2–3 weeks, being a robust marker of muscle regeneration [89].

The mature phenotype, which is successively finalized during the regenerative phase of maturation, can be then highlighted by the presence of markers including adult myosin heavy chain (MyHC) isoforms, conferring various contractile and metabolic properties to myofibers, enolase 3 (ENO3), and the muscle creatine kinase (MCK), pivotal components of terminally differentiated fibers [1,84,87].

2.3.2. The Role of "Non-Muscle" Stem Cells in Muscle Regeneration

It has been suggested that other stem cells and precursors, other than satellite cells, such as endothelial-associated cells [90], interstitial cells [91,92], bone marrow-derived side population [93,94], and fibroadipogenic progenitors (FAPs), can participate in muscle regeneration exerting a supportive role for SC activity [95]. These stem cell populations could either reside within muscle or be recruited via the circulation in response to homing signals emanating from the injured skeletal muscle. Among them FAPs, recognized as $CD45^{neg.}/CD31^{neg.}/\alpha7$-integrin$^{neg.}$ interstitial cells highly expressing Sca-1 expression [44] and PDGF receptor alpha (PDGF-R-alpha) [45], excited great interest, being involved in muscle regeneration and degeneration. Indeed, these mesenchymal progenitors are known to persist in an undifferentiated state in resting muscles, while under physiologic regenerative stimuli, FAPs undergo a transient expansion and produces paracrine factors promoting satellite cell-mediated regeneration [96]. A suite of recent findings clearly indicated that the cooperative activity of FAPs is required for muscle homeostasis and regeneration [97–99]. It has been reported that the inducible depletion of FAPs as well as the pharmacologic inhibition of their expansion in murine muscles resulted in a significant impairment of the healing process, affecting regenerative fibrogenesis and SC activity [97,98]. However, the physiologic action of FAPs is transient and finely regulated. These observations suggest that a qualitative microenvironment, generated by the balanced action of cellular and molecular players, is necessary to instruct stem cells to efficiently regenerate the injured tissue.

2.4. Tissue Remodelling and Maturation

In order to rebuild a functional muscle tissue, satellite cells and differentiating myoblasts need the structural and functional support of other cellular and molecular components. From a myogenic-centric point of view, an efficient muscle regeneration can be ratified by the formation and maturation of novel myofibers and/or the complete repair of damaged ones. This mark can be easily highlighted by the peripheralization of nuclei in mature myofibers (Figure 2). However, skeletal muscle is a multifaceted tissue with a complex cellular and molecular architecture, necessary for its functionality. Indeed, a complete muscle retrieval after injury requires the proper reconstitution of all the inner workings of the muscular machinery, namely extracellular matrix, vessels, and re-innervation. It is worth remembering that, during the degenerative and inflammatory phases following muscle injury, extracellular matrix (ECM), vascular network, and innervation undergo extensive degradation. The traumatic event, per se, can alter the ECM structure also damaging vasculature and nerves. Furthermore, several cell actors of muscle healing, including inflammatory cells and stem cells, can degrade matricellular proteins by secreting degrading agents such as metalloproteinases and elastase [100–102]. Since ECM is known to function as a scaffold to guide the formation of novel myofibers and neuromuscular junctions, the active deposition of matricellular components closely accompany muscle healing, and the remodelling of connective tissue, along with angiogenesis, defines the fourth stage of the regenerative process (Figure 1) [12,103,104]. The process starts with matrix deposition within a week post-injury, primarily due to the activity of fibroblasts in response to locally produced mediators such as TGF-β1 [105]. Although the fibrosis formation in case of self-healing injuries represents a beneficial response leading often to the efficient retrieval of muscle architecture, the overproduction of collagens within the injured area can lead to heavy scarring and the loss of muscular function.

The ECM is composed of specialized layers characterized by a variable composition of proteins, proteoglycans, and glycoproteins playing an integral role in structural support, force transmission, and regulation of the stem cell niche [46,106]. Thus, different collagen types can be labelled to evaluate the matrix composition and can be used as markers of connective tissue deposition. Indeed, although collagen I is the predominant type in the perimysium, the basement membrane is mainly comprised of laminin and collagen IV [47,48], whereas collagen I, III, and VI along with fibronectin in a proteoglycan-rich gel constitute the reticular lamina below the basement membrane (Table 1) [46–50]. The use of quantitative and qualitative high-magnification electron microscopy allowed the detailed description of the structure and composition of wild-type and fibrotic ECM. In particular, Gillies and colleagues not only clarified that collagen in the ECM is organized into large bundles of fibrils or cables but also reported that the number of the collagen cables were increased in fibrotic muscles [107]. Interestingly, since the increased number of cables but not the size was associated with an enhanced muscle stiffness, they suggested that alterations in fibrotic muscles can be related to the deregulated organization of ECM components and not only to the altered collagen content [107]. Despite the valuable and accurate results that can be obtained by using specific markers or imaging modalities, the restoration of the matrix or the excessive deposition of connective tissue can be revealed through a suite of standard histological techniques.

Trichrome staining has been frequently used to efficiently visualize connective tissue in muscle sections. The staining procedure is based on the combination of different dyes in a sequential manner. Acid fuchsin dye is used to stain muscle tissue, and although the dye can indiscriminately stain collagen, it can be removed from connective tissue by a polyacid of large molecular size such as phosphomolybdic acid. In addition, aniline blue can be used to stain collagens. Thus, in a standard Masson's Trichrome staining of muscle tissue, collagen appears blue, muscle tissue is stained red, and nuclei are stained dark brown thanks to the employment of the decolorization-resistant Weigert's hematoxylin [108].

Another sensitive method to perform qualitative and quantitative analysis of collagen network is Picrosirius red (F3BA) staining, developed by Junqueira and colleagues at the end of the 1970s [109]. The staining is based on the anionic properties of F3BA structure, which comprise sulfonate groups able to bind cationic collagen fibers, enhancing their natural birefringence under cross-polarized light [109–111]. Thus, under polarized light, collagen bundles stand out from the background appearing as green, red, or yellow. In particular, yellow-red birefringence has been associated with collagen type I bundles, whereas collagen type III has shown a weak birefringence and a green color [109–111]. Although the specificity of Picrosirius red for collagen types is controversial, this staining procedure is still considered one of the most powerful method to study and quantify collagen network [111,112].

2.5. Re-Innervation and Functional Recovery

The healing process is completed when regenerated myofibers rescue their functional performance and contractile apparatus (Figure 1). Thus, the regeneration of damaged muscles is only beneficial if the regenerated muscles become effectively innervated. Of note, this final stage of muscle regeneration must be also finely regulated. Interestingly, it has been demonstrated that, in addition to their specific role in the formation and/or repair of injured myofibers, satellite cells play a critical role in controlling myofiber innervation by upregulating the chemorepulsive semaphorin 3A expression [113]. Indeed, semaphorin 3A would prevent neuritogenesis when the regeneration of myofibers has not yet completed [113].

The first sign of a functional retrieval is the appearance of newly formed neuromuscular junctions (NMJs) between the surviving axons and the regenerated muscle fibers. The muscular terminal of NMJs can be visualized by labelling nicotinic acetylcholine receptor (nAChR) clusters on myofibers by using modified neurotoxins as probes (Table 1). In particular, α-Bungarotoxin (BTX), deriving from the venom of the banded krait, *Bungarus multicinctus*, showed the ability to bind the nAChR at the acetylcholine binding sites. Since the binding event occurs with high affinity and in a relatively irreversible manner, fluorescent α-bungarotoxin conjugates are valuable tools to localize and morphometrically analyze

NMJs [51]. Furthermore, α-BTX staining can be combined with immunolabeling of presynaptic vesicle proteins such as synaptophysin and syntaxin. Indeed, the exact overlay of BTX-derived fluorescence with the signal derived from the staining of presynaptic proteins can be considered an index of NMJ innervation [51,114]. Furthermore, it has been reported that the NMJ functionality can be indirectly evaluated through dual ex vivo electrical stimulation. In particular, we recently described an experimental protocol combining the direct electrical stimulation of muscle membrane and the stimulation through the nerve. Although the technique cannot be used to reveal morphological changes or biochemical changes in NMJs, the comparison of the muscle response to the two different stimulations can provide sensible indications about alterations in the NMJ functionality [115].

Electrical stimulations can be applied to freshly isolated muscles to evaluate the isometric contractile properties of the regenerated tissue [11,115–117]. Indeed, the recovery of the physiologic force-generating capability represents the most robust indicator of the effective muscle recovery after damage.

3. The Dynamic and the Regulation of Regenerative Phases are Altered in Pathologic Conditions: The Case of Muscular Dystrophy

The physiologic sequence of reparative phases, upon muscle injury, generally leads to the complete rescue of tissue morpho-functional properties. Unfortunately, the endogenous regenerative potential of skeletal muscle is not always sufficient to guarantee tissue restoration and/or maintenance. Pathologic conditions, including muscular dystrophies, are known to raise alterations in the dynamic and efficiency of regenerative steps. For this reason, complementary to physiologic regeneration, valuable information to clarify regenerative mechanisms can derive from models in which tissue healing is compromised because of cell-intrinsic and extrinsic defects. A well-characterized model of muscle wasting and regenerative impairment is the dystrophic mdx mouse, a classical model of Duchenne Muscular Dystrophy (DMD) pathology [118]. DMD is a degenerative disease in which the absence of the dystrophin protein leads to sarcolemma instability and fragility. The genetic defect is associated with the extensive damage of myofibers upon contraction which cannot be rescued by newly regenerated myotubes, being itself dystrophin deficient. This means that the degenerative stage of muscle healing, which is generally restricted to the first day after injury in wild-type mouse models, persists in dystrophic muscles throughout the necrotic stage of the pathology (mainly from 3 to 6 weeks of age) [119]. In this stage, EBD-injected mdx mice show high muscle permeability and dye uptake within damaged myofibers [11,120,121]. This is also associated with a sensible increase of serum CK and circulating myomiRs, further confirming the intense muscle damage in dystrophic muscle [11,120,122–128].

The continuous degeneration of dystrophin-deficient fibers represents a persistent stimulus to both inflammation and regeneration, thus inducing the alteration of the dynamic of both the inflammatory and regenerative stages. Indeed, it has been extensively described that dystrophic muscles are chronically dominated by inflammation, which can induce muscle fiber death through NO-mediated and perforin-dependent/independent mechanisms, respectively [68,119,129,130]. In accordance, Wehling and colleagues observed an improved membrane integrity upon antibody depletion of macrophages [131]. On the other hand, it has been recently reported that the local and transient depletion of macrophages in dystrophic muscle affected the balance between SC proliferation and differentiation, associated with defects in the formation of mature myofibers, inducing an exacerbation of the dystrophic phenotype [132]. Conflicting results can be associated with the technical approaches used in the studies, with reference to the persistence of the depletion and the stage of pathology in which the intervention acted. Indeed, Wehling and colleagues treated mdx mice with an anti-F4/80 antibody beginning at 1 week of age and continuing to 4 weeks of age, whereas Madaro and coworkers acted during the regenerative stage of the disease, that peaks between 9 to 12 weeks of age in mdx mice [131–133]. These observations, conflicting at first glance, provided intriguing insights about the complex impact of inflammatory events on the different stages of muscle regeneration. Thus, a better understanding of the inflammatory process in the dystrophic muscle and of the mediators involved might open novel therapeutic perspectives.

Inflammatory cells are responsible for the secretion not only of trophic factors but also of elevated levels of inflammatory mediators, influencing SC behavior. Among them, the enhanced expression of IL-6 is thought be involved in the alteration of the muscle stem cell pool by promoting the proliferation of SCs and the impairment of myoblast differentiation [11,134,135]. Interestingly, blockade of IL6 activity, using a neutralizing antibody against the IL6 receptor, conferred robustness to dystrophic muscle, impeded the activation of a chronic inflammatory response, significantly reduced necrosis, and activated the circuitry of muscle differentiation and maturation. This resulted in a functional homeostatic maintenance of dystrophic muscle. [121,136].

It is also worth to report that, in addition to maladaptive environmental signals, the altered SC behavior can be intrinsically dictated by the absence of dystrophin protein, since a defective compartmentalization of factors during asymmetric division in dystrophin deficient SCs can alter the daughter cell fate [40].

In addition, the delicate interaction between FAPs and SCs is altered in dystrophic muscles. FAPs desist from their supportive role and turn into fibro-adipocytes, which mediate fat deposition and fibrosis, contributing to the exacerbation of the dystrophic hostile microenvironment [44].

A recent study also uncovers the Wingless-related integration site (WNT)/GSK3/β-catenin axis as a new and previously unexplored pathway contributing to control FAP adipogenesis and muscle fatty degeneration, thus contributing to develop strategy to counteract intramuscular fat infiltrations in myopathies [137].

The persistence of degeneration, chronic inflammation, and defective myogenesis contribute to the alteration of the final phases of muscle healing in dystrophic muscles, resulting in the continuous attempt of defective regeneration. Altogether, these alterations lead to the progressive exhaustion of the SC pool, to accumulation of fatty/fibrotic tissue, and thus to the loss of muscle mass and functionality.

4. Technical Approaches to Induce Experimental Muscle Damage and Regeneration

The adaptative response of skeletal muscle to damage can differ in relation with the type of insult, and this is exactly coherent with the elevated plasticity of skeletal muscle tissue. Indeed, although the phases of muscle regeneration are closely interrelated and their time-dependent sequence is highly conserved in different vertebrates, the kinetic and amplitude of these procedural steps can vary depending on the organism or the extent/quality of damaging events. Indeed, a traumatic event can lead to the lesion of a single myofiber or of a localized segment of a fascicle. Furthermore, an insult can induce the degeneration of an entire fiber or can pertain to a number of myofibers dispersed throughout uninjured tissue [138,139]. Furthermore, an increasing body of evidence suggests that the events starting early after the injury profoundly influence the dynamic of tissue regeneration, affecting at various degree the different muscle components [140]. These heterogeneous events can contribute to the occurrence of doubts and difficulties in the field of clinical and experimental pathology [138]. Thus, a comprehensive understanding of the mechanisms underlining skeletal muscle adaptation to different insults can contribute to extending the current knowledge about muscle physiology and can allow the development of specific pro-regenerative therapies. To this aim, animal models of muscle injury represent a valuable and powerful tool to monitor and study muscle response to damage.

4.1. Models of Physical Injury

Murine models of acute muscle injury have been extensively studied to investigate molecular mechanisms underlining regenerative events characterizing each phase of muscle regeneration. Since the induction of an injurious assault is a prerequisite for muscle regeneration, with the necrotic phase being the first step of muscle restoration, the choice of a proper model of injury is critical for a correct interpretation of data and for the dissection of molecular mechanisms taking place in damaged muscles. A wealth of experimental procedures, adopted to induce muscle damage, have been developed and described over time, and qualitative/quantitative differences in the tissue response have been reported. Among them, the most commonly used methods are physical and chemical procedures. Most of the protocols of physical injury, which include freeze injury and crush models, are highly invasive and present technical complexities.

4.1.1. Freeze Injury

The freeze injury (FI) method mainly consists of a skin incision to expose the target muscle, and a single or repetitive action of freeze-thawing by applying for a prefixed time (10–15 s) a liquid nitrogen or dry ice cooled metallic rod [140–142]. Using this protocol, the operator can induce a diffuse necrosis in the treated muscle but the extent of muscle damage can vary not only depending on the number of freezing cycles but also with the pressure applied to the tissue with the cooled probe. The operator-dependent variability can limit the reproducibility of the data and the homogeneous use of the protocol in different laboratories. However, Hardy and colleagues, in a comparative study of muscle damage and repair, highlighted how the freeze-injury method induced a severe necrosis at the site of the lesion, destroying muscle cell components such as myofibers and satellite cells, along with basal lamina and vascular bed [140]. This can allow the study of the dynamics of infiltrating cells. Indeed, the region of damage, the so-called "dead zone", is well marked by the absence of viable cells, and the activation of regenerative events particularly requires the migration inside the lesion not only of inflammatory cells and non-myogenic supportive cells but also of myogenic progenitors [142]. Thus, viable cells infiltrating the lesion are easily identifiable since they appeared as directionally displaced from the spared tissue into the dead zone, allowing the dissection of regenerative events. In particular, the first invading population 18 h after FI is comprised of neutrophils and their presence is accompanied by an early increase of monocyte chemoattractant protein 1 (MCP-1) IL-6. The peak of expression of MCP-1 and IL-6 forewarns the second wave of cellular infiltration, characterized by F4/80[pos.] macrophages and myogenic cells, since both macrophages and muscle precursor cells express the CCR2 and are thus responsive to MCP-1 [141]. IL-6 is a pro-inflammatory cytokine with important regulatory actions on muscle stem cell functions; thus, the heightened expression of this pleiotropic factor can participate in both inflammatory and regenerative processes. This is consistent with the observation of a regenerative front of myoblasts at the periphery of the death zone at a few days after the neutrophilic peak since neutrophils are also a pivotal source of the soluble isoform of the IL-6 receptor alpha (IL6R) necessary to amplify IL-6 signal transduction [1,120,140,143]. Of note, the levels and activity of IL-6 must be finely tuned, since circulating levels of the proinflammatory cytokine IL-6 can also perturb the physiologic redox balance in skeletal muscle and can contribute to exacerbating muscle disease [143,144].

It is worth to report that the extent of tissue damage in FI model is highly elevated, and this event can profoundly affect the behavior of satellite cells from early after trauma. Indeed, it has been reported that there is a dramatic delay of satellite cells early after freeze injury (18 h), which has been quantified as about 90% of devoid cells compared to uninjured muscles. The regeneration of the damaged site is largely accomplished by progenitors deriving from outside the lesion; thus, the proliferation of SCs occurs days after damage and cycling SCs have been reported until one month after FI [140–142]. Although the histological retrieval of muscle architecture appeared complete one month after damage, the total number of SCs in FI mice returned to control levels three months after freezing.

The features of skeletal muscle response to FI were useful to study cellular actors of muscle regeneration and to clarify the involvement of the different cell populations. For instance, in 1986, Shultz and colleagues used the FI technique on the entire extensor digitorum longus (EDL) muscle to verify whether myogenic cells could migrate from adjacent muscles or could be delivered through the bloodstream [145]. Their results highlighted how muscle regeneration mainly depends on the activity of the local population of satellite cells [145]. Although extrinsic myogenic cells, such as migrating myoblasts and CD133[pos.] mononucleated cells identified in adult peripheral blood, can potentially reach the lesion, they would not be sufficient to regenerate the entire muscle [145,146].

4.1.2. Crush Injury and Ischemia-Reperfusion Damage

A muscle-crush injury occurs when high pressure is applied to skeletal muscle, which undergoes blood flow interruption, inducing the damage of myofibers. The combination of mechanical force and ischemia is known to cause an acute rhabdomyonecrosis since the profound alteration of the pressure balance can impair the volume regulation of myocytes, along with their permeability, leading to cell swelling [147].

Several experimental procedures have been developed over time to induce muscle-crush injury in rodents as a model of common trauma in humans and to study acute muscle inflammation and regeneration [148–153]. Among them, one of the most used is the opened model in which the muscle of the animal, generally the pelvic limb muscle, is surgically exposed and a force is applied by using a clamp.

Considering the invasiveness of the methodology and the needs of technical skills to perform the experiments guaranteeing the reproducibility of the data, closed noninvasive protocols have been tested. However, most of them involved dropping of weights upon the interested muscle region and such procedures can result in unwanted bone fractures. The fine-tuning of the procedure is still ongoing in order to minimize additional tissue damage induced by surgical interventions in opened models and to reduce the incidence of fractures due to dropping weights in closed models. For instance, Dobek and colleagues [148] proposed a sustained-force model of lower-extremity crush injury able to induce an acute inflammatory response, thereby reducing the extent of bone fractures. The proposed method, which has been described as a refinement of previous models, involved the use of a crush injury device platform. An air compressor activated a piston, situated in direct contact with the area to be injured, providing a contained force to the selected muscle. They reported that, although the force imposed was smaller than that applied in other studies (about 30 N in comparison with about 250 N), it was sufficient to induce muscle damage and the expected acute inflammatory response. Accordingly, it has been reported that a violent crush can destroy muscle tissue; however, even when the force is insufficient to directly wreck myofibers, the combination of mechanical force and ischemia will rapidly induce tissue degeneration [147]. Indeed, as a physiologic response to tissue injury, it has been reported that neutrophils, identified as 1A8, 7/4, and granulocyte antigen 1 (Gr1)-positive cells, rapidly invade the crushed muscle at the site of the lesion and then decreased from 24 to 48 h after injury [148]. CD68[pos.] and F4/80[pos.] macrophages followed the neutrophilic invasion increasing from 24 to 48 h after injury. However, it is plausible that the controlled force applied to the muscle would induce a mild tissue degeneration, useful to study the kinetic of inflammatory cell infiltration but probably with limitations regarding the study of regenerative events under critical conditions.

On the other hand, Criswell and colleagues [154] proposed and described a procedure of muscle crush in rats, which was able to induce tissue degeneration and to mimic the compartment syndrome (CS), a severe consequence of intense crush injuries frequently occurring in humans. Of note, the compartment syndrome occurs when the pressure within muscle fascicles dramatically increase due to posttraumatic ischemic swelling. This results in both ischemic and reperfusion insults, destroying the vasculature and the neural network and inducing the extensive necrosis of muscle tissue. In this protocol, a controlled compression of the rat hindlimb, proximal to the EDL muscle, has been cleverly obtained by using a neonatal blood pressure cuff in order to constantly maintain the pressure in a range of 120–140 mmHg for 3 h [154]. The persistent compression resulted in a composite injury of the muscular, vascular, and neural compartments. Tissue edema and disorganization were early observed 24 h after injury, and within the first 4 days, 50% of the muscle fibres underwent degeneration. Immune cell infiltration, as described in other models, occurred within 2 days after damage and persisted throughout the first week, with a peak at day four [154–156]. Following the acute inflammatory response, fibroblast and myofibroblast growth resulted in enhanced collagen deposition, also supporting the formation of newly regenerating fibers. Indeed, although early markers of satellite cell activation such as Pax7 and MyoD were observed early after damage (2 days), regenerating myofibers were detected 7 days after injury in correspondence with the phase of collagen deposition

(Figure 1) [154]. The extensive damage induced by muscle compression was also highlighted by signs of denervation, such as the dispersed localization of acetylcholine receptors around crushed myofibers and of vasculature alterations, including neo-angiogenesis preceded by the presence of enlarged vessels and hemorrhagic areas [154,156,157].

4.2. Chemical Damage Induced by Myotoxic Agents

The injection of myotoxic agents, such as the snake venom-derived toxins notexin or cardiotoxin, is one of the most frequently used methods to experimentally induce muscle damage and to study the subsequent regeneration. This is because the degeneration induced by these agents has been described as rapid, vigorous, and reproducible [139,158]. Moreover, venom toxins have been recognised as quite specific toxic agents on muscle fibers, without undermining blood vessels, basal lamina, and thus the activity of satellite cells [159–164]. This quite specific action can allow the dissection of regenerative events in a simplified model of muscle injury and study of the behavior of cellular actors and the profile of molecular players in muscle regeneration.

4.2.1. Cardiotoxin Injection

Cardiotoxins (CTX) are small polypeptides made of 60–63 amino acid residues acting as protein kinase C-specific inhibitor. Over 40 homologous cardiotoxins have been isolated and sequenced over time [165]. The purified toxin derived from the venom of the Indian cobra snake *Naja naja* or from the *Naja mossambica mossambica* is the most widely used myotoxic agent in protocols of experimental injury [140]. Although protocols can vary among laboratories, the method mainly consists of an intramuscular injection of about 20–50 µL of a 10 µM CTX working solution in sterile phosphate buffered saline (PBS). The most frequently treated muscles in murine models are hindlimb muscles such as the tibialis anterior muscle (TA) or gastrocnemius [140,166,167]. The myolytic activity of CTX involves the alteration of ion fluxes, induced by membrane depolarization, and is accompanied by the loss of protein content and organelle breakdown. Muscle degeneration occurs early after the injection, and the injured tissue is rapidly invaded by inflammatory mononucleated cells (Figure 2). Enlarged necrotic fibers in CTX-treated muscles are reached firstly by neutrophils and, later on, by macrophages which have been also described as penetrating swollen fibers [168]. Hardy and colleagues, in a benchmark work on different models of muscle injury, reported that the inflammatory response stimulated by CTX-induced necrosis was not exuberant, and it has been described that, although the kinetic of infiltrating cells is maintained, the phases are more defined and staggered if compared to other models of injury [140]. Furthermore, pro- and anti-inflammatory mediators, except for IL-6 levels showing a significant heightening, undergo a weak induction at early stages to then return to basal levels. The persistence of elevated levels of IL-6 have been detected one month after damage, possibly explaining the highly increased number of satellite cells in completely regenerated CTX-injected muscles [140]. It is worth to report that a significant myofiber hypertrophy and an increased muscle weight has been observed in muscle regenerated after CTX injection [167,169]. On the other hand, it has been postulated that CTX itself may have chemotactic properties enhancing both macrophages and satellite cell activity, thus inducing an early and efficient tissue regeneration [139,167]. Accordingly, newly regenerating myotubes with central nuclei can be observed 4 days after damage; 7 days after injury, the inflammatory response declines and the diameter of centrally nucleated fibers considerably increase [168]. Although it has been extensively described that CTX toxic action does not directly influence microvasculature, a complete destruction of the capillary network has been reported in a 3D study on CTX-injected muscles derived from Flk1$^{GFP/+}$ mice [140]. However, the initial vasculature breakdown was followed by active angiogenesis, and 1 month after the injection, the vessel network was restored [140]. The retrieval of a proper blood supply in injured muscle contributes to the efficient regeneration, without the occurrence of tissue fibrosis [164].

The ability of CTX to induce myofiber degeneration sparing the integrity of both basal lamina and satellite cells and thus inducing a controlled and rapid process of tissue reconstruction has been extensively used over time to study the role of molecular and cellular interactors in muscle regeneration. For instance, the specific action of cardiotoxin in inducing myofiber necrosis but not satellite cells (SCs) death in combination with a model of local Pax7[pos.] cell depletion contributed to clarifying the role of Pax7[pos.] cells in adult myogenesis [170]. Sambasivan and colleagues, inducing muscle damage in the presence or absence of satellite cells and monitoring the subsequent regenerative events, not only reported evidence about the essential role of SCs in skeletal muscle regeneration but also suggested the intriguing possibility that a threshold number of Pax7[pos.] cells would be required to obtain an efficient tissue reconstruction. This action would be associated not only with the proliferative rate of activated SCs but also with the potential ability of satellite cell to orchestrate the pro-regenerative action of non-myogenic cells in damaged muscle tissue. Furthermore, the cardiotoxin method was largely employed to dissect the action of inflammatory mediators in the stem cell niche after injury and to study the behaviour of satellite cell under pathologic conditions in which regeneration is known to be impaired [99,166,170–173].

4.2.2. Notexin Injection

Notexin (NTX) is a myotoxic agent contained in the venom of the *Notechis scutatus*, the Australian tiger snake, and has been described as having a more toxic effect than cardiotoxin (four times more toxic than CTX) [174]. This phospholipase A_2 presents an elevated myolytic impact, through the hydrolyzation of sarcolemma lipids, inducing the alteration of ionic fluxes, hypercontraction, and thus the degeneration of myofibers. Tissue insult provoked by notexin has been described as highly degenerative, causing myofiber breakdown and the loss of skeletal muscle functionality three days after the injection [175]. Moreover, a comparative study performed by Plant et al. reported that the maximum force of contraction recovered by notexin-injected muscles was reduced in comparison with other experimental models of muscle injury, with a percentage of force retrieval of only 10% seven days after damage and 39% after 10 days [175]. These data, along with the results from others benchmark studies, suggested that the extent and the modality of damage can influence the entity and the velocity of muscle recovery and thus the study of regenerative events [140,175–177]. For instance, myofiber regeneration, highlighted by the presence of centrally positioned nuclei, has been observed in the entire muscle injected with the toxin only 7 days after injury in contrast with the earlier observation reported in other models such as CTX-injury [140,167]. Despite the recognised action of notexin in inducing a generalized muscle damage, it is worth to report that fibers have a differential sensitivity to phospholipase A depending on the metabolism, with oxidative fibers showing an elevated susceptibility to NTX-induced damage [139].

Another important difference in the muscle response to notexin injection is the inflammatory response. Indeed, it has been described that there is a granulomatous inflammatory reaction to NTX-induced degeneration. Although the extensive necrosis produced by the myotoxic action of notexin did not activate an immediate inflammatory cell invasion, the immune response occurs with cell infiltration 4 days after damage. Instead of a typical kinetic of acute inflammatory response directed to the resolution, 12 days after injury in notexin-injected muscle, it was possible to observe multifocal calcium deposits, remains of necrotic myofibers, as a midpoint of a granulomatous reaction [140].

Interestingly, these chronically inflamed foci persist even when muscle tissue is quite completely regenerated 3–6 months after the experimental injury, potentially contributing to the establishment of an altered immune milieu. Furthermore, it has been reported that NTX can exert a neurotoxic action by blocking acetylcholine release, thereby altering the neuromuscular junctions, which must be restored for a functional tissue retrieval [178].

4.2.3. Bupivacaine Administration

Another agent used to induce reversible muscle damage with the purpose to study regenerative events is Bupivacaine (BPVC). Bupivacaine is a local anesthetic that, thanks to its highly lipophilic properties, can efficiently penetrate the sarcolemma. Although the precise mechanisms have to be fully clarified, it has been described that Bupivacaine can induce muscle degeneration by perturbing the homeostasis of mitochondria and sarcoplasmic reticulum (SR), producing a dramatic calcium efflux and a simultaneous block of calcium reuptake by the SR. This action results in the hypercontraction and rapid death of myofibers along with the mitochondria membrane depolarization and sarcoplasmic reticulum alterations, which can further induce muscle degeneration [116,179,180]. Despite the intense impact recognized on rat skeletal muscle which has been reported, Bupivacaine can induce only a faint degeneration when injected in murine muscles. Indeed, the degenerative potential of this anesthetic has been described as limited, if compared to notexin or cardiotoxin, since its injection causes the degeneration only of a 45 percentage of fibers [175]. In accordance with the low degree of muscle degeneration induced by Bupivacaine, it has been reported that the force-generating capability of injected muscle was reduced to 42% of control muscles three days after damage and that this impairment was quite completely restored ten days after the injection [175]. However, the analysis of injected muscle cross sections performed by Plant and colleagues revealed that bupivacaine can spread throughout the muscle, equally affecting both inner and peripheral regions of the muscle. In accordance with the low degree of muscle damage induced by BPVC in murine muscle, a rapid inflammatory response and regenerative phase has been described. Three days after the injection of 50–100 µL of 0.5% BPVC, a robust inflammatory infiltrate can be observed surrounding necrotic fibers, whereas small regenerating fibers appearing on day 5 seem to quite completely regenerate the lesion by day 14, when inflammatory cells are significantly reduced [181].

5. Conclusions

Muscle regeneration is one of the most important homeostatic processes of adult tissue and, as such, must be finely regulated to guarantee functional recovery and to avoid muscle alteration and diseases [182]. Skeletal muscle regeneration is a coordinate process in which several factors are sequentially activated to maintain and/or restore a proper muscle structure and function. Although the main actors of the entire process are satellite cells, a heterogenous group of other cells cooperate to reestablish muscle homeostasis after damage. Indeed, each stage of the stepwise muscle healing is dominated by a peculiar combination of cell agents and molecular signals playing a specific role in the complex framework of regeneration. However, the multifaceted nature of the regenerative process has to be still completely unveiled, and a number of pathologic conditions impairing muscle regeneration still lack an effective therapy. Thus, the comprehensive understanding of healing mechanisms still deserves further research to identify novel reliable biomarkers and to develop advanced techniques supporting the future innovation of regenerative studies.

Author Contributions: A.M. conceptualized the study; A.M. and L.F. wrote the original draft; L.F. and M.C. wrote/reviewed and edited the text and figures. All authors have read and agreed to the published version of the manuscript.

Acknowledgments: We apologize to colleagues whose studies were not cited. The authors are thankful to Carmine Nicoletti and Carmen Miano for technical support.

Abbreviations

AchR	Acetylcholine receptor
Activ.SCs	Activated SCs
ADAM	A Disintegrin and Metalloproteinase
ADAM8	A Disintegrin and Metalloproteinase Domain-Containing Protein 8
ADP	Adenosine diphosphate
ALB	Albumin
BPVC	Bupivacaine
BrdU	5-bromo-2′-deoxyuridine

BTX	α-Bungarotoxin
Cav1	Caveolin 1
CCR2	Chemokine Receptor type 2
CD11b	Cluster of Differentiation 11 b also known as Integrin Alpha M
CD133	Cluster of Differentiation 133
CD163	Cluster of Differentiation 163
CD206	Cluster of Differentiation 206 also known as Mannose receptor C-type 1
CD31	Cluster of Differentiation 31
CD34	Cluster of Differentiation 34
CD38	Cluster of Differentiation 38
CD45	Cluster of Differentiation 45
CD68	Cluster of Differentiation 68
CK	Creatine kinase
CK3 (CK-MM)	Creatine Kinase MM isoform
c-Met	Tyrosine-protein Kinase Met
c-Myc	MYC proto-oncogene, bHLH transcription factor
CS	Compartment Syndrome
CTR	Calcitonin Receptor
CTX	Cardiotoxin
CX3CR1	C-X3-C Motif Chemokine Receptor 1
CXCR4	C-X-C Chemokine Receptor type 4
DAMPs	Damage-Associated Molecular Patterns
DGC	Dystrophin-associated Glycoprotein Complex
Diff.SCs	Differentiating SCs
DMD	Duchenne Muscular Dystrophy
EBD	Evans Blue Dye
ECM	Extracellular Matrix
ED1	Monoclonal antibody staining a single chain glycoprotein of 110 kDa on the lysosomal membrane of myeloid cells, i.e., the majority of tissue macrophages (being the rat homologue of human CD68)
ED2	Monoclonal antibody reacting with a membrane antigen (175, 160, and 95 kDa) on resident rat macrophages such as monocytes and dendritic cells. ED2 discriminates between thymic cortical (positive for ED2) and medullary (negative for ED2) macrophages. The antigen is identical with CD163.
ED3	Monoclonal antibody recognizing the rat CD169 cell surface antigen, a 185 kDa molecule expressed by macrophages in lymphoid organs (no monocytes or granulocytes). In the thymus, the antigen is expressed on clusters of dendritic cells (thymic nurse cells or TNC's) in the (outer) cortex.
EDL	Extensor Digitorum Longus
EdU	5-ethynyl-2'-deoxyuridine
Egr2	Early growth response protein 2
eMyHC	embryonal Myosin Heavy Chain
ENO3	Enolase 3
F3BA	Picrosirius red
F4/80	Mouse macrophage marker. Also known as Ly71 and EMR1, the F4/80 antigen is part of the EGF-TM7 family.
FACS	Fluorescence-Activated Cell Sorting
FAPs	Fibroadipogenic Progenitors
FI	Freeze Injury
FoxK	Forkhead box protein K
Fpr2	Formyl peptide receptor 2
Gpr18	G-protein coupled receptor 18
Gr1	Granulocyte antigen 1
GSK3	Glycogen Synthase Kinase 3
H&E	Haematoxylin and Eosin staining

H2O2	Hydrogen peroxide
Hey1	Hairy/enhancer-of-split related with YRPW motif protein 1
Heyl	Hairy/enhancer-of-split related with YRPW motif protein l
IFN-β	Interferon-β
IFN-γ	Interferon-γ
IGF-1	Insulin-like Growth Factor 1
IgG	Immunoglobulin G
IL-1	Interleukin 1
IL-1β	Interleukin-1β
IL-4	Interleukin 4
IL-6	Interleukin 6
IL6R	IL-6 receptor alpha
IL-8	Interleukin 8;
Ki-67 protein (also known as MKI67)	marker of proliferation KI-67
LDH	Lactate Dehydrogenase
Ly6C	Lymphocyte antigen 6 complex, locus C
Ly6G	Lymphocyte antigen 6 complex, locus G
Ly6G-PA-GFP	Ly6Gpos. cells with a photoactivatable GFP
MAC	Macrophages
Mcad	M-cadherin
MCK	Muscle Creatine Kinase
MCP-1	Monocyte Chemoattractant Protein 1
MFs	Myogenic Factors
MyHC	Myosin Heavy Chain
miRNAs	microRNAs
MPO	Myeloperoxidase
Mrf4	Myogenic regulatory factor 4
Myf-5	Myogenic factor 5
MyoD	Myoblast determination protein
myomiRs	microRNAs involved in the regulation of myocellular processes
nAChR	nicotinic Acetylcholine Receptor
NCAM	Neural Cell Adhesion Molecule
NEU	Neutrophils
NMJs	Neuromuscular Junctions
NTX	Notexin
P38 MAP kinases	P38 mitogen-activated protein kinases
Pax3	Paired box transcription factor 3
Pax7	Paired box transcription factor 7
PBS	Phosphate Buffered Saline
PCNA	Proliferating Cell Nuclear Antigen
PDGF-R-alpha	Platelet derived growth factor receptor alpha
Prolif.SCs	Proliferating SCs
Sca-1	Stem cell antigen-1
SCs	Satellite Cells
sIL6R	soluble Interleukin-6 Receptor alpha
Sox 15	SRY-Box Transcription Factor 15
Sox 8	SRY-Box Transcription Factor 8
TA	Tibialis Anterior muscle
Ter 119 or Ly76	Lymphocyte antigen-76
TGFβ	Transforming Growth Factor beta
TNF-α	Tumor Necrosis Factor alpha
VCAM1	Vascular Cell Adhesion protein 1
WNT	Wingless-related integration site

References

1. Forcina, L.; Miano, C.; Pelosi, L.; Musarò, A. An Overview About the Biology of Skeletal Muscle Satellite Cells. *Curr. Genom.* **2019**, *20*, 24–37. [CrossRef]
2. Seale, P.; Sabourin, L.A.; Girgis-Gabardo, A.; Mansouri, A.; Gruss, P.; Rudnicki, M.A. Pax7 is required for the specification of myogenic satellite cells. *Cell* **2000**, *102*, 777–786. [CrossRef]
3. Blaauw, B.; Reggiani, C. The role of satellite cells in muscle hypertrophy. *J. Muscle Res. Cell Motil.* **2014**, *35*, 3–10. [CrossRef] [PubMed]
4. Yao, L.; Xue, X.; Yu, P.; Ni, Y.; Chen, F. Evans Blue Dye: A Revisit of Its Applications in Biomedicine. *Contrast Media Mol. Imaging* **2018**, *2018*, 18–24. [CrossRef] [PubMed]
5. Straub, V.; Rafael, J.A.; Chamberlain, J.S.; Campbell, K.P. Animal models for muscular dystrophy show different patterns of sarcolemmal disruption. *J. Cell Biol.* **1997**, *139*, 375–385. [CrossRef] [PubMed]
6. Feng, Y.; Chen, F.; Ma, Z.; Dekeyzer, F.; Yu, J.; Xie, Y.; Cona, M.M.; Oyen, R.; Ni, Y. Towards stratifying ischemic components by cardiac MRI and multifunctional stainings in a rabbit model of myocardial infarction. *Theranostics* **2014**, *4*, 24–35. [CrossRef]
7. Cona, M.M.; Koole, M.; Feng, Y.; Liu, Y.; Verbruggen, A.; Oyen, R.; Ni, Y. Biodistribution and radiation dosimetry of radioiodinated hypericin as a cancer therapeutic. *Int. J. Oncol.* **2014**, *44*, 819–829. [CrossRef] [PubMed]
8. Klyen, B.R.; Shavlakadze, T.; Radley-Crabb, H.G.; Grounds, M.D.; Sampson, D.D. Identification of muscle necrosis in the mdx mouse model of Duchenne muscular dystrophy using three-dimensional optical coherence tomography. *J. Biomed. Opt.* **2011**, *16*, 076013. [CrossRef]
9. Wooddell, C.I.; Zhang, G.; Griffin, J.B.; Hegge, J.O.; Huss, T.; Wolff, J.A. Use of Evans blue dye to compare limb muscles in exercised young and old mdx mice. *Muscle Nerve* **2010**, *41*, 487–499. [CrossRef]
10. Hamer, P.W.; McGeachie, J.M.; Davies, M.J.; Grounds, M.D. Evans Blue Dye as an in vivo marker of myofibre damage: Optimising parameters for detecting initial myofibre membrane permeability. *J. Anat.* **2002**, *200*, 69–79. [CrossRef]
11. Pelosi, L.; Berardinelli, M.G.; Forcina, L.; Spelta, E.; Rizzuto, E.; Nicoletti, C.; Camilli, C.; Testa, E.; Catizone, A.; De Benedetti, F.; et al. Increased levels of interleukin-6 exacerbate the dystrophic phenotype in mdx mice. *Hum. Mol. Genet.* **2015**, *24*, 6041–6053. [CrossRef] [PubMed]
12. Musarò, A. The Basis of Muscle Regeneration. *Adv. Biol.* **2014**, *2014*, 1–16. [CrossRef]
13. Matsuda, R.; Nishikawa, A.; Tanaka, H. Visualization of dystrophic muscle fibers in mdx mouse by vital staining with evans blue: Evidence of apoptosis in dystrophin-deficient muscle. *J. Biochem.* **1995**, *118*, 959–963. [CrossRef] [PubMed]
14. Wang, H.L.; Lai, T.W. Optimization of Evans blue quantitation in limited rat tissue samples. *Sci. Rep.* **2014**, *4*, 1–7. [CrossRef] [PubMed]
15. Morgan, J.E.; Prola, A.; Mariot, V.; Pini, V.; Meng, J.; Hourde, C.; Dumonceaux, J.; Conti, F.; Relaix, F.; Authier, F.J.; et al. Necroptosis mediates myofibre death in dystrophin-deficient mice. *Nat. Commun.* **2018**, *9*, 3655. [CrossRef]
16. Brancaccio, P.; Lippi, G.; Maffulli, N. Biochemical markers of muscular damage. *Clin. Chem. Lab. Med.* **2010**, *48*, 757–767. [CrossRef]
17. Komulainen, J.; Kytola, J.; Vihko, V. Running-induced muscle injury and myocellular enzyme release in rats. *J. Appl. Physiol.* **1994**, *77*, 2299–2304. [CrossRef]
18. Siracusa, J.; Koulmann, N.; Bourdon, S.; Goriot, M.E.; Banzet, S. Circulating miRNAs as Biomarkers of Acute Muscle Damage in Rats. *Am. J. Pathol.* **2016**, *186*, 1313–1327. [CrossRef]
19. Nishimura, D.; Sakai, H.; Sato, T.; Sato, F.; Nishimura, S.; Toyama-Sorimachi, N.; Bartsch, J.W.; Sehara-Fujisawa, A. Roles of ADAM8 in elimination of injured muscle fibers prior to skeletal muscle regeneration. *Mech. Dev.* **2015**, *135*, 58–67. [CrossRef]
20. Wang, J. Neutrophils in tissue injury and repair. *Cell Tissue Res.* **2018**, *371*, 531–539. [CrossRef]
21. Yang, W.; Hu, P. Skeletal muscle regeneration is modulated by inflammation. *J. Orthop. Transl.* **2018**, *13*, 25–32. [CrossRef] [PubMed]
22. Geissmann, F.; Jung, S.; Littman, D.R. Blood monocytes consist of two principal subsets with distinct migratory properties. *Immunity* **2003**, *19*, 71–82. [CrossRef]

23. Nahrendorf, M.; Swirski, F.K.; Aikawa, E.; Stangenberg, L.; Wurdinger, T.; Figueiredo, J.L.; Libby, P.; Weissleder, R.; Pittet, M.J. The healing myocardium sequentially mobilizes two monocyte subsets with divergent and complementary functions. *J. Exp. Med.* **2007**, *204*, 3037–3047. [CrossRef] [PubMed]

24. Kratofil, R.M.; Kubes, P.; Deniset, J.F. Monocyte Conversion During Inflammation and Injury. *Arterioscler. Thromb. Vasc. Biol.* **2017**, *37*, 35–42. [CrossRef] [PubMed]

25. Orekhov, A.N.; Orekhova, V.A.; Nikiforov, N.G.; Myasoedova, V.A.; Grechko, A.V.; Romanenko, E.B.; Zhang, D.; Chistiakov, D.A. Monocyte differentiation and macrophage polarization. *Vessel Plus* **2019**, *3*, 10. [CrossRef]

26. Jetten, N.; Verbruggen, S.; Gijbels, M.J.; Post, M.J.; De Winther, M.P.J.; Donners, M.M.P.C. Anti-inflammatory M2, but not pro-inflammatory M1 macrophages promote angiogenesis in vivo. *Angiogenesis* **2014**, *17*, 109–118. [CrossRef]

27. Jablonski, K.A.; Amici, S.A.; Webb, L.M.; de Dios Ruiz-Rosado, J.; Popovich, P.G.; Partida-Sanchez, S.; Guerau-de-Arellano, M. Novel Markers to Delineate Murine M1 and M2 Macrophages. *PLoS ONE* **2015**, *10*, e0145342. [CrossRef] [PubMed]

28. Kastenschmidt, J.M.; Avetyan, I.; Armando Villalta, S. Characterization of the inflammatory response in dystrophic muscle using flow cytometry. In *Methods in Molecular Biology*; Humana Press: New York, NY, USA, 2018; pp. 43–56. [CrossRef]

29. Crane, M.J.; Daley, J.M.; van Houtte, O.; Brancato, S.K.; Henry, W.L.; Albina, J.E. The Monocyte to Macrophage Transition in the Murine Sterile Wound. *PLoS ONE* **2014**, *9*, e86660. [CrossRef]

30. Gnocchi, V.F.; White, R.B.; Ono, Y.; Ellis, J.A.; Zammit, P.S. Further Characterisation of the Molecular Signature of Quiescent and Activated Mouse Muscle Satellite Cells. *PLoS ONE* **2009**, *4*, e5205. [CrossRef]

31. Fukada, S.I.; Yamaguchi, M.; Kokubo, H.; Ogawa, R.; Uezumi, A.; Yoneda, T.; Matev, M.M.; Motohashi, N.; Ito, T.; Zolkiewska, A.; et al. Hesr1 and Hesr3 are essential to generate undifferentiated quiescent satellite cells and to maintain satellite cell numbers. *Development* **2011**, *138*, 4609–4619. [CrossRef]

32. Maesner, C.C.; Almada, A.E.; Wagers, A.J. Established cell surface markers efficiently isolate highly overlapping populations of skeletal muscle satellite cells by fluorescence-activated cell sorting. *Skelet. Muscle* **2016**, *6*, 35. [CrossRef] [PubMed]

33. Relaix, F.; Montarras, D.; Zaffran, S.; Gayraud-Morel, B.; Rocancourt, D.; Tajbakhsh, S.; Mansouri, A.; Cumano, A.; Buckingham, M. Pax3 and Pax7 have distinct and overlapping functions in adult muscle progenitor cells. *J. Cell Biol.* **2006**, *172*, 91–102. [CrossRef] [PubMed]

34. Mechtersheimer, G.; Staudter, M.; Möller, P. Expression of the natural killer cell-associated antigens CD56 and CD57 in human neural and striated muscle cells and in their tumors. *Cancer Res.* **1991**, *51*, 1300–1307. [PubMed]

35. Tatsumi, R.; Anderson, J.E.; Nevoret, C.J.; Halevy, O.; Allen, R.E. HGF/SF is present in normal adult skeletal muscle and is capable of activating satellite cells. *Dev. Biol.* **1998**, *194*, 114–128. [CrossRef]

36. Jesse, T.L.; LaChance, R.; Iademarco, M.F.; Dean, D.C. Interferon regulatory factor-2 is a transcriptional activator in muscle where it regulates expression of vascular cell adhesion molecule-1. *J. Cell Biol.* **1998**, *140*, 1265–1276. [CrossRef]

37. Cornelison, D.D.W.; Filla, M.S.; Stanley, H.M.; Rapraeger, A.C.; Olwin, B.B. Syndecan-3 and syndecan-4 specifically mark skeletal muscle satellite cells and are implicated in satellite cell maintenance and muscle regeneration. *Dev. Biol.* **2001**, *239*, 79–94. [CrossRef]

38. Sherwood, R.I.; Christensen, J.L.; Conboy, I.M.; Conboy, M.J.; Rando, T.A.; Weissman, I.L.; Wagers, A.J. Isolation of adult mouse myogenic progenitors: Functional heterogeneity of cells within and engrafting skeletal muscle. *Cell* **2004**, *119*, 543–554. [CrossRef]

39. Volonte, D.; Liu, Y.; Galbiati, F. The modulation of caveolin-1 expression controls satellite cell activation during muscle repair. *FASEB J.* **2005**, *19*, 1–36. [CrossRef]

40. Chang, N.C.; Sincennes, M.C.; Chevalier, F.P.; Brun, C.E.; Lacaria, M.; Segalés, J.; Muñoz-Cánoves, P.; Ming, H.; Rudnicki, M.A. The Dystrophin Glycoprotein Complex Regulates the Epigenetic Activation of Muscle Stem Cell Commitment. *Cell Stem Cell* **2018**, *22*, 755.e6–768.e6. [CrossRef]

41. Relaix, F.; Zammit, P.S. Satellite cells are essential for skeletal muscle regeneration: The cell on the edge returns centre stage. *Development* **2012**, *139*, 2845–2856. [CrossRef]

42. Chen, J.F.; Mandel, E.M.; Thomson, J.M.; Wu, Q.; Callis, T.E.; Hammond, S.M.; Conlon, F.L.; Wang, D.Z. The role of microRNA-1 and microRNA-133 in skeletal muscle proliferation and differentiation. *Nat. Genet.* **2006**, *38*, 228–233. [CrossRef] [PubMed]

43. Hak, K.K.; Yong, S.L.; Sivaprasad, U.; Malhotra, A.; Dutta, A. Muscle-specific microRNA miR-206 promotes muscle differentiation. *J. Cell Biol.* **2006**, *174*, 677–687. [CrossRef]

44. Uezumi, A.; Fukada, S.I.; Yamamoto, N.; Takeda, S.; Tsuchida, K. Mesenchymal progenitors distinct from satellite cells contribute to ectopic fat cell formation in skeletal muscle. *Nat. Cell Biol.* **2010**, *12*, 143–152. [CrossRef] [PubMed]

45. Mutsaers, S.E.; Bishop, J.E.; McGrouther, G.; Laurent, G.J. Mechanisms of tissue repair: From wound healing to fibrosis. *Int. J. Biochem. Cell Biol.* **1997**, *29*, 5–17. [CrossRef]

46. Dunn, A.; Marcinczyk, M.; Talovic, M.; Patel, K.; Haas, G.; Garg, K. Role of Stem Cells and Extracellular Matrix in the Regeneration of Skeletal Muscle. In *Muscle Cell and Tissue—Current Status of Research Field*; Sakuma, P.K., Ed.; InTechOpen: London, UK, 2018.

47. Gillies, A.R.; Lieber, R.L. Structure and function of the skeletal muscle extracellular matrix. *Muscle Nerve* **2011**, *44*, 318–331. [CrossRef]

48. Kjær, M. Role of Extracellular Matrix in Adaptation of Tendon and Skeletal Muscle to Mechanical Loading. *Physiol. Rev.* **2004**, *84*, 649–698. [CrossRef]

49. Garg, K.; Boppart, M.D. Influence of exercise and aging on extracellular matrix composition in the skeletal muscle stem cell niche. *J. Appl. Physiol.* **2016**, *121*, 1053–1058. [CrossRef]

50. Sanes, J.R. The basement membrane/basal lamina of skeletal muscle. *J. Biol. Chem.* **2003**, *278*, 12601–12604. [CrossRef]

51. Tu, H.; Zhang, D.; Corrick, R.M.; Muelleman, R.L.; Wadman, M.C.; Li, Y.L. Morphological regeneration and functional recovery of neuromuscular junctions after tourniquet-induced injuries in mouse hindlimb. *Front. Physiol.* **2017**, *8*, 207. [CrossRef]

52. Kirby, T.J.; Chaillou, T.; McCarthy, J.J. The role of microRNAs in skeletal muscle health and disease. *Front. Biosci. (Landmark Ed.)* **2016**, *20*, 37–77.

53. Pelosi, L.; Coggi, A.; Forcina, L.; Musarò, A. MicroRNAs modulated by local mIGF-1 expression in mdx dystrophic mice. *Front. Aging Neurosci.* **2015**, *7*, 69. [CrossRef] [PubMed]

54. Yang, Y.; Jiang, G.; Zhang, P.; Fan, J. Programmed cell death and its role in inflammation. *Mil. Med. Res.* **2015**, *2*, 12. [CrossRef] [PubMed]

55. Roh, J.S.; Sohn, D.H. Damage-associated molecular patterns in inflammatory diseases. *Immune Netw.* **2018**, *18*, e27. [CrossRef] [PubMed]

56. Grounds, M. Phagocytosis of necrotic muscle in muscle isografts is influenced by the strain age and sex of host mice. *J. Pathol.* **1987**, *153*, 71–82. [CrossRef]

57. Tidball, J.G.; Wehling-Henricks, M. Macrophages promote muscle membrane repair and muscle fibre growth and regeneration during modified muscle loading in mice in vivo. *J. Physiol.* **2007**, *578*, 327–336. [CrossRef]

58. Summan, M.; Warren, G.L.; Mercer, R.R.; Chapman, R.; Hulderman, T.; Van Rooijen, N.; Simeonova, P.P. Macrophages and skeletal muscle regeneration: A clodronate-containing liposome depletion study. *Am. J. Physiol. Regul. Integr. Comp. Physiol.* **2006**, *290*, R1488–R1495. [CrossRef]

59. Tidball, J.G. Inflammatory processes in muscle injury and repair. *Am. J. Physiol. Regul. Integr. Comp. Physiol.* **2005**, *288*, R345–R353. [CrossRef]

60. Teixeira, C.F.P.; Zamunér, S.R.; Zuliani, J.P.; Fernandes, C.M.; Cruz-Hofling, M.A.; Fernandes, I.; Chaves, F.; Gutiérrez, J.M. Neutrophils do not contribute to local tissue damage, but play a key role in skeletal muscle regeneration, in mice injected with Bothrops asper snake venom. *Muscle Nerve* **2003**, *28*, 449–459. [CrossRef]

61. Frenette, J.; Cai, B.; Tidball, J.G. Complement activation promotes muscle inflammation during modified muscle use. *Am. J. Pathol.* **2000**, *156*, 2103–2110. [CrossRef]

62. Kishimoto, T.K.; Rothlein, R. Integrins, ICAMs, and Selectins: Role and Regulation of Adhesion Molecules in Neutrophil Recruitment to Inflammatory Sites. *Adv. Pharmacol.* **1994**, *25*, 117–169. [CrossRef]

63. Muller, W.A. Leukocyte-endothelial-cell interactions in leukocyte transmigration and the inflammatory response. *Trends Immunol.* **2003**, *24*, 326–333. [CrossRef]

64. Walzog, B.; Gaehtgens, P. Adhesion Molecules: The Path to a New Understanding of Acute Inflammation. *News Physiol. Sci.* **2000**, *15*, 107–113. [CrossRef] [PubMed]

65. Sixt, M.; Hallmann, R.; Wendler, O.; Scharffetter-Kochanek, K.; Sorokin, L.M. Cell adhesion and migration properties of β2-integrin negative polymorphonuclear granulocytes on defined extracellular matrix molecules: Relevance for leukocyte extravasation. *J. Biol. Chem.* **2001**, *276*, 18878–18887. [CrossRef] [PubMed]

66. Pizza, F.X.; Peterson, J.M.; Baas, J.H.; Koh, T.J. Neutrophils contribute to muscle injury and impair its resolution after lengthening contractions in mice. *J. Physiol.* **2005**, *562*, 899–913. [CrossRef]

67. Chazaud, B.; Brigitte, M.; Yacoub-Youssef, H.; Arnold, L.; Gherardi, R.; Sonnet, C.; Lafuste, P.; Chretien, F. Dual and beneficial roles of macrophages during skeletal muscle regeneration. *Exerc. Sport Sci. Rev.* **2009**, *37*, 18–22. [CrossRef]

68. Villalta, S.A.; Nguyen, H.X.; Deng, B.; Gotoh, T.; Tidball, J.G. Shifts in macrophage phenotypes and macrophage competition for arginine metabolism affect the severity of muscle pathology in muscular dystrophy. *Hum. Mol. Genet.* **2009**, *18*, 482–496. [CrossRef]

69. McLennan, I.S. Resident macrophages (ED2- and ED3-positive) do not phagocytose degenerating rat skeletal muscle fibres. *Cell Tissue Res.* **1993**, *272*, 193–196. [CrossRef] [PubMed]

70. Arnold, L.; Henry, A.; Poron, F.; Baba-Amer, Y.; Van Rooijen, N.; Plonquet, A.; Gherardi, R.K.; Chazaud, B. Inflammatory monocytes recruited after skeletal muscle injury switch into antiinflammatory macrophages to support myogenesis. *J. Exp. Med.* **2007**, *204*, 1057–1069. [CrossRef]

71. Silva, M.T. When two is better than one: Macrophages and neutrophils work in concert in innate immunity as complementary and cooperative partners of a myeloid phagocyte system. *J. Leukoc. Biol.* **2010**, *87*, 93–106. [CrossRef]

72. Kolaczkowska, E.; Kubes, P. Neutrophil recruitment and function in health and inflammation. *Nat. Rev. Immunol.* **2013**, *13*, 159–175. [CrossRef]

73. Nourshargh, S.; Alon, R. Leukocyte Migration into Inflamed Tissues. *Immunity* **2014**, *41*, 694–707. [CrossRef] [PubMed]

74. Wang, C.; Yue, F.; Kuang, S. Muscle Histology Characterization Using H&E Staining and Muscle Fiber Type Classification Using Immunofluorescence Staining. *Bio Protoc.* **2017**, *7*, e2279. [CrossRef]

75. Soehnlein, O.; Lindbom, L. Phagocyte partnership during the onset and resolution of inflammation. *Nat. Rev. Immunol.* **2010**, *10*, 427–439. [CrossRef] [PubMed]

76. Tonkin, J.; Temmerman, L.; Sampson, R.D.; Gallego-Colon, E.; Barberi, L.; Bilbao, D.; Schneider, M.D.; Musarò, A.; Rosenthal, N. Monocyte/macrophage-derived IGF-1 orchestrates murine skeletal muscle regeneration and modulates autocrine polarization. *Mol. Ther.* **2015**, *23*, 1189–1200. [CrossRef] [PubMed]

77. Mauro, A. Satellite cell of skeletal muscle fibers. *J. Biophys. Biochem. Cytol.* **1961**, *9*, 493–495. [CrossRef] [PubMed]

78. Scharner, J.; Zammit, P.S. The muscle satellite cell at 50: The formative years. *Skelet. Muscle* **2011**, *1*, 28. [CrossRef] [PubMed]

79. Creuzet, S.; Lescaudron, L.; Li, Z.; Fontaine-Pérus, J. MyoD, myogenin, and desmin-nls-lacZ transgene emphasize the distinct patterns of satellite cell activation in growth and regeneration. *Exp. Cell Res.* **1998**, *243*, 241–253. [CrossRef] [PubMed]

80. Yablonka-Reuveni, Z.; Rivera, A.J. Temporal expression of regulatory and structural muscle proteins during myogenesis of satellite cells on isolated adult rat fibers. *Dev. Biol.* **1994**, *164*, 588–603. [CrossRef]

81. Scholzen, T.; Gerdes, J. The Ki-67 protein: From the known and the unknown. *J. Cell. Physiol.* **2000**, *182*, 311–322. [CrossRef]

82. Mead, T.J.; Lefebvre, V. Proliferation assays (BrdU and EdU) on skeletal tissue sections. *Methods Mol. Biol.* **2014**, *1130*, 233–243. [CrossRef]

83. Ikeda, T.; Ichii, O.; Otsuka-Kanazawa, S.; Nakamura, T.; Elewa, Y.H.A.; Kon, Y. Degenerative and regenerative features of myofibers differ among skeletal muscles in a murine model of muscular dystrophy. *J. Muscle Res. Cell Motil.* **2016**, *37*, 153–164. [CrossRef] [PubMed]

84. Abmayr, S.M.; Pavlath, G.K. Myoblast fusion: Lessons from flies and mice. *Development* **2012**, *139*, 641–656. [CrossRef] [PubMed]

85. Chal, J.; Pourquié, O. Making muscle: Skeletal myogenesis in vivo and in vitro. *Development* **2017**, *144*, 2104–2122. [CrossRef] [PubMed]

86. Mizuno, Y.; Suzuki, M.; Nakagawa, H.; Ninagawa, N.; Torihashi, S. Switching of actin isoforms in skeletal muscle differentiation using mouse ES cells. *Histochem. Cell Biol.* **2009**, *132*, 669–672. [CrossRef] [PubMed]

87.   Sharma, A.; Agarwal, M.; Kumar, A.; Kumar, P.; Saini, M.; Kardon, G.; Mathew, S.J. Myosin Heavy Chain-embryonic is a crucial regulator of skeletal muscle development and differentiation. *bioRxiv* **2018**, 261685. [CrossRef]

88.   Chal, J.; Oginuma, M.; Al Tanoury, Z.; Gobert, B.; Sumara, O.; Hick, A.; Bousson, F.; Zidouni, Y.; Mursch, C.; Moncuquet, P.; et al. Differentiation of pluripotent stem cells to muscle fiber to model Duchenne muscular dystrophy. *Nat. Biotechnol.* **2015**, *33*, 962–969. [CrossRef]

89.   Guiraud, S.; Edwards, B.; Squire, S.E.; Moir, L.; Berg, A.; Babbs, A.; Ramadan, N.; Wood, M.J.; Davies, K.E. Embryonic myosin is a regeneration marker to monitor utrophin-based therapies for DMD. *Hum. Mol. Genet.* **2019**, *28*, 307–319. [CrossRef]

90.   De Angelis, L.; Berghella, L.; Coletta, M.; Lattanzi, L.; Zanchi, M.; Cusella-De Angelis, M.G.; Ponzetto, C.; Cossu, G. Skeletal myogenic progenitors originating from embryonic dorsal aorta coexpress endothelial and myogenic markers and contribute to postnatal muscle growth and regeneration. *J. Cell Biol.* **1999**, *147*, 869–877. [CrossRef]

91.   Kuang, S.; Chargé, S.B.; Seale, P.; Huh, M.; Rudnicki, M.A. Distinct roles for Pax7 and Pax3 in adult regenerative myogenesis. *J. Cell Biol.* **2006**, *172*, 103–113. [CrossRef]

92.   Wosczyna, M.N.; Biswas, A.A.; Cogswell, C.A.; Goldhamer, D.J. Multipotent progenitors resident in the skeletal muscle interstitium exhibit robust BMP-dependent osteogenic activity and mediate heterotopic ossification. *J. Bone Miner. Res.* **2012**, *27*, 1004–1017. [CrossRef]

93.   Asakura, A.; Seale, P.; Girgis-Gabardo, A.; Rudnicki, M.A. Myogenic specification of side population cells in skeletal muscle. *J. Cell Biol.* **2002**, *159*, 123–134. [CrossRef] [PubMed]

94.   Gussoni, E.; Soneoka, Y.; Strickland, C.D.; Buzney, E.A.; Khan, M.K.; Flint, A.F.; Kunkel, L.M.; Mulligan, R.C. Dystrophin expression in the mdx mouse restored by stem cell transplantation. *Nature* **1999**, *401*, 390–394. [CrossRef] [PubMed]

95.   Messina, G.; Biressi, S.; Cossu, G. Non Muscle Stem Cells and Muscle Regeneration. In *Skeletal Muscle Repair and Regeneration*; Springer: Dordrecht, The Netherlands, 2008; pp. 65–84.

96.   Joe, A.W.B.; Yi, L.; Natarajan, A.; Le Grand, F.; So, L.; Wang, J.; Rudnicki, M.A.; Rossi, F.M.V. Muscle injury activates resident fibro/adipogenic progenitors that facilitate myogenesis. *Nat. Cell Biol.* **2010**, *12*, 153–163. [CrossRef] [PubMed]

97.   Wosczyna, M.N.; Konishi, C.T.; Perez, E.E.; Gan, Q.; Wagner, M.W.; Rando, T.A.; Perez Carbajal, E.E.; Wang, T.T.; Walsh, R.A. Mesenchymal Stromal Cells Are Required for Regeneration and Homeostatic Maintenance of Skeletal Muscle In Brief Article Mesenchymal Stromal Cells Are Required for Regeneration and Homeostatic Maintenance of Skeletal Muscle. *Cell Rep.* **2019**, *27*, 2029.e5–2035.e5. [CrossRef] [PubMed]

98.   Fiore, D.; Judson, R.N.; Low, M.; Lee, S.; Zhang, E.; Hopkins, C.; Xu, P.; Lenzi, A.; Rossi, F.M.V.; Lemos, D.R. Pharmacological blockage of fibro/adipogenic progenitor expansion and suppression of regenerative fibrogenesis is associated with impaired skeletal muscle regeneration. *Stem Cell Res.* **2016**, *17*, 161–169. [CrossRef] [PubMed]

99.   Lukjanenko, L.; Karaz, S.; Stuelsatz, P.; Gurriaran-Rodriguez, U.; Michaud, J.; Dammone, G.; Sizzano, F.; Mashinchian, O.; Ancel, S.; Migliavacca, E.; et al. Aging Disrupts Muscle Stem Cell Function by Impairing Matricellular WISP1 Secretion from Fibro-Adipogenic Progenitors. *Cell Stem Cell* **2019**, *24*, 433.e7–446.e7. [CrossRef]

100.   Davis, M.E.; Gumucio, J.P.; Sugg, K.B.; Bedi, A.; Mendias, C.L. MMP inhibition as a potential method to augment the healing of skeletal muscle and tendon extracellular matrix. *J. Appl. Physiol.* **2013**, *115*, 884–891. [CrossRef]

101.   Kim, J.; Lee, J. Matrix metalloproteinase and tissue inhibitor of metalloproteinase responses to muscle damage after eccentric exercise. *J. Exerc. Rehabil.* **2016**, *12*, 260–265. [CrossRef]

102.   Arecco, N.; Clarke, C.J.; Jones, F.K.; Simpson, D.M.; Mason, D.; Beynon, R.J.; Pisconti, A. Elastase levels and activity are increased in dystrophic muscle and impair myoblast cell survival, proliferation and differentiation. *Sci. Rep.* **2016**, *6*, 1–20. [CrossRef]

103.   Grounds, M.D. Complexity of Extracellular Matrix and Skeletal Muscle Regeneration. In *Skeletal Muscle Repair and Regeneration*; Springer: Amsterdam, The Netherlands, 2008; pp. 269–302.

104.   Mann, C.J.; Perdiguero, E.; Kharraz, Y.; Aguilar, S.; Pessina, P.; Serrano, A.L.; Muñoz-Cánoves, P. Aberrant repair and fibrosis development in skeletal muscle. *Skelet. Muscle* **2011**, *1*, 21. [CrossRef]

105. Garg, K.; Corona, B.T.; Walters, T.J. Therapeutic strategies for preventing skeletal muscle fibrosis after injury. *Front. Pharmacol.* **2015**, *6*, 87. [CrossRef] [PubMed]

106. Lu, P.; Takai, K.; Weaver, V.M.; Werb, Z. Extracellular Matrix degradation and remodeling in development and disease. *Cold Spring Harb. Perspect. Biol.* **2011**, *3*, a005058. [CrossRef] [PubMed]

107. Gillies, A.R.; Chapman, M.A.; Bushong, E.A.; Deerinck, T.J.; Ellisman, M.H.; Lieber, R.L. High resolution three-dimensional reconstruction of fibrotic skeletal muscle extracellular matrix. *J. Physiol.* **2017**, *595*, 1159–1171. [CrossRef] [PubMed]

108. Dey, P. *Basic and Advanced Laboratory Techniques in Histopathology and Cytology*; Springer: Singapore, 2018.

109. Junqueira, L.C.U.; Bignolas, G.; Brentani, R.R. Picrosirius staining plus polarization microscopy, a specific method for collagen detection in tissue sections. *Histochem. J.* **1979**, *11*, 447–455. [CrossRef]

110. Montes, G.S.; Junqueira, L.C. The use of the Picrosirius-polarization method for the study of the biopathology of collagen. *Mem. Inst. Oswaldo Cruz* **1991**, *86*, 1–11. [CrossRef]

111. Lattouf, R.; Younes, R.; Lutomski, D.; Naaman, N.; Godeau, G.; Senni, K.; Changotade, S. Picrosirius Red Staining: A Useful Tool to Appraise Collagen Networks in Normal and Pathological Tissues. *J. Histochem. Cytochem.* **2014**, *62*, 751–758. [CrossRef]

112. Séguier, S.; Godeau, G.; Brousse, N. Collagen Fibers and Inflammatory Cells in Healthy and Diseased Human Gingival Tissues: A Comparative and Quantitative Study by Immunohistochemistry and Automated Image Analysis. *J. Periodontol.* **2000**, *71*, 1079–1085. [CrossRef]

113. Tatsumi, R.; Sankoda, Y.; Anderson, J.E.; Sato, Y.; Mizunoya, W.; Shimizu, N.; Suzuki, T.; Yamada, M.; Rhoads, R.P.; Ikeuchi, Y.; et al. Possible implication of satellite cells in regenerative motoneuritogenesis: HGF upregulates neural chemorepellent Sema3A during myogenic differentiation Possible implication of satellite cells in regenerative motoneuritogenesis: HGF upregulates neural che-morepellent Sema3A during myogenic differentiation. *Am. J. Physiol. Cell Physiol.* **2009**, *297*, 238–252. [CrossRef]

114. Ling, S.C.; Dastidar, S.G.; Tokunaga, S.; Ho, W.Y.; Lim, K.; Ilieva, H.; Parone, P.A.; Tyan, S.H.; Tse, T.M.; Chang, J.C.; et al. Overriding FUS autoregulation in mice triggers gain-of-toxic dysfunctions in RNA metabolism and autophagy-lysosome axis. *Elife* **2019**, *8*, e40811. [CrossRef]

115. Rizzuto, E.; Pisu, S.; Nicoletti, C.; Del Prete, Z.; Musarò, A. Measuring neuromuscular junction functionality. *J. Vis. Exp.* **2017**, *2017*, 55227. [CrossRef]

116. Rizzuto, E.; Pisu, S.; Musarò, A.; Del Prete, Z. Measuring Neuromuscular Junction Functionality in the SOD1G93A Animal Model of Amyotrophic Lateral Sclerosis. *Ann. Biomed. Eng.* **2015**, *43*, 2196–2206. [CrossRef] [PubMed]

117. Del Prete, Z.; Musarò, A.; Rizzuto, E. Measuring mechanical properties, including isotonic fatigue, of fast and slow MLC/mIgf-1 transgenic skeletal muscle. *Ann. Biomed. Eng.* **2008**, *36*, 1281–1290. [CrossRef] [PubMed]

118. Grounds, M.D.; Radley, H.G.; Lynch, G.S.; Nagaraju, K.; De Luca, A. Towards developing standard operating procedures for pre-clinical testing in the mdx mouse model of Duchenne muscular dystrophy. *Neurobiol. Dis.* **2008**, *31*, 1–19. [CrossRef] [PubMed]

119. Lagrota-Candido, J.; Vasconcellos, R.; Cavalcanti, M.; Bozza, M.; Savino, W.; Quirico-Santos, T. Resolution of skeletal muscle inflammation in mdx dystrophic mouse is accompanied by increased immunoglobulin and interferon-γ production. *Int. J. Exp. Pathol.* **2002**, *83*, 121–132. [CrossRef] [PubMed]

120. Forcina, L.; Pelosi, L.; Miano, C.; Musarò, A. Insights into the Pathogenic Secondary Symptoms Caused by the Primary Loss of Dystrophin. *J. Funct. Morphol. Kinesiol.* **2017**, *2*, 44. [CrossRef]

121. Pelosi, L.; Berardinelli, M.G.; De Pasquale, L.; Nicoletti, C.; D'Amico, A.; Carvello, F.; Moneta, G.M.; Catizone, A.; Bertini, E.; De Benedetti, F.; et al. Functional and Morphological Improvement of Dystrophic Muscle by Interleukin 6 Receptor Blockade. *EBioMedicine* **2015**, *2*, 285–293. [CrossRef]

122. Klein, S.M.; Prantl, L.; Geis, S.; Felthaus, O.; Dolderer, J.; Anker, A.M.; Zeitler, K.; Alt, E.; Vykoukal, J. Circulating serum CK level vs. muscle impairment for in situ monitoring burden of disease in Mdx-mice. *Clin. Hemorheol. Microcirc.* **2017**, *65*, 327–334. [CrossRef]

123. Liu, N.; Williams, A.H.; Maxeiner, J.M.; Bezprozvannaya, S.; Shelton, J.M.; Richardson, J.A.; Bassel-Duby, R.; Olson, E.N. MicroRNA-206 promotes skeletal muscle regeneration and delays progression of Duchenne muscular dystrophy in mice. *J. Clin. Investig.* **2012**, *122*, 2054–2065. [CrossRef]

124. Cacchiarelli, D.; Legnini, I.; Martone, J.; Cazzella, V.; D'Amico, A.; Bertini, E.; Bozzoni, I. miRNAs as serum biomarkers for Duchenne muscular dystrophy. *EMBO Mol. Med.* **2011**, *3*, 258–265. [CrossRef]

125. Vignier, N.; Amor, F.; Fogel, P.; Duvallet, A.; Poupiot, J.; Charrier, S.; Arock, M.; Montus, M.; Nelson, I.; Richard, I.; et al. Distinctive Serum miRNA Profile in Mouse Models of Striated Muscular Pathologies. *PLoS ONE* **2013**, *8*, e55281. [CrossRef]

126. Jeanson-Leh, L.; Lameth, J.; Krimi, S.; Buisset, J.; Amor, F.; Le Guiner, C.; Barthélémy, I.; Servais, L.; Blot, S.; Voit, T.; et al. Serum profiling identifies novel muscle miRNA and cardiomyopathy-related miRNA biomarkers in golden retriever muscular dystrophy dogs and duchenne muscular dystrophy patients. *Am. J. Pathol.* **2014**, *184*, 2885–2898. [CrossRef] [PubMed]

127. Zaharieva, I.T.; Calissano, M.; Scoto, M.; Preston, M.; Cirak, S.; Feng, L.; Collins, J.; Kole, R.; Guglieri, M.; Straub, V.; et al. Dystromirs as Serum Biomarkers for Monitoring the Disease Severity in Duchenne Muscular Dystrophy. *PLoS ONE* **2013**, *8*, e80263. [CrossRef] [PubMed]

128. Perfetti, A.; Greco, S.; Bugiardini, E.; Cardani, R.; Gaia, P.; Gaetano, C.; Meola, G.; Martelli, F. Plasma microRNAs as biomarkers for myotonic dystrophy type 1. *Neuromuscul. Disord.* **2014**, *24*, 509–515. [CrossRef] [PubMed]

129. McDouall, R.M.; Dunn, M.J.; Dubowitz, V. Nature of the mononuclear infiltrate and the mechanism of muscle damage in juvenile dermatomyositis and Duchenne muscular dystrophy. *J. Neurol. Sci.* **1990**, *99*, 199–217. [CrossRef]

130. Spencer, M.J.; Walsh, C.M.; Dorshkind, K.A.; Rodriguez, E.M.; Tidball, J.G. Myonuclear apoptosis in dystrophic mdx muscle occurs by perforin- mediated cytotoxicity. *J. Clin. Investig.* **1997**, *99*, 2745–2751. [CrossRef] [PubMed]

131. Wehling, M.; Spencer, M.J.; Tidball, J.G. A nitric oxide synthase transgene ameliorates muscular dystrophy in mdx mice. *J. Cell Biol.* **2001**, *155*, 123–131. [CrossRef]

132. Madaro, L.; Torcinaro, A.; De Bardi, M.; Contino, F.F.; Pelizzola, M.; Diaferia, G.R.; Imeneo, G.; Bouchè, M.; Puri, P.L.; De Santa, F. Macrophages fine tune satellite cell fate in dystrophic skeletal muscle of mdx mice. *PLoS Genet.* **2019**, *15*, e1008408. [CrossRef]

133. Turk, R.; Sterrenburg, E.; de Meijer, E.J.; van Ommen, G.J.B.; den Dunnen, J.T.; 't Hoen, P.A.C. Muscle regeneration in dystrophin-deficient mdx mice studied by gene expression profiling. *BMC Genom.* **2005**, *6*, 98. [CrossRef]

134. Pelosi, M.; De Rossi, M.; Barberi, L.; Musarò, A. IL-6 Impairs Myogenic Differentiation by Downmodulation of p90RSK/eEF2 and mTOR/p70S6K Axes, without Affecting AKT Activity. *Biomed Res. Int.* **2014**, *2014*, 206026. [CrossRef]

135. Kurosaka, M.; Machida, S. Interleukin-6-induced satellite cell proliferation is regulated by induction of the JAK2/STAT3 signalling pathway through cyclin D1 targeting. *Cell Prolif.* **2013**, *46*, 365–373. [CrossRef]

136. Wada, E.; Tanihata, J.; Iwamura, A.; Takeda, S.; Hayashi, Y.K.; Matsuda, R. Treatment with the anti-IL-6 receptor antibody attenuates muscular dystrophy via promoting skeletal muscle regeneration in dystrophin-/utrophin-deficient mice. *Skelet. Muscle* **2017**, *7*, 23. [CrossRef] [PubMed]

137. Reggio, A.; Rosina, M.; Palma, A.; Cerquone Perpetuini, A.; Lisa Petrilli, L.; Gargioli, C.; Fuoco, C.; Micarelli, E.; Giuliani, G.; Cerretani, M.; et al. Adipogenesis of skeletal muscle fibro/adipogenic progenitors is affected by the WNT5a/GSK3/β-catenin axis. *Cell Death Differ.* **2020**. [CrossRef] [PubMed]

138. Cullen, M.; Mastaglia, F. Pathological reactions of skeletal muscle. In *Skeletal Muscle Pathology*; Mastaglia, F.L., Walton, J., Eds.; Churchill Livingstone: London, UK, 1982; pp. 88–139.

139. Harris, J.B. Myotoxic phospholipases A2 and the regeneration of skeletal muscles. *Toxicon* **2003**, *42*, 933–945. [CrossRef] [PubMed]

140. Hardy, D.; Besnard, A.; Latil, M.; Jouvion, G.; Briand, D.; Thépenier, C.; Pascal, Q.; Guguin, A.; Gayraud-Morel, B.; Cavaillon, J.M.; et al. Comparative Study of Injury Models for Studying Muscle Regeneration in Mice. *PLoS ONE* **2016**, *11*, e0147198. [CrossRef]

141. Warren, G.L.; Hulderman, T.; Mishra, D.; Gao, X.; Millecchia, L.; O'Farrell, L.; Kuziel, W.A.; Simeonova, P.P. Chemokine receptor CCR2 involvement in skeletal muscle regeneration. *FASEB J.* **2005**, *19*, 1–23. [CrossRef]

142. Le, G.; Lowe, D.A.; Kyba, M. Freeze injury of the tibialis anterior muscle. *Methods Mol. Biol.* **2016**, *1460*, 33–41. [CrossRef]

143. Forcina, L.; Miano, C.; Musarò, A. The physiopathologic interplay between stem cells and tissue niche in muscle regeneration and the role of IL-6 on muscle homeostasis and diseases. *Cytokine Growth Factor Rev.* **2018**, *41*, 1–9. [CrossRef]

144. Forcina, L.; Miano, C.; Scicchitano, B.M.; Rizzuto, E.; Berardinelli, M.G.; De Benedetti, F.; Pelosi, L.; Musarò, A. Increased Circulating Levels of Interleukin-6 Affect the Redox Balance in Skeletal Muscle. *Oxid. Med. Cell. Longev.* **2019**, *2019*, 3018584. [CrossRef]

145. Schultz, E.; Jaryszak, D.L.; Gibson, M.C.; Albright, D.J. Absence of exogenous satellite cell contribution to regeneration of frozen skeletal muscle. *J. Muscle Res. Cell Motil.* **1986**, *7*, 361–367. [CrossRef]

146. Torrente, Y.; Belicchi, M.; Sampaolesi, M.; Pisati, F.; Meregalli, M.; D'Antona, G.; Tonlorenzi, R.; Porretti, L.; Gavina, M.; Mamchaoui, K.; et al. Human circulating AC133+ stem cells restore dystrophin expression and ameliorate function in dystrophic skeletal muscle. *J. Clin. Investig.* **2004**, *114*, 182–195. [CrossRef]

147. Reis, N.D.; Better, O.S. Mechanical muscle-crush injury and acute muscle-crush compartment syndrome. *J. Bone Joint Surg. Br.* **2005**, *87*, 450–453. [CrossRef] [PubMed]

148. Dobek, G.L.; Fulkerson, N.D.; Nicholas, J.; Schneider, B.S.P. Mouse model of muscle crush injury of the legs. *Comp. Med.* **2013**, *63*, 227–232. [PubMed]

149. Crisco, J.J.; Jokl, P.; Heinen, G.T.; Connell, M.D.; Panjabi, M.M. A Muscle Contusion Injury Model: Biomechanics, Physiology, and Histology. *Am. J. Sports Med.* **1994**, *22*, 702–710. [CrossRef] [PubMed]

150. Kerkweg, U.; Schmitz, D.; de Groot, H. Screening for the Formation of Reactive Oxygen Species and of NO in Muscle Tissue and Remote Organs upon Mechanical Trauma to the Mouse Hind Limb. *Eur. Surg. Res.* **2006**, *38*, 83–89. [CrossRef]

151. McBrier, N.M.; Neuberger, T.; Denegar, C.R.; Sharkey, N.A.; Webb, A.G. Magnetic resonance imaging of acute injury in rats and the effects of buprenorphine on limb volume. *J. Am. Assoc. Lab. Anim. Sci.* **2009**, *48*, 147–151.

152. Stratos, I.; Graff, J.; Rotter, R.; Mittlmeier, T.; Vollmar, B. Open blunt crush injury of different severity determines nature and extent of local tissue regeneration and repair. *J. Orthop. Res.* **2010**, *28*, 950–957. [CrossRef]

153. Takagi, R.; Fujita, N.; Arakawa, T.; Kawada, S.; Ishii, N.; Miki, A. Influence of icing on muscle regeneration after crush injury to skeletal muscles in rats. *J. Appl. Physiol.* **2011**, *110*, 382–388. [CrossRef]

154. Criswell, T.L.; Corona, B.T.; Ward, C.L.; Miller, M.; Patel, M.; Wang, Z.; Christ, G.J.; Soker, S. Compression-induced muscle injury in rats that mimics compartment syndrome in humans. *Am. J. Pathol.* **2012**, *180*, 787–797. [CrossRef]

155. Ciciliot, S.; Schiaffino, S. Regeneration of Mammalian Skeletal Muscle: Basic Mechanisms and Clinical Implications. *Curr. Pharm. Des.* **2010**, *16*, 906–914. [CrossRef]

156. Oyster, N.; Witt, M.; Gharaibeh, B.; Poddar, M.; Schneppendahl, J.; Huard, J. Characterization of a compartment syndrome-like injury model. *Muscle Nerve* **2015**, *51*, 750–758. [CrossRef]

157. Lømo, T. What controls the position, number, size, and distribution of neuromuscular junctions on rat muscle fibers? *J. Neurocytol.* **2003**, *32*, 835–848. [CrossRef] [PubMed]

158. Klein-Ogus, C.; Harris, J.B. Preliminary observations of satellite cells in undamaged fibres of the rat soleus muscle assaulted by a snake-venom toxin. *Cell Tissue Res.* **1983**, *230*, 671–776. [CrossRef] [PubMed]

159. Benoit, P.W.; Belt, W.D. Destruction and regeneration of skeletal muscle after treatment with a local anaesthetic, bupivacaine (Marcaine). *J. Anat.* **1970**, *107*, 547–556.

160. Gutiérrez, J.M.; Ownby, C.L. Skeletal muscle degeneration induced by venom phospholipases A 2: Insights into the mechanisms of local and systemic myotoxicity. *Toxicon* **2003**, *42*, 915–931. [CrossRef] [PubMed]

161. Harris, J.B.; Grubb, B.D.; Maltin, C.A.; Dixon, R. The neurotoxicity of the venom phospholipases A2, notexin and taipoxin. *Exp. Neurol.* **2000**, *161*, 517–526. [CrossRef]

162. Harris, J.B.; Vater, R.; Wilson, M.; Cullen, M.J. Muscle fibre breakdown in venom-induced muscle degeneration. *J. Anat.* **2003**, *202*, 363–372. [CrossRef]

163. Rosenblatt, J.D. A time course study of the isometric contractile properties of rat extensor digitorum longus muscle injected with bupivacaine. *Comp. Biochem. Physiol. Comp. Physiol.* **1992**, *101*, 361–367. [CrossRef]

164. Gutiérrez, J.M.; Escalante, T.; Hernández, R.; Gastaldello, S.; Saravia-Otten, P.; Rucavado, A. Why is skeletal muscle regeneration impaired after myonecrosis induced by viperid snake venoms? *Toxins (Basel)* **2018**, *10*, 182. [CrossRef]

165. Hodges, S.J.; Agbaji, A.S.; Harvey, A.L.; Hider, R.C. Cobra cardiotoxins. Purification, effects on skeletal muscle and structure/activity relationships. *Eur. J. Biochem.* **1987**, *165*, 373–383. [CrossRef]

166. Guardiola, O.; Andolfi, G.; Tirone, M.; Iavarone, F.; Brunelli, S.; Minchiotti, G. Induction of acute skeletal muscle regeneration by cardiotoxin injection. *J. Vis. Exp.* **2017**, *2017*, 54515. [CrossRef]

167. Czerwinska, A.M.; Streminska, W.; Ciemerych, M.A.; Grabowska, I. Mouse gastrocnemius muscle regeneration after mechanical or cardiotoxin injury. *Folia Histochem. Cytobiol.* **2012**, *50*, 144–153. [CrossRef] [PubMed]

168. Hirata, A.; Masuda, S.; Tamura, T.; Kai, K.; Ojima, K.; Fukase, A.; Motoyoshi, K.; Kamakura, K.; Miyagoe-Suzuki, Y.; Takeda, S. Expression profiling of cytokines and related genes in regenerating skeletal muscle after cardiotoxin injection: A role for osteopontin. *Am. J. Pathol.* **2003**, *163*, 203–215. [CrossRef]

169. El Andalousi, R.B.; Daussin, P.A.; Micallef, J.P.; Roux, C.; Nougues, J.; Chammas, M.; Reyne, Y.; Bacou, F. Changes in mass and performance in rabbit muscles after muscle damage with or without transplantation of primary satellite cells. *Cell Transplant.* **2002**, *11*, 169–180. [CrossRef]

170. Sambasivan, R.; Yao, R.; Kissenpfennig, A.; van Wittenberghe, L.; Paldi, A.; Gayraud-Morel, B.; Guenou, H.; Malissen, B.; Tajbakhsh, S.; Galy, A. Pax7-expressing satellite cells are indispensable for adult skeletal muscle regeneration. *Development* **2011**, *138*, 3647–3656. [CrossRef]

171. Ho, A.T.V.; Palla, A.R.; Blake, M.R.; Yucel, N.D.; Wang, Y.X.; Magnusson, K.E.G.; Holbrook, C.A.; Kraft, P.E.; Delp, S.L.; Blau, H.M. Prostaglandin E2 is essential for efficacious skeletal muscle stem-cell function, augmenting regeneration and strength. *Proc. Natl. Acad. Sci. USA* **2017**, *114*, 6675–6684. [CrossRef] [PubMed]

172. Siles, L.; Ninfali, C.; Cortés, M.; Darling, D.S.; Postigo, A. ZEB1 protects skeletal muscle from damage and is required for its regeneration. *Nat. Commun.* **2019**, *10*, 1–18. [CrossRef] [PubMed]

173. Sun, K.-T.; Cheung, K.-K.; Au, S.W.N.; Yeung, S.S.; Yeung, E.W. Overexpression of Mechano-Growth Factor Modulates Inflammatory Cytokine Expression and Macrophage Resolution in Skeletal Muscle Injury. *Front. Physiol.* **2018**, *9*, 999. [CrossRef] [PubMed]

174. Mirtschin, P.; Davis, R. *Dangerous Snakes of Australia. An Illustrated Guide to Australia's Most Venomous Snakes*; Rigby Publishers: Adelaide, Australia, 1982.

175. Plant, D.R.; Colarossi, F.E.; Lynch, G.S. Notexin causes greater myotoxic damage and slower functional repair in mouse skeletal muscles than bupivacaine. *Muscle Nerve* **2006**, *34*, 577–585. [CrossRef]

176. Vignaud, A.; Hourdé, C.; Butler-Browne, G.; Ferry, A. Differential recovery of neuromuscular function after nerve/muscle injury induced by crude venom from Notechis scutatus, cardiotoxin from Naja atra and bupivacaine treatments in mice. *Neurosci. Res.* **2007**, *58*, 317–323. [CrossRef]

177. Gayraud-Morel, B.; Chrétien, F.; Flamant, P.; Gomès, D.; Zammit, P.S.; Tajbakhsh, S. A role for the myogenic determination gene Myf5 in adult regenerative myogenesis. *Dev. Biol.* **2007**, *312*, 13–28. [CrossRef]

178. Baghdadi, M.B.; Tajbakhsh, S. Regulation and phylogeny of skeletal muscle regeneration. *Dev. Biol.* **2018**, *433*, 200–209. [CrossRef] [PubMed]

179. Zink, W.; Seif, C.; Bohl, J.R.E.; Hacke, N.; Braun, P.M.; Sinner, B.; Martin, E.; Fink, R.H.A.; Graf, B.M. The acute myotoxic effects of bupivacaine and ropivacaine after continuous peripheral nerve blockades. *Anesth. Analg.* **2003**, *97*, 1173–1179. [CrossRef] [PubMed]

180. Zink, W.; Graf, B.M.; Sinner, B.; Martin, E.; Fink, R.H.A.; Kunst, G. Differential effects of bupivacaine on intracellular Ca 2+ regulation: Potential mechanisms of its myotoxicity. *Anesthesiology* **2002**, *97*, 710–716. [CrossRef] [PubMed]

181. Kimura, N.; Hirata, S.; Miyasaka, N.; Kawahata, K.; Kohsaka, H. Injury and subsequent regeneration of muscles for activation of local innate immunity to facilitate the development and relapse of autoimmune myositis in C57BL/6 mice. *Arthritis Rheumatol.* **2015**, *67*, 1107–1116. [CrossRef] [PubMed]

182. Scicchitano, B.M.; Dobrowolny, G.; Sica, G.; Musaro, A. Molecular Insights into Muscle Homeostasis, Atrophy and Wasting. *Curr. Genom.* **2018**, *19*, 356–369. [CrossRef]

13

Role of Insulin-Like Growth Factor Receptor 2 across Muscle Homeostasis: Implications for Treating Muscular Dystrophy

Yvan Torrente *, Pamela Bella, Luana Tripodi, Chiara Villa and Andrea Farini *

Stem Cell Laboratory, Department of Pathophysiology and Transplantation, University of Milan,
Unit of Neurology, Fondazione IRCCS Cà Granda Ospedale Maggiore Policlinico, Dino Ferrari Center, 20122
Milan, Italy; pamelabella@hotmail.it (P.B.); tripodiluana@libero.it (L.T.); kiaravilla@gmail.com (C.V.)
* Correspondence: yvan.torrente@unimi.it (Y.T.); farini.andrea@gmail.com (A.F.);

Abstract: The insulin-like growth factor 2 receptor (IGF2R) plays a major role in binding and regulating the circulating and tissue levels of the mitogenic peptide insulin-like growth factor 2 (IGF2). IGF2/IGF2R interaction influences cell growth, survival, and migration in normal tissue development, and the deregulation of IGF2R expression has been associated with growth-related disease and cancer. IGF2R overexpression has been implicated in heart and muscle disease progression. Recent research findings suggest novel approaches to target IGF2R action. This review highlights recent advances in the understanding of the IGF2R structure and pathways related to muscle homeostasis.

Keywords: IGF2R; muscle homeostasis; inflammation; muscular dystrophy; pericytes

1. Introduction

The cation-independent mannose 6-phosphate/insulin-like growth factor 2 receptor (CI-M6P/IGF2R, hereafter IGF2R) is a type-1 transmembrane glycoprotein consisting of a large N-terminal extracytoplasmic domain, which allows it to bind to a wide variety of ligands [1,2]. The IGF2 and M6P ligands [3–5] of IGF2R have distinct but important roles in normal development and mesoderm differentiation [6]. Many studies have demonstrated the suppression action of IGF2R on insulin-like growth factor 1 receptor (IGF1R) signaling by scavenging extracellular IGF2 [7]. Furthermore, several lines of evidence demonstrate that IGF2 is highly expressed in rodent embryos, where it functions as an embryonic growth factor, while its amount is diminished at birth [8]. Smith et al. recently showed that a transgene-induced overexpression of IGF2 blocked programmed cell death, one of the main pathological features of cancer [9]. Furthermore, in some cancers such as mammary tumors, IGF2R behaves as a tumor suppressor gene [10], whereas in other cancers such as cervical tumors or glioblastomas, IGF2R acts as an oncogene [11,12]. Thus, these two traits of IGF2R might depend on cell type. Interestingly, cervical tumors and glioblastomas have common mesenchymal founders, namely myofibroblasts [13], which are also involved in muscle disease. Muscle repair is a complex and tightly regulated event that recruits different cell types, starting from macrophage and lymphocyte consecutive involvement and terminating with satellite cell (SC) activation and differentiation [14]. Among the common hallmarks of muscular dystrophy are the infiltration of immune cells into skeletal muscle fibers, and fibrotic cell proliferation [15–18].

Impaired muscle regeneration with SC pool exhaustion is considered an additional pathological feature of Duchenne muscular dystrophy (DMD) [19]. The main biological function of IGF2R is the suppression of IGF1R signaling via the deprivation of extracellular IGF2 ligands. Some studies have explained the tumor suppressive functions of IGF2R by its negative regulation of the oncogenic IGF2–IGF1R signal axis [2]. However, in muscle tissues, the IGFs bind to the IGF1R leading to conformational changes and activation of its tyrosine kinase activity, promoting muscle regeneration [20]. In injured tissues, IGF1 is secreted by SCs and mediates muscle-derived stem cell proliferation and differentiation into myoblasts, which contribute to myofiber formation for restoring normal tissue structures [21]. It has been demonstrated that prolonged expression of IGF1 causes an exaggerated protein synthesis and is responsible for muscular hypertrophy, by increasing myofiber diameter [22–25], and also preventing muscle atrophy in cases of cachexia or chronic inflammation [26]. Thus, tissue-specific IGF1 upregulation rises to the challenge of counteracting the development of muscular dystrophy.

Similar to IGF1, autocrine IGF2 is fundamental to mediate the differentiation of SCs in vitro, but little is known about its role in skeletal muscle development and regeneration in vivo [27]. The expression profile of *IGF2* is quite complicated as it depends on multiple-promoter activation, alternative translation initiation and messenger RNA (mRNA) stability. IGF2R functions as a negative regulator of IGF2 in embryonic skeletal muscles and modulates the amount of systemic IGF2 by inducing its degradation through lysosomes and clearance from the circulation [28,29].

Even if the signaling cascade that regulates the activation of IGF2 at muscular level is not determined, it has been shown that the phosphatidylinositol 3-kinase (PI3K)–the serine/threonine protein kinase B (AKT) pathway is the IGF2 downstream pathway contributing to mammalian target of rapamycin (mTOR) functions [30]. A study by Ge et al. [31] showed that the synergic activity of mTOR with miR-125b regulated *IGF2* production both transcriptionally and post-transcriptionally, and that these events positively influence myogenesis.

In muscle pathology and ageing contexts, where there is a predominant switch of the fiber phenotype from fast to slow [32,33], IGF2 was also able to orchestrate the development of fast myofibers by acting as a twitch motor unit during secondary myogenesis. The modulation of IGF2 expression had a dramatic impact on the amount of fast myofibers in the respiratory (intercostal and diaphragmatic) muscles, likely lessening cardio-respiratory dysfunction related to DMD. IGF2 targeting was suggested as a feasible therapeutic strategy, since IGF2 has a small size and consequently it could be easily distributed to a skeletal muscle target [34]. However, the IGF2R signaling pathways involved in muscle repair and disease remain to be identified.

2. Structure, Genomic Organization and Gene Imprinting of IGF2R

Imprinting genes are those whose expression is determined by one's parents. They occur in discrete clusters that are regulated by DNA elements called imprinting control regions (ICR). The two copies of one imprinted gene are characterized by methylation of cytosine–guanine base pairs. This modification originates in the paternal germ cells—after adding a methyl group, the chromatin becomes inaccessible to transcription machinery, so the gene is silenced. The IGF2/H19 locus is one of the imprinted gene clusters in human chromosome 11p15.5 or mouse distal chromosome 7 and plays a primary role in muscle cell development [35]. The expression of this cluster is regulated by a distant enhancer downstream of the H19 coding region. A recent study presents paxillin (PXN), a focal adhesion protein, as a transcriptional regulator of the IGF2 and H19 genes; in particular, it has the opposite effect on the activity of the IGF2 and H19 promoters [36]. The knockdown of PXN in human HepG2 cells allows for an increase in the activity of the H19 promoter and at the same time a decrease in the activity of the IGF2 promoter [36]. In a recent study, it was demonstrated that the loss of imprinting (LOI) in a mouse model of Beckwith–Wiedemann syndrome (BWS) results in impaired muscle differentiation and hypertrophy. It was also proposed that there is a signaling pathway in which IGF2 overexpression allows for an overactivation of mitogen-activated protein kinase (MAPK) signaling, while a loss of H19 long non-coding RNA (lncRNA) prevents the regulation of p53 levels, resulting in reduced AKT/mTOR signaling [35].

The *IGF2R* is an example of differential imprinting in the human and mouse genomes; the *IGF2R* is repressed on the paternal chromosome in the murine genome, but the same gene is expressed from both alleles in humans. For humans, the study was conducted on several tissues—adult liver, placenta, fetus, kidney, adrenal, brain, intestine, heart, tongue, skin and muscle: in all these samples both IGF2R alleles were expressed more or less at the same level. Accordingly, it was established that this character is subject to Mendelian segregation, escaping imprinting. As a plausible explanation for this phenomenon, Kalscheuer et al. suggested that the stages of initiation and maintenance of imprinting could be under the control of trans-acting factors that could act differently in mice compared to in humans [37]. They also hypothesized an alternative explanation based on the structural difference of the mouse and human *IGF2R* genes, as an "imprinting box" was previously discovered that could be modified by methylation in the female gamete and allowed maternal expression [37]. The *IGF2R* gene is located on mouse chromosome 17: it is composed of 48 exons and encoded for a 2482-amino acid protein. Exons 1–46 comprise the extracellular part of the receptor, while the transmembrane portion and the cytoplasmic region are located, respectively, on exon 46 and 46–48 [38].

3. IGF2R-Dependent Pathway

M6P/IGF2-R lacks intrinsic kinase activity, and the role of G-proteins in its downstream pathway has been investigated. Functionally, G-proteins are a class of proteins that interact with multi-spanning receptors (seven transmembrane receptors or heptahelical receptors). Some studies have speculated that M6P/IGF2-R, although characterized by a single-spanning structure, might initiate signaling cascades through G-proteins in a direct or indirect manner. It is well known that the pertussis toxin exerts its activity by binding and blocking the activation of the α subunit of the Gq/11-protein [39]. El-Shewy et al. showed that the use of this toxin is able to inhibit the function of M6P/IGF2-R, therefore suggesting the involvement of G-proteins in the downstream pathway of M6P/IGF2-R. Pre-treatment of Human embryonic kidney 293 cells (HEK-293) cells with the pertussis toxin can significantly reduce the level of extracellular signal-regulated kinase 1/2 (ERK1/2) phosphorylation resulting from the interaction of IGFs with their receptors. The indirect activity of these receptors is carried on through parallel activation of G-protein-coupled receptors (GPCR). They also observed that the administration of IGF1 and IGF2 ligands activates sphingosine kinase (SK) 4, which is translocated from the cytosol to the plasma membrane. There, it promotes an increase in extra- and intracytoplasmic levels of sphingosine-1-phosphate (S1P). S1P's interaction with its G-protein-coupled receptor represents a general mechanism for indirect G-protein-dependent signaling of M6P/IGF2-R resulting in ERK1/2 phosphorylation [40]. Conversely, the direct activity of IGF2R and G-proteins was hypothesized by Nishimoto et al. [41,42]: based on their observations, a region of the cytoplasmatic domain of M6P/IGF2-R may contain aminoacidic residues (2410–2423) that directly bind and activate G-proteins, in particular, Gi-2. This is supported by evidence that the use of both human and rat antibodies targeting aminoacidic residues is able to inhibit the activation of Gi-2 resulting from M6P/IGF2-R stimulation.

4. Functions of IGF2R

4.1. IGF2R Expression Levels Regulate Cardiac Development and Remodeling

The expression of the *IGF2R* gene is particularly abundant in embryo hearts. IGF2R-deficient mice display dramatic cardiac dysfunction and heart failure development. In adults, low levels of IGF2R expression lead to heart disease and apoptosis in cardiac myocytes [43], while upregulation determines myocardial infarction, remodeling [44] and hypertrophy [45]. In particular, the IGF2R activates phospholipase C (PLC) through the heterotrimeric G-protein-coupled receptor: this interaction is mediated by αq G subunits (Gαq) that in turn allow the function of different enzymes such as the protein kinase C-α (PKC-α), Ca^{2+}-calmodulin-dependent protein kinase II (CaMKII) and ERK kinase—all upregulated in cardiac hypertrophy [46]. Alternatively, the modulation of IGF2R can enhance cardiomyocyte apoptosis and cardiac contractility by inhibiting protein kinase A (PKA) phosphorylation [47]. A recent study showed that IGF2R expression is negatively controlled by the cardioprotective heat shock transcription factor 1 (HSF1). Antitumor drugs such as doxorubicin (DOX), meanwhile, lead to high levels of IGF2R expression in cardiomyocytes, through a decrease in HSF1, and trigger cardiac apoptotic processes [48]. IGF2R expression in the heart may also mediate increased sizes of cardiomyocytes, in a manner dependent on PKA activation, and mediate atrial natriuretic peptide (ANP), calcium-dependent channels (SERCA) and phospho-troponin I signaling, as described recently by Wang et al. [49].

4.2. IGF2R Modulates Vascular Remodeling and Skeletal Muscle Growth

IGF proteins play an essential role in skeletal muscle homeostasis and vascular mechanisms involving smooth muscle cells (SMCs). The latter are driven by IGF2 in the development and migration processes occurring during vascular growth or in response to vascular damage. A study has verified the role of IGF2 in SMC migration by studying the interaction between the cellular repressor of E1A-stimulated gene (CREG) factor and M6P/IGF2-R. Specifically, when the CREG factor binds M6P/IGF2-R, it is able to inhibit the SMC proliferation process and the migration process. Further studies showed that CREG knockdown leads to an increased release of IGF2, mitigating its internalization and partly restoring the migration process of the SMCs. Accordingly, the use of an anti-human IGF2-neutralizing antibody on a CREG knockdown population promotes the inhibition (in a concentration-dependent manner) of the SMCs' migration process [50]. Despite the shortage of detailed articles, an indirect point of view of the solid connection between vascular remodeling and IGF2R is offered by Ca^{2+} signaling. A comprehensive body of literature has already demonstrated that IGF2R triggers several intracellular signaling pathways aimed at Ca^{2+} mobilization [41]. This cascade may occur through an increase in PKC-α phosphorylation or in a Gαq-dependent manner [51], such as for controlling hypertrophy in cardiac cells, or through PLC-induced interactions between IGF2R and G(i) protein, as in endothelial progenitor cells (EPCs) [52]. In the latter case, the upstream role of IGF2R possibly affects the migration, adhesion and invasion of EPCs in the neovascular zone, therefore raising the importance of IGF2R for vessel network formation, both in embryonic and in post-ischemic vasculo-genesis. Vascular SMCs, composing the medial layer of blood vessels, are also essential for the maintenance of post-natal vascular homeostasis, and their correct functionality is subordinated to Ca^{2+} signaling. Intracellular calcium is likely to regulate the mechanical properties of SMCs through a tight modulation of $\alpha5\beta1$ integrin, α-SMA and cell–ECM interactions. The Ca^{2+} dynamic across cells may activate the elasticity and the adhesion properties of vascular SMCs, with physiologically important consequences on vascular tone and resistance, and blood flow and pressure [53].

A more complex signaling pathway underlying Ca^{2+} entry and exit from cells [54] is tuned by ATP-dependent pumps, which counterbalance the calcium ion levels and the electrolyte homeostasis. Among these pumps, sarcoplasmic/endoplasmic reticulum (SR) Ca^{2+}ATPase (SERCA) is the one in charge of the Ca^{2+} homeostasis within the reticulum, with a role susceptible to the type of cells [55,56]. There are three isoforms of SERCA characterized by tissue-specific expression. Briefly, the fast twitch skeletal muscle isoform SERCA1 has been found in the heart, and, to a lesser extent, in the liver, kidney, brain and pancreas [57]. Variants of SERCA2 have been detected preferentially in cardiac, skeletal and vascular smooth muscle [58]. SERCA3 isoforms are heterogeneously expressed through tissues and, conversely to the others, are characterized by a low affinity to Ca^{2+} [59]. Altered levels of SERCA proteins lead to aberrant calcium flux dynamics, which are responsible for the reduced contractility and dysfunction of SMCs observed in numerous diseases including cardiomyopathies, atherosclerosis, metabolic syndromes, and diabetes [60,61]. Although this evidence implies a connection between SERCA, IGF2R and calcium flux, a thorough explanation of the causal relationships is yet to be provided. Recently, we have identified a possible pathway in the context of muscular dystrophies, which are often associated with Ca^{2+} dysfunction: the contractile function of muscle fibers is dependent on the expression of many proteins involved in the calcium cycle between the cytosol and SR. Ca^{2+} signaling includes the ryanodine receptor, which is the SR Ca^{2+} release channel; the troponin protein complex, which leads to contraction; the extracellular Ca^{2+} reuptake pump, which mediates the flux of Ca^{2+} into the SR by a mechanism called store-operated Ca^{2+} entry (SOCE); and calsequestrin, the Ca^{2+}

storage protein in the SR. In addition, several Ca^{2+}-binding proteins are present in muscle tissue such as calmodulin, annexins, myosin, calcineurin and calpain [62]. In our study, we found that IGF2R expression is increased in dystrophic muscles, and IGF2R and the store-operated Ca^{2+} channel CD20 share a common hydrophobic binding motif stabilizing their association. We verified that the intravenous administration of an anti-IGF2R-neutralizing antibody facilitates IGF2/IGF1R interactions, while the occurrence of CD20 phosphorylation activation promotes the entrance of Ca^{2+} ions into the sarcoplasm [63]. Based on this evidence, we proposed a signaling pathway to explain the activation of SERCA and the Ca^{2+} flux through cells. Among the pathway proteins, STIM1 and ORAI1 are engaged in SOCE regulation and activation. STIM1 acts as a sensor of Ca^{2+} concentration in cellular stores and undergoes a horizontal movement in the SR membrane when the ER is calcium-depleted. Due to this shifting, STIM1 interacts with the membrane channel protein ORAI1 and causes calcium to enter the cell. After the replenishment of calcium stores, the ORAI1/STIM1 interaction dissolves and the Ca^{2+} influx stops. CD20 phosphorylation decreases the interaction between CD20 and ORAI1 in store-depleted myoblasts, largely in anti-IGF2R-treated myoblasts.

In dystrophic muscle, SERCA activity is reduced [64,65] leading to higher cytoplasmic levels of calcium ions. After anti-IGF2R treatment, calcium uptake is activated by CaMKII-dependent regulation of SERCA1: the blockade of IGF2R allows the activation of calcineurin, which dephosphorylates the nuclear factor of activated T cells (NFAT), which, consequently, shuttles into the nucleus, promoting activation of the genes involved in myogenic differentiation. Moreover, the binding of anti-IGF2R to domain 11 of IGF2R activates IGF2R/Gαi2 interactions, preventing the interplay with IGF2. This event increases the bioavailability of IGF2 for IGF1R and promotes the activation of PI3-K/AKT/mTOR signaling involved in expression of myogenic genes. Our results demonstrated that the blockade of IGF2R in mdx muscles rescued the murine dystrophic phenotype and increased force production. The in vivo experiments also revealed a marked vascular remodeling consisting of structural modifications resulting in higher linearization and wrapping of muscle fibers. It was conceivable that EPCs and pericyte cells accounted for the amelioration of the microvasculature and the blood supply. Adhesion and migration of EPCs could be affected directly by the IGF2R blockade, while pericytes cells, which present a contractile activity, could sense the calcium uptake activation [66]. Initially, pericytes had been discovered as mural cells able to provide capillary stability by interacting with endothelial cells. This classification was exceeded by anatomical and morphological evidence [67] demonstrating that pericytes could not only have a contractile activity, but they could regulate blood flow, capillary diameters and vascular tone [66,68,69]. In turn, pericytes' behavior in microcirculation can be regulated by upstream and downstream signaling, depending on the tissues and cell types. For instance, in healthy conditions, pericytes' coverage of the retina is essential for maintaining the contact with the endothelium and the integrity of the vascular barrier. Diabetic mice exhibit altered retinal vasal permeability caused by high levels of macrophage-secreted cathepsin D (CD). CD has been shown to disrupt the pericyte–endothelial junction either by increasing Rho/ROCK-dependent cell contractility [70] or by binding to IGF2R via 2M6P binding sites and changing PKC-α–CaMKII signaling [71].

Additional demonstrations of the association of IGF2R with insulin resistance and glucose homeostasis are based on the discovery of IGF2R genetic variants and soluble circulating IGF2R [72] in both type 1 (T1DM) and type 2 (T2DM) diabetes mellitus [73,74]. In T2DM, hyperglycemia seems to severely affect the islet capillary pericytes in terms of reduced numbers, improper islet coverage, altered calcium flux sensitivity, and relaxation phenotype shift [75]. As a response, diabetic capillaries dilate, blood pressure increases, and islets lose the ability to adapt and control their blood flow. Finally, high glucose concentrations and streptozotocin-induced diabetic conditions lead to abnormal activation of the IGF2R pathway and a downstream signaling for the expression of proteins related to hypertrophy in cardiac tissues, and to apoptosis in cardiomyocytes [76].

Taken together, this evidence suggests the importance of IGF2R in the pathogenesis or treatment of disorders related to energy metabolism, vascular remodeling and muscle homeostasis.

However, unraveling the signaling of the whole process within different tissues requires further and extensive investigation.

4.3. IGF2R Is Involved in Carcinogenesis

As described above, the proteins that constitute the IGF system—IGF1/IGF2, the surface receptors, and the IGF-binding proteins—regulate a plethora of functions related to growth and development operating through AKT1, mitogen-activated protein kinase (MAPK) and the phosphatidylinositol 3-kinase (PI3K) [77]. Consequently, dysfunction in this complex system is often associated with cancer. The upregulation of IGF2 was described in colorectal cancers (CRC) due to epigenetic mechanisms, and it was associated with poor survival [78]. In particular, IGF2 was dramatically overexpressed in tumorigenic clones related to IGF1, leading to constitutive activation of IGF1R and AKT [79] and to malignant modulation of apoptosis and stemness [80]. In addition, the loss of IGF2 imprinting was associated with esophageal adenocarcinoma [81], while the hypomethylation of one of the IGF2 promoters caused dysfunction in the transcriptional regulator Kruppel-like factor 4 (KLF4) in humane prostate cancer [82]. Genetic mutations in IGF2R can modify the bioavailability of IGF2 so that cancer cells can dramatically proliferate. Different studies demonstrated that IGF2R expression could be involved in the development of hepatocarcinoma, breast and ovarian human cancers by encoding for a tumor suppressor gene [83]. In particular, the loss of heterozygosity (LOH) at the M6P/IGF2R gene locus on 6q26–27 chromosome seemed to be associated with the invasiveness of breast cancers, while M6P/IGF2R point mutations were identified in hepatoma, gastrointestinal (mainly associated with microsatellite instability) and prostate tumors [84]. This condition likely led to uncontrolled IGF2 upregulation that enhanced cancer growth and survival by binding to IGF1R. In particular, the work of Delaine et al. [85] showed a new hydrophobic patch on the domain 11 of the IGF2R that is fundamental for the high binding affinity of IGF2/IGF2R. The first direct demonstration of IGF2R in tumor growth came from the work of Chen et al., in which they described how the downregulation of M6P/IGF2R expression in adenocarcinoma cells led to increased cell proliferation and decreased susceptibility to apoptosis, according to the bioavailability of TNFα and activated TGF-β. In addition, this condition was probably hampered by the action of IGF2 and cathepsins B and D [86]. Interestingly, ligands other than IGF2 can bind to IGF2R: among them are urokinase-type plasminogen activator receptor (uPAR) and retinoic acid, whose activity allows the internalization of IGF2 [7]. All the IGF2R-dependent pathways are summarized in Figure 1.

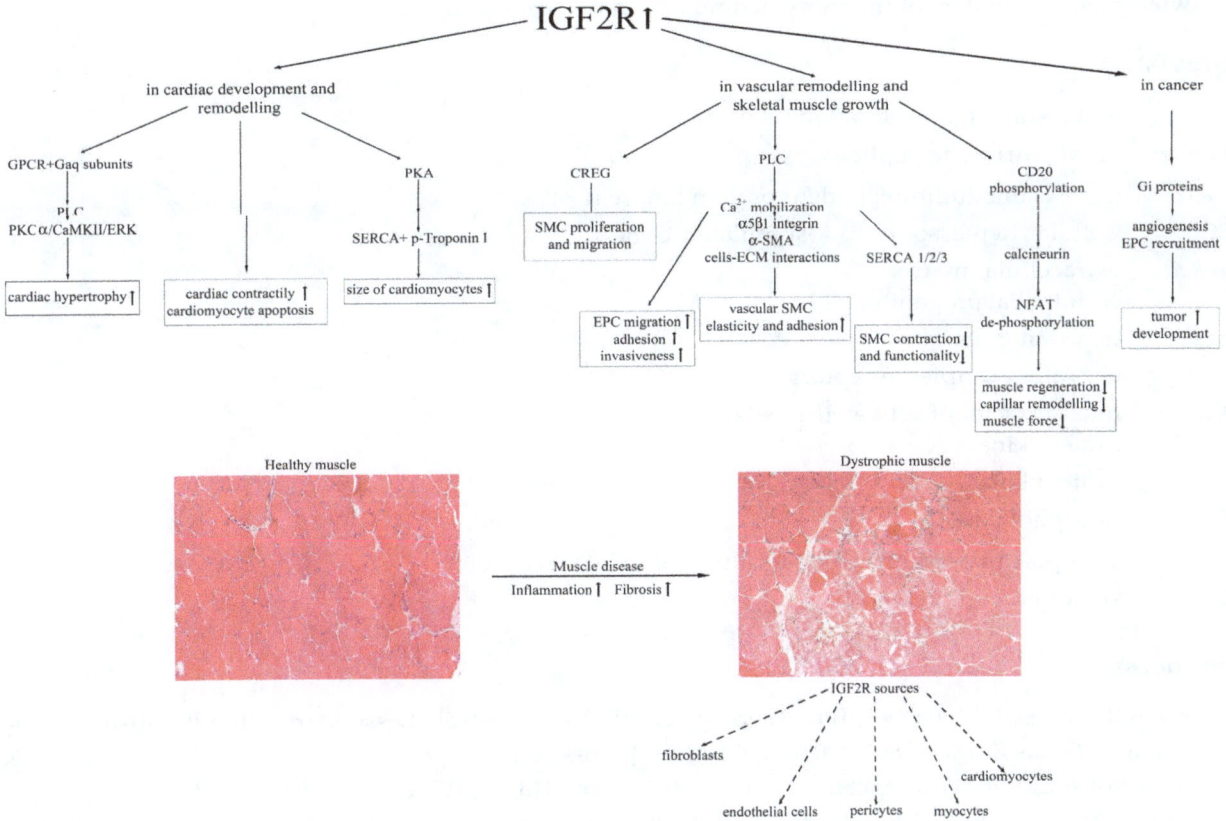

Figure 1. A schematic model of the IGF2R-dependent mechanisms leading to cardiac and skeletal muscle impairment, and cell sources of IGF2R expression in dystrophic muscle.

5. Conclusions

Fetal growth and post-natal growth are closely regulated by the insulin-like growth factor axis: alterations in the IGF signaling pathways could cause severe dysfunction in somatic growth and development and be responsible for tumor proliferation. We have recently demonstrated in mdx mice that intravenous administration of an anti-IGF2R neutralizing antibody significantly upregulated muscle regeneration and decreased fibrosis, leading to the rescue of the pathological phenotype. The inhibition of IGF2R resulted in an increase in intracellular Ca^{2+} in myoblasts and increased SERCA1 activity, possibly operating through CD20. This condition allowed NFAT dephosphorylation and its translocation into the nucleus. The dystrophic phenotype rescue activated in vivo by the anti-IGF2R antibody was further corroborated by higher numbers of structurally more linear microvessels enveloping myofibers. It is likely that anti-IGF2R acts on pericyte function, determining normalization of the vascular wall and consequent amelioration of the oxygenation of the dystrophic muscle. As contractile cells, pericytes can regulate their tone and contraction depending on the intracellular calcium concentration and consequently tune the capillary diameter and blood flow [69].

This is an exciting time in our understanding of muscular dystrophies. Increasing knowledge of IGF2R's role in muscle disease is starting to suggest new therapeutic approaches. A challenge for the future will be to understand how IGF2R interacts with other components of the muscle system to influence muscular dystrophy progression. Similarly, genetic and epigenetic changes affecting *IGF2R* need to be considered. Therefore, targeting IGF2R may be a potential therapeutic strategy for muscular dystrophies.

Author Contributions: A.F., Y.T. and C.V. wrote the paper. P.B. and L.T. prepared the original draft of the manuscript. All the authors stated were involved in the critical revision of the manuscript and approved the final version of the article, including the authorship list. The corresponding authors had final responsibility for the decision to submit for publication. All authors have read and agreed to the published version of the manuscript.

Acknowledgments: Funders of the study had no role in manuscript design.

Abbreviations

α-SMA	alpha smooth muscle actin
ANP	atrial natriuretic peptide
CaMKII	Ca^{2+-}calmodulin-dependent protein kinase II
CREG	Cellular Repressor of E1A-stimulated Gene
ECM	extracellular matrix
EPC	endothelial progenitor cell
$G\alpha q$	αq G subunits
GPCR	G-protein-coupled receptors
NFAT	nuclear factor of activated T cells
PKA	protein kinase A
PKC-α	protein kinase C-α
PLC	phospholipase C
SERCA	sarcoplasmic/endoplasmic reticulum (SR) Ca^{2+}ATPase
SMC	smooth muscle cell

References

1. Brown, J.; Jones, E.Y.; Forbes, B.E. Keeping IGF-II under control: Lessons from the IGF-II-IGF2R crystal structure. *Trends Biochem. Sci.* **2009**, *34*, 612–619. [CrossRef]

2. Livingstone, C. IGF2 and cancer. *Endocr. Relat. Cancer* **2013**, *20*, R321–R339. [CrossRef]

3. Dahms, N.M.; Brzycki-Wessell, M.A.; Ramanujam, K.S.; Seetharam, B. Characterization of mannose 6-phosphate receptors (MPRs) from opossum liver: Opossum cation-independent MPR binds insulin-like growth factor-II. *Endocrinology* **1993**, *133*, 440–446. [CrossRef] [PubMed]

4. Reddy, S.T.; Chai, W.; Childs, R.A.; Page, J.D.; Feizi, T.; Dahms, N.M. Identification of a low affinity mannose 6-phosphate-binding site in domain 5 of the cation-independent mannose 6-phosphate receptor. *J. Biol. Chem.* **2004**, *279*, 38658–38667. [CrossRef] [PubMed]

5. Williams, C.; Rezgui, D.; Prince, S.N.; Zaccheo, O.J.; Foulstone, E.J.; Forbes, B.E.; Norton, R.S.; Crosby, J.; Hassan, A.B.; Crump, M.P. Structural insights into the interaction of insulin-like growth factor 2 with IGF2R domain 11. *Structure* **2007**, *15*, 1065–1078. [CrossRef] [PubMed]

6. Morali, O.G.; Jouneau, A.; McLaughlin, K.J.; Thiery, J.P.; Larue, L. IGF-II promotes mesoderm formation. *Dev. Biol.* **2000**, *227*, 133–145. [CrossRef] [PubMed]

7. Martin-Kleiner, I.; Gall Troselj, K. Mannose-6-phosphate/insulin-like growth factor 2 receptor (M6P/IGF2R) in carcinogenesis. *Cancer Lett.* **2010**, *289*, 11–22. [CrossRef] [PubMed]

8. Rotwein, P.; Pollock, K.M.; Watson, M.; Milbrandt, J.D. Insulin-like growth factor gene expression during rat embryonic development. *Endocrinology* **1987**, *121*, 2141–2144. [CrossRef] [PubMed]

9. Smith, J.; Goldsmith, C.; Ward, A.; LeDieu, R. IGF-II ameliorates the dystrophic phenotype and coordinately down-regulates programmed cell death. *Cell Death Differ.* **2000**, *7*, 1109–1118. [CrossRef]

10. Wise, T.L.; Pravtcheva, D.D. Delayed onset of Igf2-induced mammary tumors in Igf2r transgenic mice. *Cancer Res.* **2006**, *66*, 1327–1336. [CrossRef]

11. Takeda, T.; Komatsu, M.; Chiwaki, F.; Komatsuzaki, R.; Nakamura, K.; Tsuji, K.; Kobayashi, Y.; Tominaga, E.; Ono, M.; Banno, K.; et al. Upregulation of IGF2R evades lysosomal dysfunction-induced apoptosis of cervical cancer cells via transport of cathepsins. *Cell Death Dis.* **2019**, *10*, 876. [CrossRef] [PubMed]

12. Varghese, R.T.; Liang, Y.; Guan, T.; Franck, C.T.; Kelly, D.F.; Sheng, Z. Survival kinase genes present prognostic significance in glioblastoma. *Oncotarget* **2016**, *7*, 20140–20151. [CrossRef] [PubMed]

13. Kast, R.E.; Skuli, N.; Karpel-Massler, G.; Frosina, G.; Ryken, T.; Halatsch, M.E. Blocking epithelial-to-mesenchymal transition in glioblastoma with a sextet of repurposed drugs: The EIS regimen. *Oncotarget* **2017**, *8*, 60727–60749. [CrossRef]

14. Guiraud, S.; Davies, K.E. Regenerative biomarkers for Duchenne muscular dystrophy. *Neural Regen. Res.* **2019**, *14*, 1317–1320. [CrossRef]

15. Villalta, S.A.; Nguyen, H.X.; Deng, B.; Gotoh, T.; Tidball, J.G. Shifts in macrophage phenotypes and macrophage competition for arginine metabolism affect the severity of muscle pathology in muscular dystrophy. *Hum. Mol. Genet.* **2009**, *18*, 482–496. [CrossRef]

16. Villalta, S.A.; Rosenberg, A.S.; Bluestone, J.A. The immune system in Duchenne muscular dystrophy: Friend or foe. *Rare Dis.* **2015**, *3*, e1010966. [CrossRef]

17. Kobayashi, Y.M.; Rader, E.P.; Crawford, R.W.; Campbell, K.P. Endpoint measures in the mdx mouse relevant for muscular dystrophy pre-clinical studies. *Neuromuscul. Disord.* **2012**, *22*, 34–42. [CrossRef]

18. Angelini, C.; Nardetto, L.; Borsato, C.; Padoan, R.; Fanin, M.; Nascimbeni, A.C.; Tasca, E. The clinical course of calpainopathy (LGMD2A) and dysferlinopathy (LGMD2B). *Neurol. Res.* **2010**, *32*, 41–46. [CrossRef]

19. Emery, A.E. The muscular dystrophies. *Lancet* **2002**, *359*, 687–695. [CrossRef]

20. Lawrence, M.C.; McKern, N.M.; Ward, C.W. Insulin receptor structure and its implications for the IGF-1 receptor. *Curr. Opin. Struct. Biol.* **2007**, *17*, 699–705. [CrossRef]

21. Barton-Davis, E.R.; Shoturma, D.I.; Sweeney, H.L. Contribution of satellite cells to IGF-I induced hypertrophy of skeletal muscle. *Acta Physiol. Scand.* **1999**, *167*, 301–305. [CrossRef]

22. Hennebry, A.; Oldham, J.; Shavlakadze, T.; Grounds, M.D.; Sheard, P.; Fiorotto, M.L.; Falconer, S.; Smith, H.K.; Berry, C.; Jeanplong, F.; et al. IGF1 stimulates greater muscle hypertrophy in the absence of myostatin in male mice. *J. Endocrinol.* **2017**, *234*, 187–200. [CrossRef]

23. Shavlakadze, T.; Chai, J.; Maley, K.; Cozens, G.; Grounds, G.; Winn, N.; Rosenthal, N.; Grounds, M.D. A growth stimulus is needed for IGF-1 to induce skeletal muscle hypertrophy in vivo. *J. Cell Sci.* **2010**, *123*, 960–971. [CrossRef]

24. Slusher, A.L.; Huang, C.J.; Acevedo, E.O. The Potential Role of Aerobic Exercise-Induced Pentraxin 3 on Obesity-Related Inflammation and Metabolic Dysregulation. *Mediators Inflamm.* **2017**, *2017*, 1092738. [CrossRef]

25. Yang, S.; Alnaqeeb, M.; Simpson, H.; Goldspink, G. Cloning and characterization of an IGF-1 isoform expressed in skeletal muscle subjected to stretch. *J. Muscle Res. Cell. Motil.* **1996**, *17*, 487–495. [CrossRef]

26. Clemmons, D.R. Role of IGF-I in skeletal muscle mass maintenance. *Trends Endocrinol. Metab.* **2009**, *20*, 349–356. [CrossRef]

27. Florini, J.R.; Ewton, D.Z.; Coolican, S.A. Growth hormone and the insulin-like growth factor system in myogenesis. *Endocr. Rev.* **1996**, *17*, 481–517. [CrossRef]

28. Fargeas, C.A.; Florek, M.; Huttner, W.B.; Corbeil, D. Characterization of prominin-2, a new member of the prominin family of pentaspan membrane glycoproteins. *J. Biol. Chem.* **2003**, *278*, 8586–8596. [CrossRef]

29. Spicer, L.J.; Aad, P.Y. Insulin-like growth factor (IGF) 2 stimulates steroidogenesis and mitosis of bovine granulosa cells through the IGF1 receptor: Role of follicle-stimulating hormone and IGF2 receptor. *Biol. Reprod.* **2007**, *77*, 18–27. [CrossRef]

30. Erbay, E.; Park, I.H.; Nuzzi, P.D.; Schoenherr, C.J.; Chen, J. IGF-II transcription in skeletal myogenesis is controlled by mTOR and nutrients. *J. Cell Biol.* **2003**, *163*, 931–936. [CrossRef]

31. Ge, Y.; Sun, Y.; Chen, J. IGF-II is regulated by microRNA-125b in skeletal myogenesis. *J. Cell Biol.* **2011**, *192*, 69–81. [CrossRef]

32. Deschenes, M.R. Effects of aging on muscle fibre type and size. *Sports Med.* **2004**, *34*, 809–824. [CrossRef]

33. Pedemonte, M.; Sandri, C.; Schiaffino, S.; Minetti, C. Early decrease of IIx myosin heavy chain transcripts in Duchenne muscular dystrophy. *Biochem. Biophys. Res. Commun.* **1999**, *255*, 466–469. [CrossRef]

34. Merrick, D.; Ting, T.; Stadler, L.K.; Smith, J. A role for Insulin-like growth factor 2 in specification of the fast skeletal muscle fibre. *BMC Dev. Biol.* **2007**, *7*, 65. [CrossRef]

35. Park, K.S.; Mitra, A.; Rahat, B.; Kim, K.; Pfeifer, K. Loss of imprinting mutations define both distinct and overlapping roles for misexpression of IGF2 and of H19 lncRNA. *Nucleic Acids Res.* **2017**, *45*, 12766–12779. [CrossRef]

36. Marasek, P.; Dzijak, R.; Studenyak, I.; Fiserova, J.; Ulicna, L.; Novak, P.; Hozak, P. Paxillin-dependent regulation of IGF2 and H19 gene cluster expression. *J. Cell Sci.* **2015**, *128*, 3106–3116. [CrossRef]

37. Kalscheuer, V.M.; Mariman, E.C.; Schepens, M.T.; Rehder, H.; Ropers, H.H. The insulin-like growth factor type-2 receptor gene is imprinted in the mouse but not in humans. *Nat. Genet.* **1993**, *5*, 74–78. [CrossRef]

38. Szebenyi, G.; Rotwein, P. The mouse insulin-like growth factor II/cation-independent mannose 6-phosphate (IGF-II/MPR) receptor gene: Molecular cloning and genomic organization. *Genomics* **1994**, *19*, 120–129. [CrossRef]

39. Lemamy, G.J.; Sahla, M.E.; Berthe, M.L.; Roger, P. Is the mannose-6-phosphate/insulin-like growth factor 2 receptor coded by a breast cancer suppressor gene? *Adv. Exp. Med. Biol.* **2008**, *617*, 305–310. [CrossRef]

40. El-Shewy, H.M.; Johnson, K.R.; Lee, M.H.; Jaffa, A.A.; Obeid, L.M.; Luttrell, L.M. Insulin-like growth factors mediate heterotrimeric G protein-dependent ERK1/2 activation by transactivating sphingosine 1-phosphate receptors. *J. Biol. Chem.* **2006**, *281*, 31399–31407. [CrossRef]

41. Nishimoto, I.; Hata, Y.; Ogata, E.; Kojima, I. Insulin-like growth factor II stimulates calcium influx in competent BALB/c 3T3 cells primed with epidermal growth factor. Characteristics of calcium influx and involvement of GTP-binding protein. *J. Biol. Chem.* **1987**, *262*, 12120–12126. [PubMed]

42. Nishimoto, I.; Murayama, Y.; Katada, T.; Ui, M.; Ogata, E. Possible direct linkage of insulin-like growth factor-II receptor with guanine nucleotide-binding proteins. *J. Biol. Chem.* **1989**, *264*, 14029–14038.

43. Chu, C.H.; Lo, J.F.; Hu, W.S.; Lu, R.B.; Chang, M.H.; Tsai, F.J.; Tsai, C.H.; Weng, Y.S.; Tzang, B.S.; Huang, C.Y. Histone acetylation is essential for ANG-II-induced IGF-IIR gene expression in H9c2 cardiomyoblast cells and pathologically hypertensive rat heart. *J. Cell. Physiol.* **2012**, *227*, 259–268. [CrossRef] [PubMed]

44. Chang, M.H.; Kuo, W.W.; Chen, R.J.; Lu, M.C.; Tsai, F.J.; Kuo, W.H.; Chen, L.Y.; Wu, W.J.; Huang, C.Y.; Chu, C.H. IGF-II/mannose 6-phosphate receptor activation induces metalloproteinase-9 matrix activity and increases plasminogen activator expression in H9c2 cardiomyoblast cells. *J. Mol. Endocrinol.* **2008**, *41*, 65–74. [CrossRef]

45. Chen, R.J.; Wu, H.C.; Chang, M.H.; Lai, C.H.; Tien, Y.C.; Hwang, J.M.; Kuo, W.H.; Tsai, F.J.; Tsai, C.H.; Chen, L.M.; et al. Leu27IGF2 plays an opposite role to IGF1 to induce H9c2 cardiomyoblast cell apoptosis via Galphaq signaling. *J. Mol. Endocrinol.* **2009**, *43*, 221–230. [CrossRef] [PubMed]

46. Wang, K.C.; Brooks, D.A.; Thornburg, K.L.; Morrison, J.L. Activation of IGF-2R stimulates cardiomyocyte hypertrophy in the late gestation sheep fetus. *J. Physiol.* **2012**, *590*, 5425–5437. [CrossRef]

47. Chu, C.H.; Huang, C.Y.; Lu, M.C.; Lin, J.A.; Tsai, F.J.; Tsai, C.H.; Chu, C.Y.; Kuo, W.H.; Chen, L.M.; Chen, L.Y. Enhancement of AG1024-induced H9c2 cardiomyoblast cell apoptosis via the interaction of IGF2R with Galpha proteins and its downstream PKA and PLC-beta modulators by IGF-II. *CHINESE J. Physiol.* **2009**, *52*, 31–37. [CrossRef]

48. Huang, C.Y.; Kuo, W.W.; Lo, J.F.; Ho, T.J.; Pai, P.Y.; Chiang, S.F.; Chen, P.Y.; Tsai, F.J.; Tsai, C.H.; Huang, C.Y. Doxorubicin attenuates CHIP-guarded HSF1 nuclear translocation and protein stability to trigger IGF-IIR-dependent cardiomyocyte death. *Cell Death Dis.* **2016**, *7*, e2455. [CrossRef]

49. Wang, K.C.; Brooks, D.A.; Botting, K.J.; Morrison, J.L. IGF-2R-mediated signaling results in hypertrophy of cultured cardiomyocytes from fetal sheep. *Biol. Reprod.* **2012**, *86*, 183. [CrossRef]

50. Han, Y.; Cui, J.; Tao, J.; Guo, L.; Guo, P.; Sun, M.; Kang, J.; Zhang, X.; Yan, C.; Li, S. CREG inhibits migration of human vascular smooth muscle cells by mediating IGF-II endocytosis. *Exp. Cell Res.* **2009**, *315*, 3301–3311. [CrossRef]

51. Chu, C.H.; Tzang, B.S.; Chen, L.M.; Kuo, C.H.; Cheng, Y.C.; Chen, L.Y.; Tsai, F.J.; Tsai, C.H.; Kuo, W.W.; Huang, C.Y. IGF-II/mannose-6-phosphate receptor signaling induced cell hypertrophy and atrial natriuretic peptide/BNP expression via Galphaq interaction and protein kinase C-alpha/CaMKII activation in H9c2 cardiomyoblast cells. *J. Endocrinol.* **2008**, *197*, 381–390. [CrossRef] [PubMed]

52. Maeng, Y.S.; Choi, H.J.; Kwon, J.Y.; Park, Y.W.; Choi, K.S.; Min, J.K.; Kim, Y.H.; Suh, P.G.; Kang, K.S.; Won, M.H.; et al. Endothelial progenitor cell homing: Prominent role of the IGF2-IGF2R-PLCbeta2 axis. *Blood* **2009**, *113*, 233–243. [CrossRef] [PubMed]

53. Zhu, Y.; Qu, J.; He, L.; Zhang, F.; Zhou, Z.; Yang, S.; Zhou, Y. Calcium in Vascular Smooth Muscle Cell Elasticity and Adhesion: Novel Insights Into the Mechanism of Action. *Front. Physiol.* **2019**, *10*, 852. [CrossRef] [PubMed]

54. Nance, M.E.; Whitfield, J.T.; Zhu, Y.; Gibson, A.K.; Hanft, L.M.; Campbell, K.S.; Meininger, G.A.; McDonald, K.S.; Segal, S.S.; Domeier, T.L. Attenuated sarcomere lengthening of the aged murine left ventricle observed using two-photon fluorescence microscopy. *Am. J. Physiol. Heart Circ. Physiol.* **2015**, *309*, H918–H925. [CrossRef]

55. Bers, D.M. Calcium cycling and signaling in cardiac myocytes. *Annu. Rev. Physiol.* **2008**, *70*, 23–49. [CrossRef]

56. Lipskaia, L.; Hulot, J.S.; Lompre, A.M. Role of sarco/endoplasmic reticulum calcium content and calcium ATPase activity in the control of cell growth and proliferation. *Pflug. Arch. Eur. J. Phy.* **2009**, *457*, 673–685. [CrossRef]

57. Chami, M.; Gozuacik, D.; Lagorce, D.; Brini, M.; Falson, P.; Peaucellier, G.; Pinton, P.; Lecoeur, H.; Gougeon, M.L.; le Maire, M.; et al. SERCA1 truncated proteins unable to pump calcium reduce the endoplasmic reticulum calcium concentration and induce apoptosis. *J. Cell Biol.* **2001**, *153*, 1301–1314. [CrossRef]

58. Gelebart, P.; Martin, V.; Enouf, J.; Papp, B. Identification of a new SERCA2 splice variant regulated during monocytic differentiation. *Biochem. Biophys. Res. Commun.* **2003**, *303*, 676–684. [CrossRef]

59. Bobe, R.; Bredoux, R.; Corvazier, E.; Andersen, J.P.; Clausen, J.D.; Dode, L.; Kovacs, T.; Enouf, J. Identification, expression, function, and localization of a novel (sixth) isoform of the human sarco/endoplasmic reticulum Ca2+ATPase 3 gene. *J. Biol. Chem.* **2004**, *279*, 24297–24306. [CrossRef]

60. Davies, M.G. New Insights on the Role of SERCA During Vessel Remodeling in Metabolic Syndrome. *Diabetes* **2015**, *64*, 3066–3068. [CrossRef]

61. Johny, J.P.; Plank, M.J.; David, T. Importance of Altered Levels of SERCA, IP3R, and RyR in Vascular Smooth Muscle Cell. *Biophys. J.* **2017**, *112*, 265–287. [CrossRef] [PubMed]

62. Harisseh, R.; Chatelier, A.; Magaud, C.; Deliot, N.; Constantin, B. Involvement of TRPV2 and SOCE in calcium influx disorder in DMD primary human myotubes with a specific contribution of alpha1-syntrophin and PLC/PKC in SOCE regulation. *Am. J. Physiol. Cell Physiol.* **2013**, *304*, C881–C894. [CrossRef] [PubMed]

63. Bella, P.; Farini, A.; Banfi, S.; Parolini, D.; Tonna, N.; Meregalli, M.; Belicchi, M.; Erratico, S.; D'Ursi, P.; Bianco, F.; et al. Blockade of IGF2R improves muscle regeneration and ameliorates Duchenne muscular dystrophy. *EMBO Mol. Med.* **2020**, *12*, e11019. [CrossRef] [PubMed]

64. Divet, A.; Huchet-Cadiou, C. Sarcoplasmic reticulum function in slow- and fast-twitch skeletal muscles from mdx mice. *Pflug. Arch. Eur. J. Phy.* **2002**, *444*, 634–643. [CrossRef]

65. Kargacin, M.E.; Kargacin, G.J. The sarcoplasmic reticulum calcium pump is functionally altered in dystrophic muscle. *Biochim. Biophys. Acta* **1996**, *1290*, 4–8. [CrossRef]

66. Burdyga, T.; Borysova, L. Calcium signalling in pericytes. *J. Vasc. Res.* **2014**, *51*, 190–199. [CrossRef]

67. Toribatake, Y.; Tomita, K.; Kawahara, N.; Baba, H.; Ohnari, H.; Tanaka, S. Regulation of vasomotion of arterioles and capillaries in the cat spinal cord: Role of alpha actin and endothelin-1. *Spinal cord* **1997**, *35*, 26–32. [CrossRef]

68. Borysova, L.; Wray, S.; Eisner, D.A.; Burdyga, T. How calcium signals in myocytes and pericytes are integrated across in situ microvascular networks and control microvascular tone. *Cell Calcium.* **2013**, *54*, 163–174. [CrossRef]

69. Hamilton, N.B.; Attwell, D.; Hall, C.N. Pericyte-mediated regulation of capillary diameter: A component of neurovascular coupling in health and disease. *Front. Neuroenerg.* **2010**, *2*. [CrossRef]

70. Monickaraj, F.; McGuire, P.G.; Nitta, C.F.; Ghosh, K.; Das, A. Cathepsin D: An Mvarphi-derived factor mediating increased endothelial cell permeability with implications for alteration of the blood-retinal barrier in diabetic retinopathy. *FASEB J.* **2016**, *30*, 1670–1682. [CrossRef]

71. Monickaraj, F.; McGuire, P.; Das, A. Cathepsin D plays a role in endothelial-pericyte interactions during alteration of the blood-retinal barrier in diabetic retinopathy. *FASEB J.* **2018**, *32*, 2539–2548. [CrossRef] [PubMed]

72. Chanprasertyothin, S.; Jongjaroenprasert, W.; Ongphiphadhanakul, B. The association of soluble IGF2R and IGF2R gene polymorphism with type 2 diabetes. *J. Diabetes Res.* **2015**, *2015*, 216383. [CrossRef] [PubMed]

73. McCann, J.A.; Xu, Y.Q.; Frechette, R.; Guazzarotti, L.; Polychronakos, C. The insulin-like growth factor-II receptor gene is associated with type 1 diabetes: Evidence of a maternal effect. *J. Clin. Endocrinol. Metab.* **2004**, *89*, 5700–5706. [CrossRef] [PubMed]

74. Villuendas, G.; Botella-Carretero, J.I.; Lopez-Bermejo, A.; Gubern, C.; Ricart, W.; Fernandez-Real, J.M.; San Millan, J.L.; Escobar-Morreale, H.F. The ACAA-insertion/deletion polymorphism at the 3' UTR of the IGF-II receptor gene is associated with type 2 diabetes and surrogate markers of insulin resistance. *Eur. J. Endocrinol.* **2006**, *155*, 331–336. [CrossRef] [PubMed]

75. Almaca, J.; Weitz, J.; Rodriguez-Diaz, R.; Pereira, E.; Caicedo, A. The Pericyte of the Pancreatic Islet Regulates Capillary Diameter and Local Blood Flow. *Cell Metab.* **2018**, *27*, 630–644. [CrossRef] [PubMed]

76. Feng, C.C.; Pandey, S.; Lin, C.Y.; Shen, C.Y.; Chang, R.L.; Chang, T.T.; Chen, R.J.; Viswanadha, V.P.; Lin, Y.M.; Huang, C.Y. Cardiac apoptosis induced under high glucose condition involves activation of IGF2R signaling in H9c2 cardiomyoblasts and streptozotocin-induced diabetic rat hearts. *Biomed. Pharmacother.* **2018**, *97*, 880–885. [CrossRef]

77. Kasprzak, A.; Adamek, A. Insulin-Like Growth Factor 2 (IGF2) Signaling in Colorectal Cancer-From Basic Research to Potential Clinical Applications. *Int. J. Mol. Sci.* **2019**, *20*, 4915. [CrossRef]

78. Unger, C.; Kramer, N.; Unterleuthner, D.; Scherzer, M.; Burian, A.; Rudisch, A.; Stadler, M.; Schlederer, M.; Lenhardt, D.; Riedl, A.; et al. Stromal-derived IGF2 promotes colon cancer progression via paracrine and autocrine mechanisms. *Oncogene* **2017**, *36*, 5341–5355. [CrossRef]

79. Sanderson, M.P.; Hofmann, M.H.; Garin-Chesa, P.; Schweifer, N.; Wernitznig, A.; Fischer, S.; Jeschko, A.; Meyer, R.; Moll, J.; Pecina, T.; et al. The IGF1R/INSR Inhibitor BI 885578 Selectively Inhibits Growth of IGF2-Overexpressing Colorectal Cancer Tumors and Potentiates the Efficacy of Anti-VEGF Therapy. *Mol. Cancer Ther.* **2017**, *16*, 2223–2233. [CrossRef]

80. Kessler, S.M.; Haybaeck, J.; Kiemer, A.K. Insulin-Like Growth Factor 2 - The Oncogene and its Accomplices. *Curr. Pharm. Des.* **2016**, *22*, 5948–5961. [CrossRef]

81. Zhao, R.; DeCoteau, J.F.; Geyer, C.R.; Gao, M.; Cui, H.; Casson, A.G. Loss of imprinting of the insulin-like growth factor II (IGF2) gene in esophageal normal and adenocarcinoma tissues. *Carcinogenesis* **2009**, *30*, 2117–2122. [CrossRef] [PubMed]

82. Schagdarsurengin, U.; Lammert, A.; Schunk, N.; Sheridan, D.; Gattenloehner, S.; Steger, K.; Wagenlehner, F.; Dansranjavin, T. Impairment of IGF2 gene expression in prostate cancer is triggered by epigenetic dysregulation of IGF2-DMR0 and its interaction with KLF4. *Cell Commun. Signal.* **2017**, *15*, 40. [CrossRef] [PubMed]

83. Lemamy, G.J.; Roger, P.; Mani, J.C.; Robert, M.; Rochefort, H.; Brouillet, J.P. High-affinity antibodies from hen's-egg yolks against human mannose-6-phosphate/insulin-like growth-factor-II receptor (M6P/IGFII-R): Characterization and potential use in clinical cancer studies. *Int. J. Cancer* **1999**, *80*, 896–902. [CrossRef]

84. Oates, A.J.; Schumaker, L.M.; Jenkins, S.B.; Pearce, A.A.; DaCosta, S.A.; Arun, B.; Ellis, M.J. The mannose 6-phosphate/insulin-like growth factor 2 receptor (M6P/IGF2R), a putative breast tumor suppressor gene. *Breast Cancer Res. Treat.* **1998**, *47*, 269–281. [CrossRef] [PubMed]

85. Delaine, C.; Alvino, C.L.; McNeil, K.A.; Mulhern, T.D.; Gauguin, L.; De Meyts, P.; Jones, E.Y.; Brown, J.; Wallace, J.C.; Forbes, B.E. A novel binding site for the human insulin-like growth factor-II (IGF-II)/mannose 6-phosphate receptor on IGF-II. *J. Biol. Chem.* **2007**, *282*, 18886–18894. [CrossRef]

86. Chen, Z.; Ge, Y.; Landman, N.; Kang, J.X. Decreased expression of the mannose 6-phosphate/insulin-like growth factor-II receptor promotes growth of human breast cancer cells. *BMC Cancer* **2002**, *2*, 18. [CrossRef]

Permissions

List of Contributors

Lidan Zhang
Project for Muscle Stem Cell Biology, Graduate School of Pharmaceutical Sciences, Osaka University, 1–6 Yamadaoka, Suita, Osaka 565–0871, Japan
Laboratory of Molecular and Cellular Physiology, Graduate School of Pharmaceutical Sciences, Osaka University, 1–6 Yamadaoka, Suita, Osaka 565–0871, Japan

Akiyoshi Uezumi
Muscle Aging and Regenerative Medicine, Tokyo Metropolitan Institute of Gerontology, Itabashi-ku, Tokyo 173–0015, Japan

Takayuki Kaji and So-ichiro Fukada
Project for Muscle Stem Cell Biology, Graduate School of Pharmaceutical Sciences, Osaka University, 1–6 Yamadaoka, Suita, Osaka 565–0871, Japan

Kazutake Tsujikawa
Laboratory of Molecular and Cellular Physiology, Graduate School of Pharmaceutical Sciences, Osaka University, 1–6 Yamadaoka, Suita, Osaka 565–0871, Japan

Ditte Caroline Andersen
Laboratory of Molecular and Cellular Cardiology, Department of Clinical Biochemistry and Pharmacology, Odense University Hospital, Winsloewparken 21 3rd, 5000 Odense C, Denmark
Clinical Institute, University of Southern Denmark, Winsloewparken 21 3rd, 5000 Odense C, Denmark

Charlotte Harken Jensen
Laboratory of Molecular and Cellular Cardiology, Department of Clinical Biochemistry and Pharmacology, Odense University Hospital, Winsloewparken 21 3rd, 5000 Odense C, Denmark

Satoshi Oikawa, Minjung Lee and Takayuki Akimoto
Faculty of Sport Sciences, Waseda University, Saitama 359-1192, Japan

Hye-Won Yang
Department of Marine Life Science, School of Marine Biomedical Sciences, Jeju National University, 1 Ara 1-dong, Jejudaehak-ro, Jeju 63243, Korea

Myeongjoo Son, Junwon Choi and Kyunghee Byun
Department of Anatomy & Cell Biology, Gachon University College of Medicine, Incheon 21936, Korea
Functional Cellular Networks Laboratory, College of Medicine, Department of Medicine, Graduate School and Lee Gil Ya Cancer and Diabetes Institute, Gachon University, Incheon 21999, Korea

Seyeon Oh
Functional Cellular Networks Laboratory, College of Medicine, Department of Medicine, Graduate School and Lee Gil Ya Cancer and Diabetes Institute, Gachon University, Incheon 21999, Korea

You-Jin Jeon and BoMi Ryu
Department of Marine Life Science, School of Marine Biomedical Sciences, Jeju National University, 1 Ara 1-dong, Jejudaehak-ro, Jeju 63243, Korea
Marine Science Institute, Jeju National University, Jeju 63333, Korea

Roberta Squecco, Rachele Garella and Eglantina Idrizaj
Department of Experimental and Clinical Medicine, Section of Physiological Sciences, University of Florence, 50134 Florence, Italy

Flaminia Chellini, Alessia Tani, Sofia Pancani, Sandra Zecchi-Orlandini and Chiara Sassoli
Department of Experimental and Clinical Medicine, Section of Anatomy and Histology, University of Florence, 50134 Florence, Italy

Paola Pavan and Franco Bambi
Transfusion Medicine and Cell Therapy Unit, "A. Meyer" University Children's Hospital, 50134 Florence, Italy

Cheng-long Jin, Chun-qi Gao, Hui-chao Yan and Xiu-qi Wang
College of Animal Science, South China Agricultural University/Guangdong Provincial Key Laboratory of Animal Nutrition Control/National Engineering Research Center for Breeding Swine Industry, Guangzhou 510642, China

Jin-ling Ye
Institute of Animal Science, Guangdong Academy of Agricultural Sciences, Guangzhou 510642, China

Jinzeng Yang
Department of Human Nutrition, Food and Animal Sciences, University of Hawaii, Honolulu, HI 96822, USA

Hai-chang Li
Department of Surgery, Davis Heart and Lung Research Institute, The Ohio State University, Columbus, OH 43210, USA

Ornella Cappellari, Paola Mantuano and Annamaria De Luca
Section of Pharmacology, Department of Pharmacy-Drug Sciences, University of Bari "Aldo Moro", via Orabona 4—Campus, 70125 Bari, Italy

Jean-Philippe Leduc-Gaudet
Meakins-Christie Laboratories and Translational Research in Respiratory Diseases Program, Research Institute of the McGill University Health Centre, Department of Critical Care, McGill University Health Centre, Montréal, QC H4A 3J1, Canada
Division of Experimental Medicine, McGill University, Montréal, QC H4A 3J1, Canada
Département des sciences de l'activité physique, Faculté des Sciences, UQAM, Montréal, QC H2X 1Y4, Canada
Groupe de recherche en Activité Physique Adaptée, Montréal, QC H2X 1Y4, Canada
Département des sciences biologiques, Faculté des Sciences, UQAM, Montréal, QC H2X 1Y4, Canada

Dominique Mayaki and Tomer J. Chaffer
Meakins-Christie Laboratories and Translational Research in Respiratory Diseases Program, Research Institute of the McGill University Health Centre, Department of Critical Care, McGill University Health Centre, Montréal, QC H4A 3J1, Canada

Olivier Reynaud
Division of Experimental Medicine, McGill University, Montréal, QC H4A 3J1, Canada
Département des sciences de l'activité physique, Faculté des Sciences, UQAM, Montréal, QC H2X 1Y4, Canada
Groupe de recherche en Activité Physique Adaptée, Montréal, QC H2X 1Y4, Canada
Département des sciences biologiques, Faculté des Sciences, UQAM, Montréal, QC H2X 1Y4, Canada

Felipe E. Broering and Sabah N. A. Hussain
Meakins-Christie Laboratories and Translational Research in Respiratory Diseases Program, Research Institute of the McGill University Health Centre, Department of Critical Care, McGill University Health Centre, Montréal, QC H4A 3J1, Canada
Division of Experimental Medicine, McGill University, Montréal, QC H4A 3J1, Canada

Gilles Gouspillou
Division of Experimental Medicine, McGill University, Montréal, QC H4A 3J1, Canada
Département des sciences de l'activité physique, Faculté des Sciences, UQAM, Montréal, QC H2X 1Y4, Canada
Groupe de recherche en Activité Physique Adaptée, Montréal, QC H2X 1Y4, Canada
Département des sciences biologiques, Faculté des Sciences, UQAM, Montréal, QC H2X 1Y4, Canada
Centre de Recherche de l'Institut Universitaire de Gériatrie de Montréal, Montréal, QC H3W 1W5, Canada

Marielle Saclier, Michela Lapi, Chiara Bonfanti, Giuliana Rossi, Stefania Antonini and Graziella Messina
Department of Biosciences, University of Milan, via Celoria 26, 20133 Milan, Italy

Anna Picca and Riccardo Calvani
Fondazione Policlinico Universitario "Agostino Gemelli" IRCCS, 00168 Rome, Italy

Raffaella Beli, Cecilia Bucci and Flora Guerra
Department of Biological and Environmental Sciences and Technologies, Università del Salento, 73100 Lecce, Italy

Hélio José Coelho-Júnior
Università Cattolica del Sacro Cuore, 00168 Rome, Italy

Francesco Landi, Roberto Bernabei and Emanuele Marzett
Fondazione Policlinico Universitario "Agostino Gemelli" IRCCS, 00168 Rome, Italy
Università Cattolica del Sacro Cuore, 00168 Rome, Italy

Eun Ju Lee, Sibhghatulla Shaikh, Dukhwan Choi, Khurshid Ahmad, Mohammad Hassan Baig, Jeong Ho Lim and Inho Choi
Department of Medical Biotechnology, Yeungnam University, Gyeongsan 38541, Korea

Yong-Ho Lee
Department of Biomedical Science, Daegu Catholic University, Gyeongsan 38430, Korea

Sang Joon Park
College of Veterinary Medicine, Kyungpook National University, Daegu 41566, Korea

Yong-Woon Kim and So-Young Park
Department of Physiology, College of Medicine, Yeungnam University, Daegu 42415, Korea

Michèle M. G. Hillege, Ricardo A. Galli Caro, Carla Offringa, Gerard M. J. de Wit, Richard T. Jaspers and Willem M. H. Hoogaars
Laboratory for Myology, Department of Human Movement Sciences, Faculty of Behavioural and Movement Sciences, Vrije Universiteit Amsterdam, Amsterdam Movement Sciences, 1081 BT Amsterdam, The Netherlands

Laura Forcina, Marianna Cosentino and Antonio Musarò
Laboratory affiliated to Istituto Pasteur Italia—Fondazione Cenci Bolognetti, DAHFMO-Unit of Histology and Medical Embryology, Sapienza University of Rome, Via Antonio Scarpa, 14, 00161 Rome, Italy

Yvan Torrente, Pamela Bella, Luana Tripodi, Chiara Villa and Andrea Farini
Stem Cell Laboratory, Department of Pathophysiology and Transplantation, University of Milan, Unit of Neurology, Fondazione IRCCS Cà Granda Ospedale Maggiore Policlinico, Dino Ferrari Center, 20122 Milan, Italy

Index

www.ingramcontent.com/pod-product-compliance
Lightning Source LLC
Chambersburg PA
CBHW080411190526
45161CB00003B/199